Veterinary & Animal Ethics

The Universities Federation for Animal Welfare

UFAW, founded in 1926, is an internationally recognised, independent, scientific and educational animal welfare charity that promotes high standards of welfare for farm, companion, laboratory and captive wild animals, and for those animals with which we interact in the wild. It works to improve animals' lives by:

- Funding and publishing developments in the science and technology that underpin advances in animal welfare;
- Promoting education in animal care and welfare;
- Providing information, organising meetings and publishing books, videos, articles, technical reports and the journal *Animal Welfare*;
- Providing expert advice to government departments and other bodies and helping to draft and amend laws and guidelines;
- Enlisting the energies of animal keepers, scientists, veterinarians, lawyers and others who care about animals.

'Improvements in the care of animals are not now likely to come of their own accord, merely by wishing them: there must be research ... and it is in sponsoring research of this kind, and making its results widely known, that UFAW performs one of its most valuable services.'

Sir Peter Medawar CBE FRS, 8th May 1957
Nobel Laureate (1960), Chairman of the UFAW Scientific Advisory Committee (1951–1962)

UFAW relies on the generosity of the public through legacies and donations to carry out its work, improving the welfare of animal now and in the future. For further information about UFAW and how you can help promote and support its work, please contact us at the address below:

Universities Federation for Animal Welfare
The Old School, Brewhouse Hill, Wheathampstead, Herts AL4 8AN, UK
Tel: 01582 831818 Fax: 01582 831414 Website: www.ufaw.org.uk
Email: ufaw@ufaw.org.uk

UFAW's aim regarding the UFAW/Wiley-Blackwell Animal Welfare book series is to promote interest and debate in the subject and to disseminate information relevant to improving the welfare of kept animals and of those harmed in the wild through human agency. The books in this series are the works of their authors, and the views they express do not necessarily reflect the views of UFAW.

Veterinary & Animal Ethics

PROCEEDINGS OF THE FIRST INTERNATIONAL CONFERENCE ON VETERINARY AND ANIMAL ETHICS, SEPTEMBER 2011

Edited by Christopher M. Wathes,
Sandra A. Corr, Stephen A. May,
Steven P. McCulloch and
Martin C. Whiting

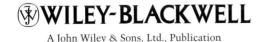

WILEY-BLACKWELL

A John Wiley & Sons, Ltd., Publication

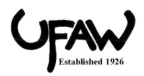

UFAW

Established 1926

69.99

Registered Office
John Wiley & Sons, Ltd, The Atrium, Southern Gate, Chichester, West Sussex, PO19 8SQ, UK

Editorial Offices
9600 Garsington Road, Oxford, OX4 2DQ, UK
The Atrium, Southern Gate, Chichester, West Sussex, PO19 8SQ, UK
2121 State Avenue, Ames, Iowa 50014–8300, USA

For details of our global editorial offices, for customer services and for information about
how to apply for permission to reuse the copyright material in this book please see our website
at www.wiley.com/wiley-blackwell.

Library of Congress Cataloging-in-Publication Data

International Conference on Veterinary and Animal Ethics (1st : 2011 : London, England)
Veterinary and animal ethics : proceedings of the First International Conference on Veterinary and
Animal Ethics, September 2011 / edited by C M Wathes ... [et al.].
      p.   cm.
   Includes bibliographical references and index.
   ISBN 978-1-118-31480-7 (hardcover : alk. paper)   1. Veterinarians–Professional
ethics–Congresses.   2. Animal welfare–Congresses.   I. Wathes, Christopher M.   II. Title.
   SF756.39.I58 2011
   179'.3–dc23
                                    2012010187

A catalogue record for this book is available from the British Library.

Cover image: top left: © Sharon Redrobe; top right and bottom left and right: © Shutterstock.com
Cover design by Sandra Heath

Set in 10/12.5pt Sabon by SPi Publisher Services, Pondicherry, India
Printed and bound in Singapore by Markono Print Media Pte Ltd

1   2013

Contents

Contributors

Michael C. Appleby
World Society for the Protection of Animals
London

Patrick Bateson
University of Cambridge
Cambridge

Madeleine Campbell
Hobgoblins Equine Reproduction Centre
Duddleswell

Sandra A. Corr
University of Nottingham
Nottingham

Björn Forkman
University of Copenhagen
Copenhagen

Marie Fox
University of Birmingham
Birmingham

Nigel Gibbens
Department for Environment, Food and Rural Affairs
London

Colin Gilbert
The Babraham Institute
Cambridge

Sophia Hepple
Department for Environment, Food and Rural Affairs
London

Peter Jinman
Royal College of Veterinary Surgeons
London

Carolyn Johnston
King's College and Kingston University
London

Karsten Klint Jensen
University of Copenhagen
Copenhagen

James K. Kirkwood
Universities Federation for Animal Welfare
London

Judy MacArthur Clark
Home Office
London

Stephen A. May
Royal Veterinary College
London

Steven P. McCulloch
Royal Veterinary College
London

John McInerney
University of Exeter
Exeter

David J. Mellor
Massey University
Palmerston North

Kate Millar
University of Nottingham
Nottingham

Bernard E. Rollin
Colorado State University
Colorado

Peter Sandøe
University of Copenhagen
Copenhagen

John Webster
University of Bristol
Emeritus

Martin C. Whiting
Royal Veterinary College
London

Sarah Wolfensohn
Seventeen Eighty Nine
Swindon

Abigail Woods
Imperial College
London

James Yeates
RSPCA
Horsham

Foreword

Ethics is synonymous with Moral Philosophy, which implies much more than just trying to do the right thing; it forces such questions as what is right, right for whom and why? This conference on veterinary and animal ethics asks us to consider our duties to the animals, primarily in our care, not excluding animals in the wild where their welfare is directly or indirectly affected by man or his activities. It explores how these duties may be reconciled with our other duties of care not only to human society but to the entire living environment. It recognises that if these ethical principles are to be put into practice, rather than act merely as aids to a sense of moral superiority, they have to accommodate both the realities of politics and economics and the biology of human motivation.

Veterinary ethics is a clearly defined subset of this general duty of care. Veterinarians have to reconcile their responsibilities to their animal patients, their human clients, their own welfare and that of their families. However, the ethical principles that apply to veterinary practice do not differ in essence from those that apply to anyone who uses animals, whether directly as a farmer or pet owner, or indirectly as food, clothing or for new drugs.

A useful way to address our complex ethical responsibilities to all parties is through application of the ethical matrix, described here by Kate Millar. This (in my interpretation) sets out two fundamental principles of ethics (input factors). The first is the consequentialist principle of beneficence/non-maleficence, which equates to the utilitarian promotion of general well-being. The second is the principle of autonomy, which equates to the duty to 'do as you would be done by'. In veterinary and animal ethics, these principles are applied to four concerned parties: society at large, direct animal users (farmers, veterinarians, scientists), domestic animals (used by us) and finally all the fauna and flora that make up the living environment. Balanced application of these two moral principles to recognise and address the needs of all concerned parties should achieve the desired outcome, which is the best approximation to justice for all. If this requires a descent into moral relativism, then so be it.

Direct and indirect users of animals, for example farmers and consumers, respectively, are moral agents with the duty to balance rights and responsibilities; rights to safe food and drugs against our responsibilities to the animals involved in their production. The animals (and the environment) are the moral patients. They have no responsibilities to us. One can conclude from this that they have no rights either although this is a very one-sided conclusion since they cannot argue their case. What is certain is that we all share the responsibility to ensure that those to whom we entrust the duty of care have both the competence and the compassion to do it well. It is very easy to care *about* animals; caring *for them* takes skill and it takes patience.

The invited papers, debate and discussion contained within this book may be seen as variations on three main themes:

- History and evolution of human attitudes to animals, the environment and professionalism in human and veterinary medicine.
- Ethical analysis of current practice with regard to the use of animals on farm, in the home, for science and for sport.
- Practical application of ethical principles through the law, political action and the economics of the free market.

Classic moral philosophy (e.g. Plato) may define *the good* according to absolute and unchanging paradigms. However, our interpretation of these paradigms is in a state of constant flux. Papers by Woods, Johnson, May and Appleby explore changing attitudes within and between cultures to the human and animal patients that come within our care. When I was young it was deemed perfectly acceptable to drown kittens at birth; now we agonise over whether it is an insult to its *telos* to spay a cat. The shifting sands of practical morality should engender a sense of caution. We cannot assume that we who attended a meeting in London, UK, in 2011 are necessarily more moral now than those who came before or those in other cultures who live far away. Neither can we assume that our current concepts of middle-class morality will survive the impact of unforeseen future knowledge and future pressures on society. The principle of 'judge not, that ye be not judged' has an excellent provenance.

Papers by Mellor, Gilbert, Campbell and Corr examine ethical issues arising from the way we currently treat the animals which bring us direct benefits in the form of food, medicine, entertainment and love. James Kirkwood considers our responsibilities to wildlife. These papers, explicitly or by implication, acknowledge at the outset the principles of beneficence and autonomy then proceed to explore the extent to which animal owners fulfil their duties to promote the general well-being and individual freedoms of animals in their care in the light of current knowledge of their physiological and behavioural needs. The moral strength of these papers lies in their recognition of the need to seek a better understanding of what they, the animals, would like from us, as distinct from what we would like from them.

The third and most pragmatic series of papers address problems of acting according to ethical principles within the real world. The law defines the limits of acceptable and unacceptable conduct. Laws defined in broad terms such as 'unacceptable suffering' are essential and flexible enough to accommodate changing concepts of what is meant by care and suffering. Governments interpret the law through regulations that seek to describe in detail just what one should and should not do in specific circumstances. When drafting regulations, the aim should be to strike a balance between carrot and stick, while avoiding pettifogging intrusions on personal liberties and lengthy expositions of the blindingly obvious. The paper by Hepple and Gibbens on the ethical basis of UK Government (Defra) policy is refreshingly true to these aims. However, the main limitation of laws and regulations is that they can do little more than seek to ensure that we comply with current standards of acceptability. If we are to encourage the spread of higher standards of animal care than those permitted within the law, we need to harness the power of the people. In the final paper, John McInerney presents a cool economist's evaluation of the things that determine the value we give to animals. He points out that every time we make a value judgement, we make an ethical decision and, in these matters, we are probably getting better. There have in recent years been some spectacular improvements in standards of animal care, and this has come about largely through the power of the people rather than through legislation. The markets (specifically the supermarkets) have responded to increased public demand for higher welfare (e.g. free range eggs) with an impressive range of measures and quality control procedures that are bringing about real improvements. Many of us for many years have been calling for justice for the animals. Progress has been slow and our ideals are probably unachievable, but now, more than ever before, I believe that we are limping in the right direction.

John Webster
University of Bristol

Preface

This book contains the extended proceedings of the First International Conference on Veterinary and Animal Ethics (ICVAE). The conference was held at the Royal College of Physicians, London, from 12 to 13 September 2011. It was organised by the Editors and sponsored by:

The Wellcome Trust
The Royal Veterinary College
The Animal Care Trust
Universities Federation for Animal Welfare, UFAW

The guest at the reception was Jim Paice, MP, Minister for Food and Farming, Defra, London.

In the original preamble, we said:

We have seen dramatic changes over the last few decades in the way we live alongside and interact with animals. Extraordinary advances have been made in our understanding of animal behaviour, physiology and disease. Fifteen years ago, the first mammal was successfully cloned from an adult cell and Dolly the sheep was born. Advances in animal breeding have created dairy cows that can produce 50 litres of milk per day at a metabolic cost of five times maintenance (in comparison a Tour de France cyclist has a demand of 2.7 times maintenance). The selective breeding of chickens has created a modern broiler that has undergone a 300% increase in growth rate. Advances in veterinary surgery enable us to prolong animal life using heart by-pass procedures and renal transplants and to give routinely artificial joints to arthritic dogs.

Yet there is an increasing sense that these developments have not been scrutinised ethically and that such review is overdue. This conference aims to present and encourage stimulating, challenging, thought-provoking and sometimes controversial discussion. We encourage you to participate in the debate wholeheartedly.

The organisers recognise that we need to ask the right questions. We hope that the conference will agree on the questions, even if the answers are not to hand, yet. As starters, we suggest:

a. *To whom does the veterinarian owe primary obligation: the owner or their animal?(Rollin 2006)*
b. *Have veterinarians lost their direction or in some way defaulted on their responsibility for animal welfare?*
c. *How should we decide when animal suffering is necessary?*
d. *Do animals have moral status and, if so, what should this mean?*
e. *How should a balance sheet of harms (to the animal) and benefits (usually to another species) be drawn up when the animal's and human interests are in conflict?*
f. *Does quantity of life, as opposed to quality of life, matter to an animal?*

The conference was separated into four sessions, each containing four or five papers. Questions and answers after each paper were recorded and transcribed and these are presented here too. In addition, each author has availed themselves of the opportunity to write a commentary after they had reviewed their paper and answers.

The debate included a debate with the motion 'Is it better to have lived and lost than never to have lived at all?' This was also recorded and transcribed. The conference programme described it thus: '*Banner's principles of animal ethics mix the approaches of duties-based ethics and consequence-based ethics. This pragmatic solution is often used when humans have to make difficult moral choices about the treatment of animals in our care. Often we have to weigh up issues relating to an animal's quality and quantity of life. This balance lies at the heart of the moral – as well as the welfare – debate. During this discussion, delegates will consider a proposal, which can be interpreted variously, e.g. in terms of moral principles, specific issues such as population control, or illustrative examples.*' James Kirkwood, Bernard Rollin and James Yeates spoke to the motion before it was opened to registrants from the floor.

The Editors, 2012

Principles of Veterinary and Animal Ethics

PATRICK BATESON

University of Cambridge

The first session of this excellent symposium consisted of an eclectic group of lectures. The first was given by a historian, Abigail Woods; the next by a philosopher, Peter Sandøe; the third by a lawyer, Carolyn Johnston; and the final one by a veterinarian, Stephen May. The organiser, Christopher Wathes, had allowed 10 min for discussion after each lecture. I had worried that this might prove too much, especially as each speaker was going to be kept strictly to time. I thought that I might have to keep the session going with chairman-like remarks and contrived questions. I need not have been concerned. The audience were splendid and generated first-rate discussion. So much so, indeed, that hands were still being raised when the allotted time for discussion came to an end. This attentiveness by the audience to a broad range of issues augured well for the rest of the meeting.

In his book *Man and the Natural World*, Keith Thomas described how the moral concerns of those who had preached and pamphleteered against cruelty to animals had remained remarkably constant in England from the fifteenth to the nineteenth century. Humans are fully entitled to domesticate animals and to kill them for food and clothing, but they are not to tyrannise or cause *unnecessary suffering* to animals. Domestic animals should be allowed food and rest and their deaths should be as painless as possible. Wild animals could be killed if they were needed for food or thought to be harmful. Even though game could be shot and vermin hunted, it was wrong to kill for mere pleasure.

Veterinary & Animal Ethics: Proceedings of the First International Conference on Veterinary and Animal Ethics, September 2011, First Edition. Edited by Christopher M. Wathes, Sandra A. Corr, Stephen A. May, Steven P. McCulloch and Martin C. Whiting.

Moral philosophers have made major contributions to the ethical problems raised by the treatment of animals. Even so, all their adopted positions require careful thought. *Utilitarians* often have problems trading off animal suffering against the benefits humans derive from animals because the costs and benefits of any action are not measured in the same terms. Those who confer rights on animals do not reveal what responsibilities animals have in return in the same way that humans have when they make an implicit contract in return for their rights. To my mind, even Bernard Rollin, who spoke in the second session, had too inflexible a notion of what animals should be allowed to experience. After all, adaptability is as much part of the animal's *telos* as anything else it is adapted to do.

Those concerned with human medicine considered the ethical and legal issues raised by medical care long before the veterinarians thought formally about the *ethics* of their care of animals. Informed consent does not arise with animals but, even in humans, the issue has proved much more difficult to deal with than was at first thought. It is widely believed that the veterinarians should always have the welfare of animals at the forefront of their minds. The sheer expense of running an expensive practice does mean, however, that conflicts of interest arise. I felt therefore that this meeting, which started so well, was especially welcome in addressing the ethical problems faced by the veterinary profession.

The History of Veterinary Ethics in Britain, ca.1870–2000

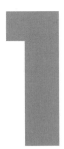

ABIGAIL WOODS

Imperial College

Abstract: This paper examines the history of veterinary ethics in Britain over the period 1870–2000. It lays aside present-day normative conceptions of veterinary ethics in order to understand how veterinarians in the past perceived this issue and the social, economic and political factors that influenced their thinking. This analysis reveals the changing nature and scope of veterinary ethics. Prior to 1948, when anyone could legally practice veterinary surgery, veterinarians argued that treating animals ethically meant placing them under veterinary care: The interests of the veterinarian, owner, animal and society were best served by ensuring full veterinary discretion in treatment. The state acknowledged this claim with the passage of the 1948 Veterinary Surgeons Act, which restricted the practice of veterinary surgery to qualified veterinarians. Veterinary ethical priorities then shifted to professional conduct. However, later in the century, as the social and economic climate grew more hostile to professional power and privileges, and animal welfare moved up the political agenda, veterinarians began to recognise potential conflicts in interest between animals, owners, society and the profession, and to navigate them using new forms of ethical thinking. No longer concerned with extending their power to treat animals, they focussed on the appropriate exercise of that power within the clinical encounter. Previously regarded as a matter of individual clinical freedom, how veterinarians treated animals became an ethical problem that attracted both professional and public concern.

Keywords: Britain, conduct, concern, ethics, ewe, owner, veterinarian, veterinary ethics, veterinary history, veterinary surgeon, Veterinary Surgeons Act, welfare

Veterinary & Animal Ethics: Proceedings of the First International Conference on Veterinary and Animal Ethics, September 2011, First Edition. Edited by Christopher M. Wathes, Sandra A. Corr, Stephen A. May, Steven P. McCulloch and Martin C. Whiting.
© 2013 Universities Federation for Animal Welfare. Published 2013 by Blackwell Publishing Ltd.

1.1 Introduction

Veterinarians have always encountered ethical dilemmas in the course of their work. The nature of these dilemmas and how veterinarians perceived and responded to them has changed over time. Focusing on Britain, from the late nineteenth century to the very recent past, this paper provides a preliminary analysis of these changes. Its short length precludes a detailed examination of particular ethical issues. Rather, the aim is to identify broad trends in how veterinarians conceptualised and approached veterinary ethics in their practice and politics.

There is little existing literature on this topic. Histories of medical ethics do not examine the veterinary field (Rothman 1991; Cooter 2002) and veterinarians rarely feature in histories of animal ethics, which focus on key thinkers, scientists, politicians and campaigners (Kean 1998; Guerrini 2003; Boddice 2009). Tannenbaum's (2005) textbook on veterinary ethics does not attempt a historical account, while Legood's (2000) is restricted to the history of animal welfare. Only Rollin (2006) engages seriously with the history of veterinary ethics. His purpose is to show that veterinarians have an under-developed sense of ethics. Drawing on lived experience in the USA, he argues that veterinary ethical concerns were traditionally confined to matters of professional conduct. Only in the later 1970s and 1980s did veterinarians respond – albeit belatedly and reluctantly – to society's emerging concern for animal ethics.

This paper presents a quite different account of the history of veterinary ethics. Using a standard historical method to analyse documentary evidence, it aims to situate and understand veterinary ethics within its historical context. Instead of hunting, retrospectively, for the roots of present-day ethical thinking, it adopts a prospective view, in which veterinary ethics is regarded as whatever veterinarians at the time believed it to be. Their views are not judged against present-day norms or ideals but rather explained in reference to the broader social, political and economic milieu.

This approach reveals that while, as Rollin (2006) argued, professional conduct was a major veterinary preoccupation, veterinarians also had a long history of concern for animal ethics. The nature of that concern and the contexts in which it was expressed changed over time, as did the solution proposed. The first half of the paper reveals how, from the late nineteenth century until the 1948 Veterinary Surgeons Act, veterinarians worked to convince animal owners and the state that treating animals ethically meant placing them under veterinary care and ensuring full veterinary discretion in treatment. In the immediate post-war years, this ambition was largely achieved and the veterinary focus shifted to professional ethics. Later in the century, animal ethics returned to the forefront of veterinary agendas. However, it was now approached in a quite different way. Veterinary priorities shifted away from winning the power to treat animals towards the appropriate exercise of that power. Previously regarded as a matter of individual clinical freedom, how veterinarians treated animals within the clinical setting became an ethical problem that attracted both professional and public concern.

1.2 Professional Conduct and the Relief of Animal Suffering, 1870–1919

For most of the nineteenth century, the British veterinary profession was a small, insecure and highly fragmented body. More of a trade than a profession, its members received a very basic level of training at the London-based Royal Veterinary College (RVC, established 1791) or William Dick's school in Edinburgh (1823), before entering into the highly competitive field of animal doctoring. Reformers battled to improve the status and income of the profession and achieved some success with the 1844 foundation by royal charter of a corporate body, the Royal College of Veterinary Surgeons (RCVS). However, the RCVS was unable to abolish the competition posed by unqualified individuals, who often assumed the title 'veterinary surgeon' (Pattison 1984).

One strategy that veterinarians used to counter this competition was to assert their ethical superiority over unqualified men. They claimed that the latter inflicted cruelty on animals, while they were expert in relieving it. They carved out roles as expert witnesses in prosecutions for animal cruelty, participated in the 1870s campaign against vivisection and gave evidence on proposed legislation to improve the welfare of animals in transit. Supported by the Royal Society for the Prevention of Cruelty to Animals (RSPCA), they argued that much animal suffering could be prevented by substituting veterinary for lay intervention (Editorial 1876; Walley 1876; Poyser 1877; Discussion 1881; Harrison 1973).

If treating animals ethically meant placing them under veterinary care, then to encourage such behaviour on the part of owners and the state, the profession had to conduct itself in a particular way. Animal ethics and professional ethics were therefore linked. Using the medical profession as a model, veterinary reformers urged veterinarians to adopt gentlemanly habits, abandon trade-like practices such as horse dealing, and charge properly for services rather than relying on drug sales. Veterinarians should also improve their dress, stop advertising and behave considerately and courteously to fellow veterinarians instead of stealing their cases and badmouthing them to clients. Such reforms would enable the public to differentiate qualified men from fraudulent quacks (Woods & Matthews 2010).

These efforts met with only partial success. On the one hand, they helped to persuade Parliament to pass the 1881 Veterinary Surgeons Act. This gave veterinarians a monopoly over the title 'veterinary surgeon' and also formalised professional ethics by creating a register from which veterinarians could be removed for 'disgraceful professional conduct'. On the other hand, unqualified practice remained legal and some animal owners and local authorities continued to preferentially employ unqualified animal doctors (Woods & Matthews 2010). The grassroots of the profession interpreted this outcome in different ways. Some claimed that the standards of professional conduct were still too low for veterinarians to win respectable employment. Others, practising in rural areas, complained that RCVS strictures on advertising had left them unable to compete effectively with unqualified healers (Dellagana 1900–1901; Onlooker 1905–1906). The RCVS's sympathies lay with the former view. Throughout the late nineteenth and first half of the twentieth centuries, it sought to set distance between the veterinary profession and other animal healers by policing professional conduct and prosecuting those who illegally assumed the title veterinary surgeon (Bullock 1927).

Meanwhile, veterinary attention was drawn to questions of animal ethics, such as the docking of horses' tails. Justified on the basis that it prevented horses from getting their tails caught under the reins, docking was a routine operation usually performed without anaesthesia by veterinarians, farriers and horse dealers. During the 1880s, the RSPCA supported by RCVS President, George Fleming, proclaimed docking a cruel act, performed only for reasons of fashion and monetary gain. In the ensuing intra-professional debate, majority opinion held that docking should be judged on the basis of utility, not sentimentality. Veterinarians were the people best qualified to make this judgement and to perform the operation effectively and without cruelty (Editorial 1883, 1884; Correspondence and reports 1884). Consequently, the RSPCA had no reason to '*plunge promiscuously into prosecutions, seriously interfering with rights and privileges which certainly ought to be enjoyed by respectable veterinary surgeons*' (Briggs 1885).[1]

This belief that placing animals under veterinary care guaranteed their ethical treatment paralleled doctors' concurrent claims about the ethical status of the doctor–patient relationship, which they invoked in an attempt to defend medical autonomy against threats from the laymen and the state (Cooter 2002). It manifested repeatedly in subsequent veterinary discussions. For example in 1910, when the RSPCA alleged widespread cruelty in the export of decrepit horses, members of the Central Veterinary Society concluded that the best means of preventing cruelty was to appoint veterinarians to supervise the trade (Central Veterinary Society 1909–1910).

The same thinking featured in discussions on the 1912 Animals (Anaesthetics) Bill 'to make further provision for the prevention of cruelty to animals'. Brought before Parliament by Walter Guinness, MP, this sought to make anaesthetics compulsory for certain veterinary operations (Parliamentary 1912–1913).[2] While recognising that the bill would enable veterinarians to override owners' resistance to anaesthesia, to the benefit of their patients, leading veterinarians nevertheless opposed it. This was partly because its lay promoters had failed to seek veterinary

---

[1] The RSPCA did not agree and continued its attempts to secure the prosecution of a veterinary surgeon for docking (Editorial 1896–1897). The procedure was not outlawed until 1949.

[2] These operations included the castration and spaying of dogs and the castration and firing of horses. Local anaesthetic was required for neurectomy, enucleation and trephining. Although anaesthetics had been used in human medicine since the 1840s, the use of chloroform in veterinary surgery did not become routine until the turn of the twentieth century (Editorial 1905–1906).

input. Also, the bill would constrain veterinary freedom of action, and because it did not restrict anaesthetic use to veterinarians, it would enable untrained men to attempt it, resulting in poorly anaesthetised animals and much suffering (Correspondence 1912–1913; Hobday 1913–1914). These complaints had little effect, and in 1919, after several revisions to the schedule of operations, the bill became law (Memo 1918–1919). Although viewed as an overall advance in humanity to animals, leading veterinary surgeon and future RVC principal, Frederick Hobday, was not alone in feeling that, '*It rather galls on the veterinary surgeon to be told that he is not to have it left to his discretion in all operations and we are apparently told that by the laity*'. The best interests of the animal were served by placing it under veterinary care and granting veterinarians full discretion in treatment (Hobday 1919–1920).

1.3 The Ethical Nature of Veterinary Work, 1919–1948

Similar views of veterinary ethics were expressed repeatedly during the inter-war period as veterinarians sought to carve out new niches in agriculture and small animal medicine. These efforts were stimulated by threats to traditional sources of employment. Horse numbers were declining with the rise of mechanised transport; scientific thinking had shifted to favour preventive and hygienic measures over bleeding, firing and drugging; and veterinarians faced increasing competition from patent medicine vendors, whose advertising practices were not constrained by professional ethics (Onlooker 1905–1906; Woods 2007).[3]

Veterinarians' growing exposure to farm animals caused them to reflect on the ethics of new production practices that arose in response to the deepening agricultural depression. In dairy farming – which proved popular due to its immunity from foreign competition – producers established so-called 'intensive' units in suburban areas, where cows were kept indoors, fed on imported cattle cake and replaced with new purchases. Elsewhere, low cereal prices encouraged the production of pigs within indoor 'factory-style' units. Veterinarians often moralised about these practices and their implications for livestock health (Woods 2007, 2012). Typical comments included those of practising veterinarian, Lesley Pugh, and pig specialist, D. J. Anthony. Pugh complained that '*Too often the cow becomes a mere machine for the provision of milk. As a result of our ignorance of the machinery we fail sooner or later to maintain its efficiency. The machine fails and sterility ensues*' (Pugh 1924). Anthony criticised the growing tendency '*to regard the pig as more of a machine than a live animal*'. Warning of a vengeful nature who '*exacts a penalty for any violation of her laws*', he argued that producers '*must try to adopt scientific methods while still having due regard for Mother*

---

[3] The number of horses in Great Britain fell from 3.07 million in 1911 to 1.89 million in 1924 (Thompson 1976).

Nature' (Anthony 1940). The proposed solution to all of these problems was for veterinarians to play a more extensive role in the prevention and management of livestock disease.

Similar thinking can be identified in the profession's concurrent conflict with the People's Dispensary of Sick Animals (PDSA). Founded in 1917, this charitable organisation offered free treatment to the sick animals of the poor. Treatment was performed by 'skilled experts', who were laymen trained through lectures and experience in the PDSA's hospital. As the charity grew wealthier and its network of clinics and hospitals extended, it attracted criticism from veterinarians keen to increase their own activities in pet medicine. Decrying the sentimentalism of the PDSA's promoters and advertising the profession's own tradition of providing cheap treatment to poor clients, veterinarians argued that they were best able to judge whether an animal was suffering and whether its owner merited charity. They also argued that on moral grounds, all animals deserved the best possible care, which meant placing them under expert veterinarians, not untrained quacks. Such claims, which overlooked the in-depth training received by PDSA officers, won little public support during the inter-war years (Gardiner 2010).

1.4 The Eclipse of Animal Ethics, 1948–1975

The first half of this paper has shown that prior to World War II, veterinary reflections on ethical issues ranging from professional conduct to the treatment of animals centred on the need to place animals under veterinary care and to ensure full discretion in treatment. These actions would not only serve the interests of the animal but also those of the owner, state and society. This thinking was shaped by the profession's overlapping ambitions to relieve animal suffering, overcome market competition and extend the scope, autonomy and status of veterinary work.

In the immediate post-war decades, these ambitions were largely achieved. New confidence in science (which had played a crucial role in winning the war), respect for professional expertise and the vital veterinary contribution to feeding the nation in wartime facilitated the passage of the 1948 Veterinary Surgeons Act, which made it illegal for unqualified persons to practice veterinary surgery. This resolved the long battle with the PDSA in the profession's favour (Gardiner 2010). In 1954, veterinary dissatisfaction with anaesthetics legislation was overcome by the passage of a new act of Parliament. Promoted by the British Veterinary Association (BVA), this granted veterinarians full discretion over anaesthetic agents and techniques (Editorial 1954).

Veterinary services to farmers were also increasing on account of the post-war emphasis placed on domestic food production. In helping farmers to tackle disease, veterinarians enabled them to develop more efficient, intensive systems of production, as demanded by Government policy. Public criticism of these systems erupted in 1964 with the publication of *Animal Machines*, Ruth Harrison's expose of factory farming (Harrison 1964). Veterinary reactions to changing agricultural practices reveal a shift in their ethical thinking since the inter-war years. Leaving behind their earlier concerns about going against nature, many argued that if veterinarians were to maintain their 'rightful place' on the farm, they had to embrace and assist intensification (Hignett 1956; Sainsbury 1965). Dismissing lay criticisms of factory farming as 'sentimental anthropomorphism', they asserted the profession's moral responsibility for and expertise in humane practices (BVA 1965). In defining health as a state of 'maximum economic production commensurate with economy and humanity' (Editorial 1969) and equating disease with poor welfare (BVA 1965), veterinarians proclaimed their ability to make livestock farming both productive and ethical.

Veterinarians continued to equate the ethical care of animals with veterinary care. This view shaped their claims that veterinarians were the experts best qualified to oversee and regulate the use of animals in experiments (The Littlewood Committee 1964–1965). It also caused them to affix the label 'ethical' to pharmaceutical companies that restricted drug sales to veterinarians. 'Unethical' companies sold direct to farmers. These labels disappeared when the 1968 Medicines Act granted veterinarians privileges in the sale and supply of drugs (MacKellar 1963).

As the scope, autonomy and status of veterinary work increased and the spectre of unqualified competition disappeared, veterinarians ceased to proclaim an ethical 'deficit' in the treatment of animals. At the same time, their perceived need to justify the privileges awarded to them under the 1948 Veterinary Surgeons Act pushed professional conduct to the forefront of veterinary ethical concerns. In 1951, the RCVS published its first *Guide to Veterinary Professional Conduct* (RCVS 1951). This contained headings such as: 'the status and dignity of the veterinary profession' (which laid down strictures on advertising), 'relationships between practitioners' (which emphasised honour, faith and mutual trust) and 'relationships between veterinarians and laypersons' (laymen must not carry out veterinary work).

The term 'ethics' did not appear until the 1961 edition of the guide, which defined unethical behaviour as that 'undesirable and unbecoming to a professional man' (RCVS 1961). Subsequent updates, which appeared every 3 years, reveal the emergence of new ethical concerns thrown up by the changing nature of veterinary employment, practice organisation and therapeutic interventions. By the early 1970s, the code had grown to encompass standards for veterinary hospitals, claims to specialisation, relationships between veterinarians in practice and in industry, and guidance on employing veterinary nurses. This period also saw administrative changes, introduced under the 1966 Veterinary Surgeons Act, to the RCVS's procedure for disciplining members who infringed the code (RCVS 1961, 1964, 1967, 1971).

1.5 The Reshaping of Veterinary Ethical Thought, 1975–2000

During the last quarter of the twentieth century, the professional, political and public consensus that managing animals ethically meant placing them under veterinary care began to fracture, and new questions arose about the conduct of that care. Formerly, clinical intervention had been viewed as a private veterinary matter: the veterinarian's professional expertise and code of conduct meant that he or she could be trusted to act in the interests of all parties. Now, however, there was growing recognition within and outwith the profession of the potential conflicts of interest between veterinarians, animals, owners, society and state. This led to new public, political and professional scrutiny of veterinary conduct both within and beyond the clinical setting.

Commentators past and present often link these developments to the operation of financial constraints in the care of large animals, and conversely, to the lack of such constraints in small animal practice, a rapidly expanding field in which major technical advances offered many new prospects for treatment. In both cases, ethical reflection was required to decide what forms of veterinary intervention were necessary and justifiable (Orpin 1984; News 2010). This argument has strength. However, it overlooks the fact that economics have always constrained farmers' actions to a greater or lesser extent and that many new clinical techniques were developed prior to the 1970s without inspiring this kind of ethical scrutiny. In order to make sense of the late twentieth century reshaping of veterinary ethical thought, it is necessary to move beyond the clinical encounter, to explore its broader social and political contexts.

From the 1970s, trust in all the professions diminished and their privileges, practices and expertise were subjected to challenge. The origins of this challenge lay in the 1960s and 1970s counter-culture, the women's and civil rights movements, and the rise of consumerism and the free market (Cooter 2002). While the medical profession was singled out for particular criticism (Szasz 1961; Foucault 1965; Freidson 1970; Illich 1975), veterinarians did not escape the fallout. The first direct threat came from the Monopoly Commission's 1976 report on the veterinary profession. One of a set of government-commissioned enquiries into the professions, it claimed that the RCVS's 'ethical' restrictions on advertising contravened the public interest by withholding vital information from customers and preventing competition between practices (News and reports 1976). For RCVS registrar, Alistair Porter, the report signalled that the state no longer trusted the profession to manage its own affairs and to act in the interests of its clients (Porter 1976).

Most veterinarians did not want to permit advertising. They viewed it as a commercial practice at odds with their professional image (Comment 1984). However, in 1984 the RCVS was forced to lift its restrictions. By then, consumer bodies had begun to attack veterinary fees, and the media to scrutinise the profession's privileges. Animal owners were demanding higher levels of veterinary competence, ethical conduct and value for money (Society of Practising Veterinary Surgeons

1984; Comment 1986; Cripps 1986; Napley 1987) and were *'fast moving away from the attitude that the word of the professional man ... has to be accepted without question'* (Comment 1985). This shift was reflected in their increasing employment of laymen to perform traditionally 'veterinary' tasks like foot trimming and equine dentistry (Comment 1995).

Veterinarians faced other challenges to their claims to be acting in the public good. On account of their services to livestock farmers, they were implicated in mounting criticisms of intensive agricultural practices. Critics highlighted the detrimental effects of indiscriminate antibiotic and pesticide use on the health of humans and the environment, and the impact of factory farming systems on livestock health and welfare (The Swann Committee 1969–1970). Welfare, in particular, achieved a high political profile following a 1978–1979 campaign by animal welfare societies 'to put animals into politics' (Hollands 1985).

Critics both within and outwith the profession claimed that veterinarians were failing to take the lead in improving animal welfare. This failure was attributed firstly to veterinarians' resistance to anthropomorphism, which set them apart from a public that related to animals on largely subjective terms. Secondly, veterinarians were reluctant to engage in general ethical reflection on welfare, instead insisting on objective scientific evidence before acknowledging the existence of a problem. Thirdly, veterinarians' continuing tendency to equate welfare to health and productivity ran counter to the growing emphasis placed by animal welfare scientists on the animal's subjective state. Their insights challenged veterinary claims to welfare expertise and encouraged critics in their belief that veterinarians were privileging the interests of livestock owners over the welfare of their animals (Anon 1977; Gee & Meischke 1982; Various 1983; Fox 1984; Broom 1987; Hollands 1987; Carter *et al.* 1990; Comment 1992).[4]

Implicit in these developments was the realisation that the interests of veterinarians, animals, owners, state and society did not necessarily align. In order to maintain public trust, their legal privileges, social status and market share, veterinarians had to rethink their responsibilities and relationships (Comment 1986; Wooley 1994) and their assumption that veterinary care was, by definition, ethical. While they continued to claim ethical superiority when defending veterinary practices against lay encroachment, in other contexts veterinarians began to reflect more critically on the nature of the care they provided and whose interests it served.

The *RCVS Guide to Professional Conduct* (1975, 1978, 1984, 1993, 2000) offers preliminary insights into the changing nature of veterinary ethical thinking.[5] Over

---

[4] This period saw the rise of the philosophy of animal rights, which awarded animals' intrinsic worth and viewed welfare initiatives as attempts to justify the unjustifiable keeping of animals for human ends (Regan 1989).

[5] A more detailed exploration of this issue – which is beyond the scope of this paper – requires further research into the role of ethics within veterinary education, the debates it stimulated in veterinary meetings and the veterinary press, the rationales for disciplinary investigations performed by the RCVS and the profession's attempts to assert itself within the field of animal welfare, most notably through the 1984 establishment of the BVA Animal Welfare Foundation.

successive editions, it has shifted from a profession-centred, to an owner-centred, to an animal-centred view of veterinary obligations. In 1975, the rationale for the code was 'preventing members from harming each other'. The 1978 version claimed that rules were formulated not to confer financial or other benefits on the profession but 'with the interests of animals and their owners clearly in mind'. In 1984, this state- ment was included in a new section entitled 'Duty to the public'. In 1993, it was replaced by a section entitled 'Duty to animals and their owners'. Later in this edition, the RCVS stated that in formulating ethical guidance, its overriding consideration was to ensure animal welfare. By 2000, veterinarians reading the guide were informed that they must make animal welfare their first consideration. In the list of professional responsibilities, 'responsibilities to patients' came first, followed by responsibilities to clients, to the general public and then to professional colleagues.

Concurrently, the RCVS began to pronounce on the ethical status of particular clinical interventions. In 1987, its disciplinary committee made the landmark decision to strike a veterinarian off the register for performing treatment that caused a pony unnecessary suffering and distress. Formerly, the College's disciplinary apparatus had confined its attention to allegations of unprofessional conduct such as fraud. Clinical interventions had been viewed as a private matter, to be decided by the individual veterinarian in accordance with the circumstances and needs of the animal and its owner. Owners who alleged clinical incompetence or negligence had been left to pursue the matter through the courts, which alone could award compensation. However, the precedent set by the 1987 case showed that the RCVS was now willing to consider such cases. In this way, it broadened its definition of 'conduct disgraceful in a professional respect' to include veterinary clinical conduct (Editorial 1987; RCVS 1987).

The 1993 *Guide to Professional Conduct* reveals the RCVS's expanding surveillance over clinical practice. It defined the docking of dogs' tails (which had been debated within the profession since 1969 (Singleton 1970)) as unethical and frowned upon the firing of horses (controversial since 1979 (McCullagh 1979)) to such an extent as to warn that its performance could be used as evidence in disciplinary procedures. The RCVS also noted its intention, *'from time to time [to] give guidance to the profession in relation to specific procedures which current scientific evidence shows to be ineffective and/or inhumane'* (RCVS 1993). More positive welfare measures were included in its 2000 guide, which stated the veterinarian's responsibilities to ensure humane treatment, adequate pain control, relief of suffering and the avoidance of neglect.

Meanwhile, the RCVS decided that veterinary ethics was a sufficiently complex and important topic to merit dedicated training. It added a certificate and then a diploma in veterinary ethics, welfare and law to its existing suite of postgraduate qualifications.[6] Problem-based education in veterinary ethics entered the mainstream

---

[6] This move did not go unchallenged. Various members of the profession argued that the topics were sufficiently covered by existing clinically oriented programmes (Correspondence 1994).

veterinary curriculum, while the profession's continuing education journal, *In Practice*, began to publish articles on ethical dilemmas encountered in clinical settings (Mullan & Main 2001). These developments set the seal on the reshaping of veterinary ethical thought. Instead of assuming that the veterinary care of animals was, by definition, ethical, veterinarians now recognised the multiple ethical dilemmas it posed.

1.6 Conclusion

This paper has traced the history of veterinary ethics in Britain over the period 1870–2000. It approached this problem by laying aside present-day normative conceptions of veterinary ethics, in order to understand how veterinarians in the past perceived this issue. This mode of analysis reveals the changing nature, scope and importance of professional and animal ethics. It also shows that veterinary ethical thinking is essentially a product of its time, shaped by veterinary prospects, ambitions and practices; methods of animal management; scientific advances; and the relationships between veterinarians, animals, society and the state.

Prior to 1948, when anyone could legally practice veterinary surgery, qualified veterinarians sought to distinguish themselves from the competition by their ethical credentials. Motivated by a mix of humanitarianism, business interests and the desire to increase the profession's influence, they claimed that veterinary codes of conduct and expertise in relieving suffering meant that the veterinary treatment of animals equated to their ethical treatment. The interests of animal, owner, profession and society were best served by awarding full clinical discretion to the vet concerned.

The passage of the 1948 Veterinary Surgeons Act signalled the state's recognition of this claim and removed the veterinary need to assert it. Veterinarians then focussed on their professional conduct in an attempt to justify the award of a market monopoly. However, in the later twentieth century, the social and economic climate grew more hostile to the exercise of professional power. In this context, veterinarians began to recognise the potential conflicts in interest between animal, owner, society and profession and to navigate them using new forms of ethical thinking. The key issue was no longer the provision of veterinary care but the manner in which it was performed. In this way, the care provided within the clinical encounter, and its implications for animal welfare, became the focus of veterinary ethical concern.

Acknowledgements

I would like to thank Dr Alastair Porter and Dr Andrew Gardiner for their valuable insights and advice.

References

Anon. (1977) BVA congress: Veterinarians on animal welfare. *Veterinary Record*, **101**, 357.

Anthony, D.J. (1940) *Diseases of the Pig and Its Husbandry*. Bailliere Tindall and Cox, London.

Boddice, R. (2009) *A History of Attitudes and Behaviours toward Animals in Eighteenth and Nineteenth-Century Britain: Anthropocentrism and the Emergence of Animals*. Edwin Mellen Press, Lewiston, Maine.

Briggs, T. (1885) The prevention of cruelty to animals. *Veterinary Journal*, **21**, 63.

Broom, D.M. (1987) The veterinary relevance of farm animal ethology. *Veterinary Record* **121**, 400–401.

Bullock, F. (1927) *Handbook for Veterinary Surgeons*. Taylor & Francis, London.

BVA. (1965) Evidence to Brambell committee. *Veterinary Record*, **77**, 180–189.

Carter, H., Sainsbury, D. & Ewbank, R. (1990) BVA policy on animal welfare. *Veterinary Record*, **127**, 251.

Central Veterinary Society. (1909–1910) Exportation of decrepit horses. *Veterinary Record*, **22**, 698–701.

Comment. (1984) Remember King Canute? *Veterinary Record*, **115**, 529.

Comment. (1985) Advertising of fees. *Veterinary Record*, **117**, 321.

Comment. (1986) Professions at risk. *Veterinary Record* **119**: 257.

Comment. (1992) Shaping policy on welfare. *Veterinary Record*, **131**, 352.

Comment. (1995) Professional activities: Protecting animals and the public. *Veterinary Record*, **136**, 549.

Cooter, R. (2002) The ethical body. In: *Companion to Medicine in the 20th Century* (eds R. Cooter & J. Pickstone), pp. 451–468. Routledge, London.

Correspondence. (1912–1913) Anaesthetics bill. *Veterinary Record*, **25**, passim.

Correspondence. (1994) *Veterinary Record*, **134**, passim.

Correspondence and Reports of Veterinary Meetings. (1884). *Veterinary Journal*, **18**, passim.

Cripps, Y. (1986) The professions: A critical review. *Veterinary Record*, **119**, 277–280.

Dellagana, W. (1900–1901) Some reflections on 'unprofessional conduct' and suggested reforms. *Veterinary Record*, **13**, 711–714.

Discussion. (1881) Cruelty to animals from a veterinary point of view. *Veterinary Journal*, **13**, 355–357.

Editorial. (1876) The protection of the veterinary profession and the public. *Veterinary Journal*, **3**, 448–450.

Editorial. (1883) The ethics of veterinary surgery. *Veterinary Journal*, **17**, 88–90.

Editorial. (1884) The fashionable mutilation of domestic animals. *Veterinary Journal*, **18**, 114–115.

Editorial. (1896–1897) Docking. *Veterinary Record*, **9**, 681.

Editorial. (1905–1906) Anaesthesia. *Veterinary Record*, **18**, 429.

Editorial. (1954) Protection of animals (anaesthetics) bill. 1954. *Veterinary Record*, **66**, 123.

Editorial. (1969) An exercise in preventive medicine. *Veterinary Record*, **84**, 25.

Editorial. (1987) New grounds for 'misconduct.' *Veterinary Record*, **120**, 121.

Foucault, M. (1965) *Madness and Civilisation*. Pantheon, New York.

Fox, M.V. (1984) Towards a philosophy of veterinary medicine. *Veterinary Record*, **115**, 12–13.

Freidson, E. (1970) *Profession of Medicine.* Dodd, Mead & Co, New York.

Gardiner, A. (2010) The development of small animal veterinary practice in 20th-century Britain. Unpublished PhD thesis. University of Manchester, Manchester.

Gee, R.W. & Meischke, H.R.C. (1982) The veterinarian and animal welfare. *Veterinary Record,* **110,** 86.

Guerrini, A. (2003) *Experimenting with Animals: From Galen to Animal Rights.* John Hopkins University Press, London.

Harrison, R. (1964) *Animal Machines: The New Factory Farming Industry.* V Sykes, London.

Harrison, B. (1973) Animals and the state in nineteenth century England. *English Historical Review,* **88,** 786–820.

Hignett, S. (1956) Farm health problems – Where does Britain stand today? *Veterinary Record,* **68,** 887–900.

Hobday, F. (1913–1914) The veterinary profession and the anaesthetics bill. *Veterinary Record,* **16,** 56–58, 76–79.

Hobday, F. (1919–1920) Anaesthetics. *Veterinary Record,* **32,** 344.

Hollands, C. (1985) Animal rights in the political arena. In: *In Defense of Animals* (ed. P. Singer), pp. 168–178. Basil Blackwell, New York.

Hollands, C. (1987) What the animal welfare movement expects of the veterinarian. *Veterinary Record,* **121,** 367–371.

Illich, I. (1975) *Medical Nemesis.* Calder and Boyers, London.

Kean, H. (1998) *Animal Rights: Political and Social Change in Britain Since 1800.* Reaktion, London.

Legood, G. (ed.) (2000) *Veterinary Ethics: An Introduction.* Continuum, London.

MacKellar, J.C. (1963) The role of the veterinary surgeon in British agriculture. *Veterinary Record,* **75,** 1444–1445.

McCullagh, K.G. (1979) Tendon injuries and their treatment in the horse. *Veterinary Record,* **105,** 54–57.

Memo. (1918–1919) Animals (anaesthetics). *Veterinary Record,* **31,** 439–441, 452.

Mullan, S. & Main, D. (2001) Principles of ethical decision-making in veterinary practice. *In Practice,* **23,** 394–401.

Napley, D. (1987) The professions in today's society: The Wooldridge memorial lecture. *Veterinary Record,* **121,** 281.

News (2010) BVA congress: Where do you draw the line on treatment? *Veterinary Record,* **167,** 636–637.

News and Reports. (1976) Veterinarians should be allowed to advertise. *Veterinary Record,* **99,** 114–115.

Onlooker. (1905–1906) Optimism v pessimism. *Veterinary Record,* **18,** 534.

Orpin, P. (1984) Philosophy of veterinary medicine. *Veterinary Record,* **115,** 72.

Parliamentary. (1912–1913) Animals (anaesthetics) bill. *Veterinary Record,* **25,** 670.

Pattison, I. (1984) *The British Veterinary Profession, 1791–1948.* JA Allen, London.

Porter, A. (1976) Wooldridge memorial lecture: Look forward to posterity: The challenge to the professions. *Veterinary Record,* **99,** 243–249.

Poyser, R. (1877) Cruelty to animals in India. *Veterinary Journal,* **4,** 316–323.

Pugh, L. (1924) The sterility of forced lactation in the cow. *Veterinary Record,* **36,** 87.

RCVS, (1951, 1961, 1964, 1967, 1971, 1975, 1978, 1984, 1987, 1993, 2000) Guide to professional conduct. RCVS, London.

Regan, T. (1989) The case for animal rights. In: *Animal Rights and Human Obligations* (eds T. Regan & P. Singer), 2nd edn., pp. 105–114. Prentice-Hall, London.

Rollin, B. (2006) *An Introduction to Veterinary Medical Ethics: Theory and Cases*, 2nd edn. Blackwell, Oxford.

Rothman, D. (1991) *Strangers at the Bedside*. Basic Books, New York.

Sainsbury, D. (1965) Intensive livestock production. *Veterinary Record*, 77, 1249–1250.

Singleton, W.B. (1970) The ethics of certain surgical procedures in the dog. *Veterinary Record*, 86, 332–335.

Society of Practising Veterinary Surgeons. (1984) Countering attacks on the profession. *Veterinary Record*, 114, 530.

Szasz, T. (1961) *The myth of mental illness*. Harper and Row, New York.

Tannenbaum, J. (2005) *Veterinary Ethics*, 2nd edn. Mosby, London.

The Littlewood Committee. (1964–1965) *Report of the Departmental Committee on Experiments on Animals* (Command 2651). HMSO, London.

The Swann Committee (1969–1970) *Report of the Joint Committee on the Use of Antibiotics in Animal Husbandry and Veterinary Medicine* (Command 4190). HMSO, London.

Thompson, F.M.L. (1976) Nineteenth-century horse sense. *Economic History Review*, 29, 80.

Various. (1983) Animal welfare correspondence. *Veterinary Record*, 112, passim.

Walley, T. (1876) Edinburgh veterinary college: Opening of winter session. *Veterinary Journal*, 3, 461–463.

Woods, A. (2007) The farm as clinic: Veterinary expertise and the transformation of dairy farming, 1930–1950. *Studies in the History and Philosophy of the Biological and Biomedical Sciences*, 38, 462–487.

Woods, A. (2012) Rethinking the history of modern agriculture: British pig production, c.1910–1965. *Twentieth Century British History*, 23, 165–191.

Woods, A. & Matthews, S. (2010) 'Little, if at all, removed from the illiterate farrier or cow-leech': The English veterinary surgeon, c. 1860–1885, and the campaign for veterinary reform. *Medical History*, 54, 29–54.

Wooley, P. (1994) The future role of the RCVS. *Veterinary Record*, 134, 552–554.

Questions and Answers

Q: We always tend to be rather UK-centric in the way in which we view this. This is an international conference and I just wondered if, indeed, being so UK-centric is a marker that we've led this debate, or have we trailed it? And, indeed, with the benefit of so many international members here, perhaps a little input of their particular situations would be quite helpful.

A: Yes, I completely agree. Unfortunately, this was, by necessity, a UK-centric account, first of all because no one had written on this issue before, which meant I had no jumping off point, and secondly because writing a paper just on Britain involved months of work. I had to look through the index of every *Veterinary Record*, searching under multiple headings because there was nothing listed under ethics. So, I would really welcome perspectives from history in other countries.

Q: You ended up with a question: moral progress or product of historical circumstances? Well, couldn't it be both? Couldn't it be the case that we actually do have things that we would describe as moral progress, even though we shouldn't be so proud about it, because we had the opportunity? Now, you said you wouldn't, as a historian, take a moral stance, but you ended up being relativistic and nihilistic. Couldn't you allow more progress?

A: Obviously, we wouldn't be here today if we didn't feel that there was scope to make progress in ethical thinking. I want to guard against people dismissing the past as irrelevant and viewing our forebears as stupid and immoral. I want to show that history is important and did inform how we got to where we are today.

Q: When I became a veterinarian, I said that my prime concern was the welfare of animals entrusted to my care. Has that always been what people have sworn or when did that come in? There's obviously an ethical background to it.

A: I can't give a firm answer. The term 'welfare' was used very little prior to *Animal Machines*, the *Brambell Report* and the 1968 Agriculture Act. That might give some indication of when the oath was introduced, but I would need to research that further.

Q: It would be very interesting to know when the RCVS oath originated and what differences there are between different countries. One person who has written on this from an international perspective is Caroline Hewson, Professor of Animal Welfare at the Veterinary College in Prince Edward Island, Canada. She wrote a nice article called 'Veterinarians Who Swear'.

C: Can you clarify for those who don't know? Is there a kind of Hippocratic Oath for veterinarians?

A: Yes there is, and as far as I'm aware it's compulsory in the UK, but just for one contrast, the American Veterinary Medical Association oath is voluntary. It's also taken voluntarily by Canadian veterinarians but is worded differently which suggests some interesting differences in perspective.

C: Just to comment on that particular point. It is not an oath; it is a declaration in this country. There's a legal difference between the two.

Q: I wonder if it might be possible to see how many people here are veterinarians. You were saying that the veterinary profession considered itself or aimed to become the authority on animal welfare, but from looking around this conference, I think that today this debate doesn't just involve veterinarians. There are a lot of expert animal welfarists here.

A: The issue of veterinarians coming into animal welfare is quite interesting because in the early years, when welfare was becoming a political issue, veterinarians had little to do with it. I looked through the *Veterinary Record* in the years that *Animal Machines* and the Brambell report came out, and there's very little comment, apart from a few derogatory remarks about Ruth Harrison. I think the BVA's evidence to the Brambell committee had to be drafted by the president of the day, because virtually no veterinarians responded to his invitation to contribute. By the mid-1970s, though, veterinarians were suddenly realising that they'd missed the boat. That's when they founded the BVA Animal Welfare Foundation and decided to sponsor a chair. But certainly early on they were left behind and maybe, as you imply, they're still being left behind now.

Q: I've thought about this idea of moral progress and history and of course the main concern I have is that even if we think it is moral progress, we may, ourselves, be the product of our history. From the point of view of people a 100 years from now, what we think may be complete moral degradation.

Q: It is not my place to defend veterinarians but I just want to make the point that when phrases are used like 'veterinarians did not consider animal welfare before such and such date', that is more a question of terminology than practical impact. It is quite clear that there are different views of what is important in animal welfare. Veterinarians have always considered that health and the physical state of the animal is the most important thing. The question then arises of other aspects of animal welfare and what view veterinarians and others have taken of that. We are now in a different position from 50 years ago, because views of what is important in animal welfare have emerged and changed.

A: I disagree with you to some extent because when the term animal welfare began to be used in the 1960s, and certainly by 1970, it meant something quite different from the straightforward prevention of cruelty. However, veterinarians weren't much interested in the new concept of welfare or in its definition.

Q: I wouldn't phrase it that they were not interested. They didn't see the necessity for these additional concepts to health and growth and physical well-being, but there were clearly some aspects of animal welfare which were integral to their profession.

A: Clearly, they cared for animal well-being, but welfare, as we all know, is a slippery concept and it's very difficult to use it with precision.

The Idea of Animal Welfare – Developments and Tensions

2

PETER SANDØE AND KARSTEN KLINT JENSEN

University of Copenhagen

Abstract: This paper focuses on developments and tensions within the idea of animal welfare. There is divergence among those who believe in the idea of animal welfare. First, we discuss what it takes for farm animal welfare to be good enough. How far should society go beyond the starting point of the Brambell Committee, which was to prevent avoidable suffering? Secondly, we turn to the tricky question of how welfare should be distributed between animals. Here, a tension within the concept of animal welfare, between a focus on the individual animal and on the herd, flock or shoal, is pointed out. Finally, the role of economic considerations is considered, given that animal production takes place in a global market with free trade between countries with various standards of animal welfare.

Keywords: animal welfare, animal welfare legislation, avoidable suffering, Brambell Committee, market, production, unnecessary suffering

2.1 Background – The Modern Idea of Animal Welfare and the Brambell Report

The modern idea of animal welfare was given its first clear statement in the Brambell report (Brambell 1965). Although the term 'welfare' has been applied to animals since the eighteenth century (Radford 2001, p. 261), the Brambell report signalled a change in the rationale towards animal protection. Earlier, animal

Veterinary & Animal Ethics: Proceedings of the First International Conference on Veterinary and Animal Ethics, September 2011, First Edition. Edited by Christopher M. Wathes, Sandra A. Corr, Stephen A. May, Steven P. McCulloch and Martin C. Whiting.

protection was specifically set up to protect animals from pointless (i.e. wanton) cruelty. This meant that constructive uses of animals – specifically in agricultural production – were not hindered by legislation at this time. Animal welfare, in the modern sense of the word, on the other hand, aims to protect animals in farm animal production against rational overuse.

The Brambell Committee was set up by the British government following the public outcry about intensive livestock farming prompted by Ruth Harrison's book *Animal Machines*, published in 1964. The recommendations of the committee formed the basis of subsequent British and European animal welfare legislation. Intensification of animal production in western countries was encouraged by public policies put in place immediately before, during and after World War II. These promoted the development of abundant, cheap food. As a result, animal production became much more efficient, as measured by the cost of producing each egg, kilogram of meat or litre of milk. The pressure for efficiency subsequently became market-driven, with competition between producers and between retailers to sell food as cheaply as possible, and thereby acquired its own momentum. In some ways, this can be viewed as a success story.

At the same time, as Ruth Harrison pointed out, the advances gave rise to conflicts between productivity and the interests of the animals, and the animals invariably paid the price. Typically, they were given less space per individual than previously, and many were reared in barren environments and were unable to exercise their normal range of behaviours. Also, as has now become clear, higher productivity was boosted by genetic selection, which has in many cases been accompanied by production-related diseases.

The Brambell report focused mainly on the negative effects that modern intensive production systems can have on animals, particularly suffering. The fact that such suffering was seen as a moral problem was nothing new, however. Rather, the new developments were as follows: first, efficient production and animal suffering were seen as two sides of the same coin, whereas earlier it had been argued by producers that increased productivity entails good welfare (Rollin 2005, p. 16); second, demand for cheap food was no longer assumed to override concerns about the welfare of farm animals.

Another new and influential idea presented in the Brambell report was that farm animals have *behavioural urges*, often frustrated in intensive confinement systems, which they need to perform to avoid suffering (Mench 1998). This led to the statement of a general principle of animal welfare according to which farm animals should be free 'to stand up, lie down, turn around, groom themselves and stretch their limbs' (the so-called Brambell freedoms) (Brambell 1965, p. 13).

Brambell broadened the received conception of what counts as suffering. The committee insisted that suffering covers much more than pain, and should include discomfort and stress (understood to cover a wide range of mental states including frustration and fear). In this, the Brambell report, besides presenting its own ideas on behavioural needs, drew on results presented earlier that year in the Littlewood *Report of the Departmental Committee on Experiments on Animals* (Littlewood 1965).

A final and very influential thought found in the Brambell report was that studies based on methods from physiology and ethology were necessary elements of animal welfare assessment. This was given great weight when the report's conclusions were implemented. By requiring agricultural reform to be underpinned by scientific evidence, the British Government, on the one hand, undertook to set up new research, and on the other, bought time before having to embark on controversial legislation.

The Brambell report and similar initiatives in other European countries set off a process of legal reform, which have improved the conditions of farm animals in the UK and the rest of Western Europe. However, the early formulations of animal welfare, beginning with the Brambell report, remained loyal to the basic idea of farm animal production as a legitimate human endeavour. This in many ways curbed the criticisms that were levelled against modern intensive animal production, as we shall now try to explain.

First, the focus was mainly on the *absence* of suffering; there was little mention of positive welfare. Even the central principle of the Brambell report, that animals require certain basic freedoms (later developed into the Farm Animal Welfare Council's Five Freedoms (FAWC 2009)), was understood to be violated only when the infringement of a freedom leads to suffering. Second, the protection from suffering secured in most animal welfare legislation applied only to so-called unnecessary suffering. This in practice allowed a number of welfare problems to be accepted as necessary, for example those related to keeping laying hens in battery cages. Third, claims regarding animal welfare could only be made on the basis of solid scientific evidence, so the burden of proof lay with those who claimed that animal welfare was threatened. Fourth, the whole idea that intensive animal production was the right solution to food production was not being questioned.

In the past, a significant amount of literature has focused on the limitations about the definition of animal welfare. It has been argued that a correct definition presupposes an ideal of what counts as a *good* animal life and that there is conceptual space for alternatives to this kind of negative hedonism, that is the view that only prevention of suffering matters as described above (Fraser 1997, 1999; Appleby and Sandøe 2002; Sandøe and Christiansen 2008, ch. 3). This shows that animal welfare is not just based on science but also has an underpinning in values.

For example, it can be claimed that animals should be able to perform natural behaviour not only for the reason that this prevents suffering (the key rationale presented in the Brambell report), or because doing so generates pleasure, but also because this is of value in its own right. This kind of perfectionist view, focusing on animals *doing* well rather than just *feeling* well, seems to be ignored in the dominant conception of animal welfare. In fact, studies of popular perceptions show that the ordinary person's view of animal welfare is more perfectionist than the dominant expert view (in which there is an almost exclusive focus on suffering and disease (Lassen *et al.* 2006)).

In this paper, we focus on developments and tensions within the idea of animal welfare. We ask what it takes for farm animal welfare to be good enough, how this welfare should be distributed between animals and how animal welfare can be promoted in a globalised world with free trade of animal products.

There seems to be a difference between people who have concerns about animal welfare, yet believe in the permissibility of animal use as long as those concerns are fulfilled, and animal rights advocates (and others) who question the very legitimacy of human use of animals. However, even among those in the first of these groups – call them 'welfarists' – differences have developed over the ideal balancing of animal welfare and human benefits.

In the following sections, we outline three lines of discussions showing divergences among welfarists. First, we discuss how far to go beyond the starting point of the Brambell Committee, which was to prevent avoidable suffering. Second, we discuss a tension within the concept of animal welfare, between a focus on the individual animal and one on the herd, flock or shoal. Finally, we touch upon the role of economic considerations in efforts to improve animal welfare, given that animal production takes place in a global market with free movement of products across borders between countries with varying standards of animal welfare.

2.1.1 From 'no unnecessary suffering' to 'a good life' for animals

The Brambell report recommended that animal welfare legislation 'should make it an offence to cause, or permit to continue, avoidable suffering' (Brambell 1965, p. 61). Here, suffering should be understood in a broad sense, including not only pain but also discomfort and the feeling of stress. Few would deny that this is a laudable goal. However, it seems perfectly reasonable to ask, first, how is avoidable to be defined, and second, why we should not go further than that.

There is an element of truth in the idea that some animal suffering is unavoidable: the only completely effective way of preventing suffering in animals is not to bring them into existence. To experience the good moments of life, every animal (including humans) will invariably have to experience some of the bad ones too.

However, there is much more to the idea of unavoidable suffering than just that. What is at issue here is suffering that is necessary *given* the goal of efficient animal production. For example, the Brambell report did not recommend a ban on battery cages, but only that there should be a limit on stocking densities in such cages. This was not because cages do not cause suffering, but because other production systems which were commercially viable had similar problems. The more fundamental question, whether there ought to be commercial mass production of cheap eggs, was not asked.

British legislation, following Brambell, uses the term 'unnecessary suffering'. But again, there are different ways of understanding what qualifies as *necessary* suffering. At one end of the scale, all suffering that is due to factors that enhance the efficiency of production will be deemed necessary. Here, unnecessary suffering could be called a remnant of the old notion of wanton cruelty. At the other end of the scale, only suffering that is necessary for the greater good of the animals, such as living through periods of disease or inter-group fighting for rank, will count as necessary. Most animal welfare legislation draws the line somewhere between these two extremes. For example, in British legislation one of the criteria that must be met for suffering to be deemed necessary is that what causes the suffering must be for a legitimate purpose and proportionate to that purpose (Animal Welfare Act 2006, Section 4, Sub-section 3). Hence, the term 'unnecessary suffering' is not useful here, but rather serves to cloud underlying ethical issues about how to balance animal welfare against efficient animal production. Of course, this problem does not go away when the term is avoided, for example as in the current EU legislation and in the national legislation of some Member States, including Denmark.

Turning to the question of whether to be more progressive, one can ask why the focus is on avoiding unnecessary suffering. Why should we not also focus on the unnecessary withholding of positive welfare? If, at no significant cost, it is possible to give animals opportunities to explore, eat preferred food or otherwise engage in behaviours which give pleasure, it seems wrong not to enable this.

In a report published in 2009, the Farm Animal Welfare Council (FAWC) raised the issue of the level of animal welfare to aim for. FAWC drew a distinction between three levels of quality of life that can be achieved by an animal: *a life not worth living*, *a life worth living* and *a good life*. The first is a life where suffering outweighs pleasure and therefore a life that should be terminated for the sake of the animal in question (or husbandry changed for the better). In *a life worth living*, the good moments outweigh the bad ones, and therefore such a life is worthwhile. However, to aim to give animals lives worth living is not to aspire very high. A life worth living will cover a range from a life *barely* worth living to a life full of happy and pleasurable moments, and the lower end of that range is really not very good.

FAWC recommended, as a minimal condition, that '*the intention of British policy should be that an animal kept in full compliance with the law should have a life worth living*' (FAWC 2009, p. 19). This would mean that it is enough, legally speaking, to provide animals with conditions ensuring that it would not be better for the animal to be euthanised than to go on living. It is not entirely clear whether this goal signalled real progress or, if taken literally, mandated serious deterioration relative to the *status quo*.

However, an important subject is raised here, which is that however good the law is there will always be room for improvement – and there will probably have to be different levels of welfare. Besides the legal minimum, which ideally will guarantee the animals more than a life barely worth living, there will be room also for production systems that guarantee a higher level of welfare. An issue here, also addressed by FAWC, is how to safeguard that products sold with a claim to enhance animal welfare deliver on what they promise.

To deal with this issue, a new wave of animal welfare research has developed since the 1990s. The focus of this work is on measuring animal welfare at the farm or group level. Whereas earlier studies of animal welfare focused chiefly on the environment in which the animals are raised, new methods have been developed which allow one to gauge welfare outcomes. These methods may turn out to be instrumental in raising welfare standards in a way that genuinely benefits affected animals. However, they also give rise to challenging questions about how the interests of the individual are to be balanced against those of the herd. To this we now turn.

2.1.2 From the individual to the herd

According to Brambell's recommendations – and indeed many subsequent initiatives in European countries and at the EU level – the main vehicle for improving farm animal welfare is regulation. To date, European regulation has focused largely on minimum standards for housing and animal handling, but it is recognised that variations in management can lead to welfare problems even on farms satisfying the legal minimum.

Attempts to deal with the management factor through higher minimum standards may lead to a bureaucratic system of rules and controls. It is not clear that this benefits the animals. Except in certain clear-cut areas, like the handling of some diseases, management regulation has, therefore, tended to rely on a somewhat vague notion of good practice. However, since, to attract penalties, violations of good practice must be severe and made with intent or gross negligence, this has created a grey zone in which the regulatory authorities encounter poor welfare *within* the rules. Naturally, this generally is not received well when explained to the public.

Currently, therefore, the regulation of farm animal production is undergoing a transformation. One influential idea is to motivate farmers to improve welfare with incentives linked to welfare outcomes. Rather than telling the farmer how to manage his animals, a limit is set on the prevalence of a certain welfare problem. Using measures of welfare on-farm or at slaughter, the authorities can then check whether a given farm is within the limits. When the prevalence of the problem on a farm is too high, the farmer can be required to develop a plan to improve matters. In severe cases, the farmer can be fined or face a restriction on production.

In some countries, certain welfare problems – notably, foot-pad dermatitis in broilers and shoulder lesions in sows – have been successfully managed by this approach. At the same time, there is a change of focus from the protection of each individual to the minimisation of welfare problems at the group level. For example, in Denmark, at slaughter 100 chicken feet from each batch of broiler chickens are inspected for foot-pad dermatitis. Each foot is evaluated on a point-scale: 'no foot-pad lesions' scores 0 points, 'few and minor lesions' scores 1 point and 'many or severe lesions' scores 2 points.

Using this information, batches are divided into three categories: category A, up to 40 points; category B, between 41 and 80 points; and category C, between 81 and 200 points. Farms with birds in category A are given the all-clear. When a batch is in category B, a warning is given to the farmer. When a batch is in category C (or there are repeated cases of category B), then the farmer is reported to the authorities. Reported farmers receive an instruction to improve the situation. They will then be under increased surveillance and may eventually be required to decrease stocking density.

The system, originally developed in Sweden (Ekstrand *et al.* 1998), has had a substantial effect on broiler welfare in Denmark: between 2002 and 2005 the number of batches in category C decreased from around 50% to about 10%. So, in that respect, the legislation has been very successful. However, this system potentially neglects individual animals with severe problems; for as long as a small number of animals suffer from foot-pad dermatitis, the system will pass that batch of animals.

Traditional animal welfare legislation, which stipulates minimum requirements for husbandry, treats all animals as equals. However, even on very good farms, there have always been animals that suffer, but they have not done so, as it were, in full view. The recent focus on the prevalence of problems may have the implication that some prevalence of a problem is explicitly deemed acceptable, even though it might be said to violate the minimal requirements for treatment of each individual animal. It is not a solution to this dilemma to stop measuring animal welfare at farm level and thereby allow severe but preventable animal welfare problems to occur, which is what happens where authorities do not require assessments of foot-pad dermatitis. To avoid a welfare problem by not measuring it is to stick one's head in the sand.

Proposals to deal with welfare at a group level should, however, give rise to serious ethical reflection on the relation between concern about the least well-off animals and those with 'average' levels of welfare. The issues are similar to those that arise about humans in a modern welfare state, for example in the distribution of health care resources.

In the EU's recent Welfare Quality® project, an attempt was made to aggregate the welfare of animals on a farm into a grade that could be compared across farms. Here, the dilemma was how to weigh severe welfare problems against mild ones. The researchers chose to give priority to the worst-off animals with the implication that of two farms with the same average level of welfare, one would score lower than the other if it had more animals with severe problems (Veissier *et al.* 2011).

In general, developments of this kind illustrate the need to add the ethical dimension of *justice* to discussions of animal welfare, to focus on the distribution of welfare among the animals. A recent paper by Houe *et al.* (2011) makes an attempt to do this in relation to the assessment of welfare in diseased dairy cattle.

Another obstacle to the improvement of animal welfare is the effect of international free trade. This will be discussed next.

2.1.3 Role of economic considerations in animal welfare

The Brambell Committee saw national legislation as a main tool to secure animal welfare. However, since the remit of the committee extended only to affairs and arrangements in the UK, its report focused exclusively on British legislation. Hence,

Brambell's recommendations relate to changes in British animal welfare legislation. Some of them concern changes in statutory provision; others are about codes of good practice, which also play a key role in British legislation.

The committee was aware of a lack of scientific knowledge about farm animal welfare. For this reason, and to allow for flexibility to deal with new developments in agriculture, it argued that,

> 'It must be possible to modify any standards laid down without the necessity for constantly amending the main legislative instrument. Therefore we recommend that any Act necessary to make our recommendations effective should be in the form of an enabling Act, so that Statutory Instruments can be made to implement them and to give early effect to desirable changes which may prove necessary.' (Brambell 1965, p. 60)

In this way, the committee ingeniously suggested a flexible legal structure of animal welfare legislation, which has subsequently been adopted in many European countries.

The principal idea is that animal welfare is regulated by legislation–stipulating requirements that guarantee a decent minimum standard of animal welfare. The committee was aware that given the extra costs imposed on domestic farmers by the legislation, and given the risk of imports of animal products from countries with less stringent standards of animal welfare, this policy could have problems. However, it deferred this issue to the British Government:

> '... we recognise that the effect of some of our recommendations may be to increase costs in certain sectors of the industry, at least in the initial stages. We believe that public concern about animal welfare on farms is such that this will be understood and consumers will be prepared to meet any marginal extra costs. We would, however, be concerned if the standards we have recommended for adoption in this country had the result of encouraging imports produced overseas under systems contrary to these. This might largely invalidate the intention of our Report; we therefore recommend that the Government take such steps as may be practicable to ensure that it does not happen.' (Brambell 1965, p. 62)

This may have been something that a British government could deal with in 1965. However, with the rules governing international trade today, this is certainly no longer the case. Since the 1970s, the EU has placed limits on what the British government can do to regulate trade; and more recently, through international trade agreements, limits have restricted what the EU can do. Even though in theory the World Trade Organization (WTO) allows for non-discriminatory measures to protect animal life and health (see GATT article XX), in practice animal welfare is not recognised as a legitimate concern allowing trade restrictions, and animal products are sold freely across continents.

In the recent FAWC report (2009), a strategy for improving farm animal welfare is presented. The focus is not only on farm animal production in Great Britain, but also on imported animal products. Again, the tool of choice is no longer, at any rate, primarily legislation. Instead, the report looks carefully at how to bring about change in the supply sources of retailers, and how to encourage consumers to demand products with high standards of animal welfare.

With this development, animal welfare can no longer be regarded as an issue to be dealt with solely by traditional experts in the field of animal welfare. When, in 1965, the Brambell Committee suggested that the British government should set up what became FAWC, they envisaged a need for the following kinds of experts on the council: *'a veterinarian, an expert on animal behaviour or comparative psychology, a zoologist, or physiologist, persons knowledgeable in animal husbandry and farm buildings and a legal expert'* (Brambell 1965, p. 62). What is clearly missing here is mention of experts understanding the role of markets and trade.

It was an understandable limitation of the foresight of the Brambell Committee to overlook, or downplay, the role of economics and other social sciences in the project of improving farm animal welfare. This, however, has had a lasting negative effect on the understanding of animal welfare. Luckily things now seem to be changing for the better. Thus, for example, for a number of years FAWC has had economists and other kinds of social scientists on board.

2.2 Conclusions

The work of the Brambell Committee has undoubtedly had an enormously positive effect on the welfare of billions of animals in Britain and elsewhere. This is an achievement that cannot be overstated.

However, with hindsight it can be seen that the vision of animal welfare presented in the report has some limitations. Earlier work exposed limitations in the implicit negative hedonist view on animal welfare. In this paper, we have discussed aspects of animal welfare regulation and assessment, including what is a fair distribution of welfare, and on how to most effectively promote animal welfare.

Briefly, we have argued that (1) discussions about animal welfare should move away from the exclusive focus on unnecessary suffering to the ideal of good welfare; (2) there is an often overlooked issue about the fair distribution of animal welfare across animals within a herd which need to be explicitly addressed; and (3) in promoting animal welfare in today's world, legislation is not a sufficient tool, and those working for animal welfare should also be concerned about changing minds and moving markets.

Acknowledgements

Thanks are due to Clare Palmer, Paul Robinson, Geir Tveit and two anonymous referees for useful comments on an earlier version of this paper, and to Thorkil Ambrosen and Mie Nielsen Blom for information on the foot-pad dermatitis case.

References

Appleby, M.C. & Sandøe, P. (2002) Philosophical Debate on the Nature of Well-being: Implications for Animal Welfare. *Animal Welfare*, **11**, 283–294.

Brambell, F.W.R. (1965) *Report of the Technical Committee to Enquire into the Welfare of Animals Kept under Intensive Livestock Husbandry Systems* (Command Report 2836). Her Majesty's Stationery Office, London.

Ekstrand C., Carpenter, T.E., Andersson, I. & Algers, B. (1998) Prevalence and control of foot-pad dermatitis in broilers in Sweden. *British Poultry Science*, **39**, 318–324.

FAWC (2009) *Farm Animal Welfare in Great Britain: Past, Present and Future*. Farm Animal Welfare Council, London.

Fraser, D. (1997) Science in a value-laden world: keeping our thinking straight. *Applied Animal Behaviour Science*, **54**, 29–32.

Fraser, D. (1999) Animal ethics and animal welfare science: bridging the two cultures. *Applied Animal Behaviour Science*, **65**, 171–189.

Harrison, R. (1964) *Animal Machines: The New Factory Farming Industry*. Vincent Stuart, London.

Houe, H., Sandøe, P. & Thomsen P.T. (2011) Welfare Assessments Based on Lifetime Health and Production Data in Danish Dairy Cows. *Journal of Applied Animal Welfare Science*, **14**, 255–264.

Lassen, J., Sandøe, P. & Forkman, B. (2006) Happy pigs are dirty! – conflicting perspectives on animal welfare. *Livestock Science*, **103**, 221–230.

Littlewood, S. (1965) *Report of the Departmental Committee on Experiments on Animals* (Command Report 2641). Her Majesty's Stationery Office, London.

Mench, J.A. (1998) Thirty Years After Brambell: Whither Animal Welfare Science? *Journal of Applied Animal Welfare Science*, **1**, 91–102.

Radford, M. (2001) *Animal Welfare Law in Britain: Regulation and Responsibility*. Oxford University Press, Oxford.

Rollin, B.E. (2005) Animal Agriculture and Social Ethics for Animals. In *Encyclopedia of Animal Science* (eds W.G. Pond & A.W. Bell). Marcel Dekker, New York.

Sandøe, P. & Christiansen S.B. (2008) *Ethics of Animal Use*. Blackwell, Oxford.

Veissier, I., Jensen, K.K., Botreau, R. & Sandøe, P. (2011) Highlighting ethical decisions underlying the scoring of animal welfare in the Welfare Quality® scheme. *Animal Welfare*, **20**, 89–101.

Questions and Answers

Q: As a philosopher, you will be aware of the phrase 'All philosophy is footnotes to Plato'. I have often thought much animal welfare science is similarly footnotes to the Brambell report. There is much in Brambell's report that is radical. I paint a different picture and urge people to read the report, which is a pleasure to read as well as a mine of information. You mentioned Brambell's report as putting the burden on science, which you expressed as a normative position, but it can be interpreted as a non-philosophical, practical or pragmatic position, that is science will affect policy, which is the case generally today with evidence-based policy making in government.

My other point is about the WTO. Although it is certainly a big challenge, it is also an opportunity because if we could change WTO rules or the interpretation of them, then its application would be international and it would affect animal welfare universally.
A: Perhaps I overemphasised the burden that Brambell puts on science; it's more a matter of interpretation by government. I'm a great admirer of animal welfare science, but often it hasn't got anything new or relevant to say. For example, in the case of stocking densities of broilers, there is, apart from at the very extremes, a linear correlation without a tipping point. Scientific evidence can be an illusion: the idea that science can solve all the problems has, unfortunately, been encouraged within the EU.

On the WTO, I agree that we should go for a big change. However, so far we've got nowhere. There was a meeting in Sweden a few years ago where a representative of WTO said something like the following, '*Well in theory you can get through but in practice you will get nowhere*'. When I talked with those concerned with trade in the Danish civil service, they said, '*Well forget it*'. I would love to share your optimism but have found no reason that I should.

Q: I'm a great fan of the role of the free market in helping society to work towards improved standards of welfare for as many animals as possible, since by definition, legislation can never define standards that are any better than acceptable. In that context we've raised the role of the animal welfare scientist, who has to recognise public opinion. Our responsibility as animal welfare scientists is to work towards systems of animal husbandry in which the public's perception of animal welfare of the food animals is as close as possible to the animal's perception of its welfare. This means, for example, that it's not terribly helpful for animal welfare scientists to say, 'Science says that the improved cage for laying hens is better than a free range system that allows maximum freedom of choice', because, by definition, that will never become better than acceptable and the public won't buy it. We have a responsibility to achieve this compromise between what the public needs and what the animals need.
A: I agree. Sometimes animal welfare scientists could learn from the public because they may be right and see things that others have overlooked. For example, in the current debate about grazing for dairy cows, maybe the public didn't have all the answers but they actually seem to have seen something in their own naive way. For a long time, I have thought that aesthetics is important: if you can't show someone a picture of a farming circumstance, then there's a problem.

Q: You asked the question, when is enough, enough and used *the good life* in that context. I would suggest that the good life is not very good at drawing a line. It is just a positive value of saying, this is the goal or these are ideal states. There are many regulatory structures to define what is enough, but there isn't is a framework for the good life.
A: The good life is a continuum. We have to find a middle way and need to bring in public perception because there isn't a natural place to cut the line, so to speak, even though I still think that just being barely suicidal is not the right place.

Q: The predictions are that there's going to be an increasing demand for meat in other parts of the world, for example China. How strongly do you think welfare will be respected if meat starts disappearing from supermarket shelves?

A: What needs to be done is to link animal welfare to some of the agendas that people are concerned about, for example climate. If you buy, for example, organic produce you buy less meat: going for a diet of less meat and more quality could deal with climate and environmental issues, as well as human health. There's a need for a more rounded approach; Danish ministers listen as soon as food safety, health or climate are mentioned, whereas they often won't talk about animal welfare. Animal welfare is mostly low on their agenda; you must, therefore, link animal welfare with other agendas.

Q: I don't understand your dilemma about inspecting for welfare. You talked about welfare being a continuum, moving towards improvement, moving in the right direction, etc. Why does this not apply to inspecting for welfare? If the current criterion for finding – or not finding – is less than 10% foot damage and this is achieved, can you not move towards a much stronger criterion, potentially no damage at all?

A: The dilemma is that certain things are allowed which, strictly according to the legislation, are not permitted, for example some broiler chickens walk around in pain. If you only consider the bird's environment, everything appears to be okay.

Q: Part of my point is that telling people that this is a temporary issue is part of moving in the right direction and also part of not fooling them that there is an ideal world that we can reach in three year's time with nothing needed to change thereafter.

A: The issue will never be temporary. The question is the prevalence, not just the incidence.

Q: The Swedes and the Danes measured foot-pad dermatitis as part of a business improvement programme on each farm. I disagree with others here that you should only use law for minimum standards. The EU's Broiler Directive has done much more by requiring governments to put in place monitoring schemes in the abattoir, requiring feedback and action plans and introducing a culture of continuous improvement. There are other examples, such as the Healthy Feet programme in the UK. We're already using social scientists and business improvement ways to progress at a speed that the livestock industry can cope with.

A: Some schemes are ingenious examples of using the market's mechanism on farmers rather than consumers. It's a pity that the EU's Broiler Directive didn't use either the Danish or the Swedish model because billions of broiler chickens in Europe could have a much better life than they do have now.

Q: You mentioned involving economists, sociologists and psychologists in altering people's minds. This is related to the debate between animal welfare and animal liberation. Animal welfare is trying to improve the conditions for animals within the present framework while animal liberation is trying to alter the framework. In a way, our discussion is about how far to go. In terms of distributive justice and the problems with the differences between different countries, if people change their own minds about these issues, then supply and demand will help to push things in the right direction. I appreciate that governments have to make rules and regulations but in a democracy it's the general public that places demands on governments.

A: The contrast between animal welfare and animal rights is, as far as I can see, getting smaller. In terms of animal welfare, people start to think about animals being able to show pleasure and have a good life. This may engage those rightists who are not in principle against the killing of animals but consider that standards of animal welfare should be much higher. The polarised debate between animal welfare and animal rights may diminish significantly.

Lessons from Medical Ethics

3

CAROLYN JOHNSTON

King's College and Kingston University

Abstract: Like veterinary medicine, human medicine raises ethical issues, – what can be done and what should be done, across a spectrum from the patient, to business and commercial considerations. However, medical ethics is a better-developed discipline and may provide insights to some of the dilemmas confronting the modern veterinarian.

Keywords: law, medical ethics, medicine, patient, veterinarian, veterinary ethics

3.1 What Can Veterinary Ethics Learn from Medical Ethics (and *Vice Versa*)?

Members of both professions have undergone lengthy training, giving rise to specialist expertise and privileges that ordinary members of society do not have (Rollin 2006). Both types of practitioners hold vital positions in society and are in positions of trust. Membership of the respective professional bodies aims to ensure certain standards and appropriateness of behaviour and there is normally an assumption that, given the technical nature of their professions and specialised knowledge, both professions will be able to deal appropriately with ethical dilemmas arising in clinical practice. But, of course, there are differences in practice, not least the nature of the relationship between the professional and the patient/client, giving rise to different priorities in the duties and obligations owed. The aim of

Veterinary & Animal Ethics: Proceedings of the First International Conference on Veterinary and Animal Ethics, September 2011, First Edition. Edited by Christopher M. Wathes, Sandra A. Corr, Stephen A. May, Steven P. McCulloch and Martin C. Whiting.
© 2013 Universities Federation for Animal Welfare. Published 2013 by Blackwell Publishing Ltd.

this paper is to highlight some differences and similarities arising in the practice of the two professions and to consider what can be learnt when appraising professional and ethical dilemmas.

3.2 The Relevance of Medical/Veterinary Ethics and Its Place in the Undergraduate Curriculum

Ethics can be loosely defined as a system of moral principles to enable value judgments about what course of action is 'good' or 'bad', 'right' or 'wrong'. Of course, this definition belies the complexity and variety of dilemmas arising, but nevertheless principles and frameworks can be useful in a process of transparent decision making using relevant factors in a coherent and uniform manner. As Mullan and Main (2001) note, '*While using the ethical frameworks described may not change the actual decisions made by clinicians, an understanding of ethical issues is important for client communication, improving job satisfaction and maintaining a positive public profile – for both the individual vet and the profession at large*'.

Medical ethics and law are considered 'core' parts of the undergraduate medical curriculum. The General Medical Council (GMC) in its document *Tomorrow's Doctors* (2009) requires that medical graduates '*will be able to behave according to ethical and legal principles*'. In 2010, the Institute of Medical Ethics published a revised curriculum to put flesh to the bare bones of the GMC requirements (Stirrat *et al.* 2010). The Royal College of Veterinary Surgeons (RCVS) requires similar, although not equivalent, learning (RCVS 2006).

Of course, that is not to say that students nor qualified doctors and veterinarians necessarily remember, understand or apply these principles. Although medical ethics and law are core subjects, they are often seen by students as marginal to their medical studies. '*Medical students find themselves prioritising the basic science subjects over perceived "fluffy" topics, such as professionalism, ethics, and the social context of medicine*' (Leo & Eagen 2008). A questionnaire survey of medical students at King's College London School of Medicine across 4 years indicated that, although most students gave positive responses regarding their interest and experiences of learning ethics and law, a small minority (6.5%) said that they were not interested in the topic. In giving reasons for their lack of interest, a number of students said they found it *difficult* and *complicated* (Johnston & Haughton 2007). In a recent study of medical students in two UK medical schools, Preston–Shoot *et al.* (2011) state that '*the majority of students lack confidence in their knowledge and skills across many areas of medical law*' and they may not be adequately prepared for practice.

Ethics and law are included in the curricula for veterinary and medical undergraduates and it is encouraging that new curricula to teach ethics to veterinary undergraduates have increased instruction on this important discipline. However, we should be clear about what is being taught, why and how effective it may be in achieving the desired aims. This requires attention to curriculum planning for ethics, law and professionalism, clear objectives, and interesting and relevant teaching methods. Cowley (2005) considers that medical students will already have encountered ethical dilemmas as a part of everyday life and that *'there is a real risk that spurious technocratic jargon will be deployed by teacher and student alike in the futile search for intellectual respectability, culminating in a misplaced sense of having "done" the ethics module'*. Nevertheless, as Rhodes and Alfandre (2007) note *'an understanding of the basic principles and concepts of medical ethics is critically important for navigating the ethical dilemmas that arise in clinical medicine'*. We should also be clear that acting within the law and acting ethically do not necessarily lead to the same conclusion. Our students could be challenged when they perceive that the only relevant question to be answered is 'is it lawful?'

Ethics teaching should enable medical and veterinary practitioners to recognise ethical problems in clinical practice and to be confident in the appropriate use of ethical principles and frameworks to come to consistent, robust and defensible decisions which can thus be respected by patients/clients and peers. There is a need for lifelong learning and engagement to counterbalance the effects of 'ethical erosion' (Feudtner *et al.* 1994).

3.3 Role of Medical Ethics in Driving Legal Change

Reflection on medical ethical principles may act as a driver for legal change and perhaps professional attitudes.

Entrenchment of human rights in law, reflecting the important principle of respect for patient autonomy. Two examples in medical practice illustrate this proposition. Let us first consider the doctrine of 'informed consent'. The legal requirement that patients are informed about the risks of and alternatives to treatment options has shifted over the years from the reasonable doctor standard, that is what risks the doctor thinks is reasonable to disclose, to the prudent patient standard, that is what a reasonable person in that patient's position would want to know. The shift has come about because of the priority given to respect for autonomy. As Lord Hope stated in Chester v Afshar (2005), *'the law of informed consent works as a means of protecting patient autonomy'*. So respect for patient autonomy has driven the change for the *nature* of the information to be disclosed, that is the risks and alternative treatments, and also the *manner* in which it is given. The High Court's decision (Al Hamwi v Johnston (2005) recognised that in explaining risks of treatment, *'a clinician must take reasonable care to give a warning which is adequate in scope, content and presentation, and take steps to see that the warning is understood'*.

In veterinary medicine, the client (normally the owner of the animal) making the choice for treatment is not the patient. Nevertheless there is a duty to communicate and disclose risks. Whether the sort of information being disclosed has or will change in veterinary medicine does not rest on the notion of 'patient autonomy' but rather on the wider concept that truthful open discussion with the client enables better informed choices.

Perhaps more challenging is the way the law may respond to the demand for respect for patient autonomy in end-of-life decision making, particularly assisted suicide. Competent adults may refuse life-sustaining treatment but currently assisted suicide is unlawful in the UK, although in other jurisdictions such as Oregon (USA), the Netherlands and Belgium, physician-assisted suicide (PAS) is lawful within certain boundaries. Generally, these are that a competent patient has made a non-coerced choice for PAS to avoid unbearable suffering in the face of a terminal illness. In 2009, Debbie Purdy argued that a lack of clarity about the circumstances in which the Crown Prosecution Service would prosecute relatives, who had taken loved ones to Dignitas in Switzerland, interfered with her human rights, that is her right under Article 8 of the European Convention on Human Rights to choose the way in which she lived which 'included the way in which she chose to pass the closing moments of her life'. As a result, in 2010, the Director of Public Prosecutions issued guidance clarifying the factors tending towards and against prosecution for assisting a suicide. We are now in interesting times as there is a groundswell of public opinion in favour of legalising PAS. Indeed, in 2012 the Commission on Assisted Dying – an independent body – reported on its review of a wide range of expert opinion in the field.

A recent empirical study of Swedish veterinary surgeons towards PAS showed that their response pattern to questions on PAS was very similar to the general public (Lerner *et al.* 2011). Physicians by contrast had a more restrictive attitude to PAS. The authors note that '*there are similarities between veterinary surgeons and physicians even if the patients differ.... Their common goal is to prevent disease, to promote the health and well-being of their patients and to provide treatment where possible*'. The general public tended to stress the respect for autonomy argument in favour of PAS, whilst veterinarians used the 'minimise suffering' argument. Yeates (2010) argues that '*non-human animals are – and, on welfare grounds, should be – euthanased when it is considered that their predicted overall quality of life is worth avoiding and cannot be avoided in any other (practical) way*'. It is perhaps possible that the 'minimise suffering' argument may give rise to a degree of paternalism in respect of the animal: the veterinarian may restrict treatment options to the owner when under pressure to perform euthanasia, which the veterinarian may consider to be unnecessary.

Nevertheless in a study by Yeates and Main (2011), the most common justification given by respondent veterinarians why they had refused euthanasia was a lack of legitimate reasons for euthanasia, that is the animal was young and not suffering or there were only mild health problems. Although some 'owner-based' reasons, such as financial circumstances of the client were considered relevant to the decision for euthanasia, Yeates and Main found that animal-based reasons were given more frequently than owner-based reasons in arguments for and against euthanasia. '*In general, these findings suggest that a concern for the patient has more influence on the decision of whether or not to euthanase than a concern for the owner*', although refusing euthanasia was reported as an uncommon issue for most respondents.

Euthanasia of a suffering and untreatable animal patient may be ethically defensible on the basis of its welfare to prohibit unnecessary suffering, although it should be remembered that euthanasia is not the only 'treatment' option for suffering; palliative care is possible but needs to be justified and not cause more distress. In medical practice, euthanasia is unlawful even if the patient is suffering. A high priority is given to the principle of sanctity of human life, although this does not mean that everything must be done to preserve life. The General Medical Council (2010) considers the *overall benefit* of the treatment. At this stage, a useful discussion could be had about the moral differences between human and non-human animals justifying differences of treatment, but I will not take this point further, for fear of diverting away from the main theme of this paper.

End of life decision-making in medical ethics has a strong focus on the principle of respect for autonomy. Indeed, respect for (human) patient autonomy and the 'right' to choose how to pass the closing moments of life has opened the debate for legalisation of PAS. In comparison of course, animals are not fully autonomous in the sense that they cannot choose the method – or timing – of their death and so the choice is made in their best interests to avoid suffering, although longevity maybe dictated by the purpose of the animal (eg. farm animal).

Whilst the law may push for respect for human patient autonomy where he/she is autonomous, it is also very clear to protect the interests of the vulnerable and those who lack the capacity (autonomy) to make decisions. Some may argue that a greater priority should be accorded to avoidance of suffering in the medical arena. This is a complicated area involving resources and, most importantly, professional attitudes and behaviours.

3.4 Professional Ethics – Behaviour and Regulation

The General Medical Council (2006) states, '*Patients must be able to trust doctors with their lives and health. To justify that trust you must show respect for human life*'. Professionals through knowledge and expertise are in positions of power with respect to the patient/client yet trust is at the heart of both professions. In the (human) medical arena, patients divulge personal and confidential information in order to receive optimal care. But this often is the case in veterinary medicine too, as many diseases are transmissible between pets and owners and the client's health may be disclosed as this may influence treatment. Veterinarians also may hear about an owner's personal finances when treatments costs are high.

There may be slightly different commercial concerns in veterinary medicine: is the proposed treatment necessary and can the client afford optimum care for a much loved animal? But is this power used appropriately and adequately checked? To justify this trust, professionals must behave in accordance with norms and standards of their profession and the public must be assured that there are robust processes in place to ensure those standards are met.

Much has been written and discussed on medical professionalism in the past decade. The Royal College of Physicians (2005) reflects on the changing role of the medical profession. In 2005 and 2006, the King's Fund and the Royal College of Physicians ran a series of 'road shows' to further explore and explain these issues, and the findings from these events have been reported (Levenson *et al.* 2008). The Institute of Medical Ethics has updated its core content of learning for medical law and ethics (Stirrat *et al.* 2010) and highlights the need for medical students to

> '*demonstrate an understanding of: i) the importance of trust, integrity, honesty and good communication in all professional relationships; ii) the need to accept personal responsibility and be aware of limitations of their practical skills or knowledge and to know how and where to seek appropriate help iii) the need to maintain professional boundaries with patients; iv) issues raised by the religious beliefs of patients, students and other healthcare professionals and the role and limits of conscientious objection; v) the need to recognise and avoid all forms of unfair discrimination in relation to patients, colleagues and other healthcare professionals; and vi) areas of potential conflict of interest, e.g., the pharmaceutical and medical equipment industries.*'

Many of these learning outcomes directly relate to the practice of veterinary medicine. The core content of learning also identifies the need for understanding of reporting adverse incidents.

The veterinary profession remains largely self-regulating across the world, for example by the RCVS in the UK. Cases involving challenges to professionalism and duty of care are largely dealt with via the veterinary governing bodies (see Chapters 4 and 17, this volume). The GMC has authority to review fitness to practice and has the role of revalidating and relicensing doctors registered in the UK.

It is also worth reflecting on the professional duties owed in the different professions. A doctor has a clear duty towards his patient. In veterinary medicine, the veterinarian has a duty towards the client and the animal and may also have a duty to the public to ensure their safety (e.g. methicillin- resistant Staphylococcus aureus (MRSA) from pets, tuberculosis or brucellosis in milk, rabies from dogs or bats and meat hygiene issues such as listeriosis, *Escherichia coli*, salmonellosis or campylobacter infection). This might give rise to conflicts of duty raising real ethical concerns. Outside the public health arena, doctors would consider their primary duty to do the best for their patient. The General Medical Council (2009) states that doctors must '*protect and promote the health of patients and the public*', although clearly it may not be possible for these duties to be fulfilled with limited resources. So both professions are grappling with concerns around professional duties and responsibilities and the ethical tensions that arise.

3.5 Ethical Approaches to Dilemmas Confronting the Modern Veterinarian – Can We Learn from Clinical Ethics Frameworks?

Education in clinical ethics and professional ethics is essential to enable future practitioners to identify, engage with and acquire the skills to deal with difficult ethical dilemmas arising in veterinary and medical practice. The driver for increased attention to veterinary ethics may result in a heightened '*scrutiny from animal owners and the media over ethical issues*' (Mullan and Main 2001).

Whilst the detail of the dilemmas will depend on the profession and the facts of each case, an ability to know about and use ethical principles and frameworks will provide the tools to grapple with these issues. Ethical dilemmas arise when there is uncertainty or a conflict about what to do and this will often centre on a difference of values or perspectives. In the medical setting, this difference of views may arise between members of the healthcare team and the patient or the patient's family, and the law; indeed, resources will have an impact too. For the veterinary practitioner, public health concerns throw up ethical dilemmas but so too does the perception of animal suffering or cruelty.

The four principles coined by the American bioethicists Beauchamp and Childress (2009) have caught the imagination of doctors and those training them for their simplicity and scope. Principlism refers to respect for patient autonomy, beneficence, non-maleficence and justice. Although these principles are assumed to be non-hierarchical, respect for patient autonomy has perhaps gained particular significance when set against the backdrop of human rights discourse. In my experience, these principles can be trotted out by medical students and doctors alike, without real engagement with the underlying concerns. Alternative, or indeed additional approaches, might include virtue ethics, narrative ethics, consequences and rule-based ethics (deontology). No single theory or framework will provide an answer and nor should they. It is the garnering of different perspectives and views that enables an informed and rounded approach. Martje Fentener van Vlissingen has stated that 'codes of ethics for veterinarians focus mainly on professional conduct in relation to colleagues and clients, such as advertising and the adoption of one another's clients. Meanwhile, the interests of animals are considered implicit rather than being discussed explicitly' (Fentener van Vlissingen 2001). The patient – whether a human or animal – is at the heart of the decision-making process and we should be clear that ethical frameworks explicitly reflect that importance.

How useful is this approach to veterinary ethics? Fentener van Vlissingen noted that

'for very obvious reasons veterinary ethics are more complicated than medical ethics: i) the informed opinion of the animal in question is never available; ii) to sustain the life of an individual animal is not a central issue because most domestic animals do not complete their natural life span; and iii) at best, the reasons for keeping animals are not contradictory to their interests.'

I am not sure I fully agree with this view. First, it is often the values expressed through the informed opinion of the patient or the relatives/carers that give rise to the ethical dilemma. Secondly, as we have seen, the principle of sanctity of (human) life presents physicians with a dilemma where that principle may seem to be at odds with quality of life assessments. Finally, rearing animals for slaughter is against their best interests where they would have 'a life worth living', although of course I accept that other justifications can be advanced for livestock farming. Best interests of a patient may be very difficult to assess because it is not just the clinical outcomes that are relevant but also the wishes and values expressed by the patient and those who are close to him/her. Nevertheless, the law clearly prevents a deliberate action taken to end human life, even where a competent adult patient, suffering through the pain and indignity of terminal illness, does not consider it is in his/her own best interests to continue living.

Fentener van Vlissingen (2001) suggests that an analysis of a case, 'with a view to developing a model for decision-making and identifying the relevant professional responsibilities, might lead to the following scheme, which summarises the interests of all parties concerned':

1. animals' interests: 'the availability of therapy and its likely success and quality of life after treatment';
2. owners' interests: 'the consideration for the health and well-being of the animal, the emotional bond with the animal and the costs of treatment';
3. veterinarians' interests: 'consideration for the health and well-being of the animal, his relationship with the client and the professional challenge, the commercial interest; and
4. interest of the population to which the animal belongs and issues of inheritable conditions causing serious defects'.

This seems to be a very good approach, reflecting upon case-based analysis which is popular in the medical setting. The inclusion of perspectives of all the stakeholders can also ensure the maintenance of public trust.

Finally, I should like to draw your attention to Clinical Ethics Committees (which are different from Research Ethics Committees you will be familiar with) which provide a multi-disciplinary forum for discussion of cases raising ethical concerns. They can also have the remit for input into policy and teaching. They may provide a useful dimension for the discussion of ethical issues arising in a particular case to consideration of the ethical concerns raised through commercial considerations and wider policy matters.

References

Al Hamwi v Johnston and the North West London Hospitals NHS Trust (2005) EWHC 206.

Beauchamp, T.L. & Childress, J.F. (2009) *Principles of Biomedical Ethics*, 6th edn. Oxford University Press, New York.

Chester v Afshar (2005) 1 AC 134, para 57.

Cowley, C. (2005) The dangers of medical ethics. *Journal of Medical Ethics*, **31**, 739–742.

Fentener van Vlissingen, M. (2001) Professional ethics in veterinary science – Considering the consequences as a tool for problem solving. *Veterinary Sciences for Tomorrow*, **1**, 1–8.

Feudtner, C., Christakis, D.A. & Christakis, N.A. (1994) Do clinical students suffer ethical erosion? Students' perceptions of their ethical and personal development. *Academic Medicine*, **69**, 670–679.

General Medical Council. (2006) Good medical practice. Available at: http://www.gmc-uk. org/guidance/good_medical_practice.asp.Accessed on 28 May, 2012.

General Medical Council. (2009) Tomorrow's doctors. Available at: http://www.gmc-uk. org/education/undergraduate/tomorrows_doctors.asp.Accessed on 28 May, 2012.

General Medical Council. (2010) Treatment and care towards the end of life: Good practice in decision making. Available at: http://www.gmc-uk.org/End_of_life.pdf_32486688.pdf. Accessed on 28 May, 2012.

Johnston, C. & Haughton, P. (2007) Medical students' perceptions of their ethics teaching. *Journal of Medical Ethics*, **33**, 418–422.

Leo, T. & Eagen, K. (2008) Professional education, the medical student response. *Perspectives in Biology and Medicine*, **15**, 508–516.

Lerner, H., Lindblad, A., Algers, B. & Lynoe, N. (2011) Veterinary surgeons' attitudes towards physician assisted suicide: An empirical study of Swedish experts on euthanasia. *Journal of Medical Ethics*, **37**, 295–298.

Levenson, R., Dewar, S. & Shepherd, S. (2008) *Understanding Doctors: Harnessing Professionalism*. Royal College of Physicians of London, London.

Mullan, S. & Main, D. (2001) Principles of ethical decision-making in veterinary practice. *In Practice*, **23**, 394–401.

Preston-Shoot, M., McKimm, J., Kong, W. M. & Smith, S. (2011) Readiness for legally literate medical practice? Student perceptions of their undergraduate medico-legal education. *Journal of Medical Ethics*, **37**, 616–622.

RCVS. (2006) Essential competences required of the veterinary surgeon. Part 1 A1.9. Available at: http://www.rcvs.org.uk/document-library/day-and-year-one-competences/ day_and_year_one_competences.pdf

Rhodes, R. & Alfandre, D. (2007) A systematic approach to clinical moral reasoning. *Clinical Ethics*, **2**, 66–70.

Rollin, B.E. (2006) *An Introduction to Veterinary Medical Ethics*, 2nd edn. Blackwell Publishing, Ames, Iowa.

Royal College of Physicians. (2005) Doctors in society: Medical professionalism in a changing world. *Report of a Working Party of the Royal College of Physicians of London.* Royal College of Physicians, London.

Stirrat, G., Johnston, C., Gillon, R. & Boyd, K. (2010) Medical ethics and law for doctors of tomorrow: The 1998 Consensus Statement updated. *Journal of Medical Ethics*, **36**, 55–60.

Yeates, J. (2010) Death is a welfare issue. *Journal of Agricultural and Environmental Ethics*, **23**, 229–241.

Yeates, J. & Main, D. (2011) Veterinary opinions on refusing euthanasia: Justifications and philosophical frameworks. *Veterinary Record*, **168**, 263–267.

Questions and Answers

Q: One of the areas in which veterinary ethics differs from medical ethics is the dual obligations a veterinarian has to the client (as the animal's owner) and the animal *per se*. How should best interests be judged? The law has not always dealt very well with best interest, for instance, in the family context. Are there lessons to be drawn, for example from the way that law deals with children?

A: Parents do take healthcare decisions on behalf of their children; they have authority to do so, as do animal owners in respect of the animal. In both cases, the remit is to make such decisions in the best interests of those who are the subject of the decision. Ethical conflicts may arise where the parents/animal owner and the doctor/veterinarian have different perspectives of best interests. Medicine can impose normative concepts, e.g. the idea that a minimum state of health or a certain level of suffering is (un)acceptable. This may also be true in the veterinary arena. It is relevant to consider how much weight should be attributed to the more holistic, less clinically identifiable concepts which the animal owner/parents can contribute to the discussion of best interests of the animal/child.

Q: Medical ethics is less pluralist than veterinary ethics; in the latter, some may say, 'Well there are different opinions'. People are allowed to have very different views about how to treat farm animals: the role of ethics is not to tell what's right and wrong but rather to make people understand veterinarians, that is a client may have a completely different view to the veterinarians. It's about understanding different viewpoints. What are your comments on the balance between showing different viewpoints and allowing people to see different perspectives rather than telling them what to do? Some of veterinary ethics is about seeing different viewpoints. Veterinary ethics is much more preoccupied by actually allowing different viewpoints to be seen rather than telling people what's good practice.

A: 'Patient centred care' recognises the importance of providing care that is respectful of and responsive to individual patient preferences, needs and values (Institute of Medicine). The core content of learning for medical ethics and law in the medical curriculum places emphasis on patient narrative, patients' moral and legal rights and the views of carers. There is acknowledgement in law and ethics that patients and their relatives and carers have an important part in the decision making process. Of course there is room for disagreement on what treatment options are in the 'best interests' of a patient' but good medical practice requires that differing viewpoints and perspectives are taken into account.

Q: I wanted to come back to the issue of consent. A veterinarian commented to me that the regime of chemotherapy for dogs is much less harsh than would be used for humans because the animal can't consent to the treatment. Is that the norm in the veterinary profession or was his comment unusual? Whereas I expected a justification on the basis of welfare, the justification was because an animal can't consent to harsh treatment.
A: Does that mean that a human patient can consent to particular harms as long as he/she is given sufficient information of the risks and alternatives of treatment? There must be a *de minimis* point where we would say that very harmful treatments, even if there is no realistic alternative, should not be offered even if a patient is informed and consents.

Q: At what point do you think veterinarians should get involved in the development of research, using the examples of chemotherapy and transplant technologies? Should veterinarians be involved to put on an 'ethical brake' on some developments, such as organ regeneration? Just because medical colleagues can do it with humans, should we be following that line in the veterinary field? Should there be a point at which we say that's a road we shouldn't go down?
A: There is a tension between scientists wanting to prove a particular point and the application or the benefit that might be achieved in the future. There is always a sense of pushing the boundaries to benefit future medical science. This will be constrained by research ethics approval and the nature of the benefit to be achieved over the harm. There is a responsibility to consider how far research should go: there could be a useful comparison between the two professions.

Author's Commentary

There is much that can be learned from a dialogue between veterinary and medical ethics. As we have seen from the questions raised, appropriate professional behaviour, the limits of consent and the balance between benefits and harms both for the individual patient and the wider community are common to both professions.

The issue of patient welfare highlights the values that are apparent in veterinary and medical ethics discourse. Consideration of the value that is attributed to human and animal life, and perceptions of quality of life and the desire to avoid harm, highlights the similarities and differences of the professions and the justifications for making decisions that can have a profound effect on individual patients, their families/owners and society.

Veterinary Ethics, Professionalism and Society

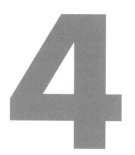

STEPHEN A. MAY

Royal Veterinary College

'... *any understanding of professional practice and values must take account of the embeddedness of professionals in a broader cultural context. It may be suggested that the acceptance of the authority of professional knowledge is a hard won cultural and political achievement, and one that is threatened in contemporary society.*'

Edgar (2011). Used with permission.

Abstract: Veterinary ethics embraces all the behaviours of veterinarians and their decisions in practice. However, it is more than etiquette! It involves the principles that underlie professional reasoning, and the processes that govern the veterinarian's intentions and actions, ensuring that each aspect is appropriately weighted so as to arrive at rational and defensible judgements. This paper explores the 'contract' that exists between society and the profession, its implications for professional education, values and conduct, the clash between the self-regulated professional model and the current fashion for the externally regulated, free market model and concludes by considering the relevances of professionalism and the professional model for twenty-first century society.

Keywords: agency, conduct, ethics, hidden curriculum, market, professionalism, rights, social contract, value, veterinarians, veterinary ethics

Veterinary & Animal Ethics: Proceedings of the First International Conference on Veterinary and Animal Ethics, September 2011, First Edition. Edited by Christopher M. Wathes, Sandra A. Corr, Stephen A. May, Steven P. McCulloch and Martin C. Whiting.
© 2013 Universities Federation for Animal Welfare. Published 2013 by Blackwell Publishing Ltd.

4.1 Introduction

A certain amount of confusion surrounding the term 'veterinary ethics' has been created, particularly in the UK, by its narrow application to animal welfare–related discussions (Legood 2000; Thornton *et al.* 2001; Schneider 2002; Felipedia 2011) and the relative lack of specific attention to professional ethics in curricula of professional programmes throughout the world. A focus on animal suffering is understandable; it is part of the promise that every veterinarian in the UK makes when they are admitted to the veterinary profession (RCVS 2010) but, together with the suggestion that professional ethics is no more than 'etiquette' (Thornton *et al.* 2001; Main *et al.* 2005), it detracts from the broader definition of veterinary ethics embracing the various behaviours of veterinarians and their decisions in practice (Tannenbaum 1995; Rollin 2006; Free Dictionary 2011; Wikipedia 2011).

The advent of the knowledge society and the increased complexity of decisions relating to animal management and therapy mean that, as in other areas (Tulgan 2001), there has been a marked shift away from the professional role of transmission of knowledge to judgement as the key professional attribute. In addition, judgements that may involve a balance of animal, client, societal, professional and individual interests are increasingly subject to challenge, or at least scrutinised for their underlying rationale that will often involve decision making across several ethical dimensions. If professional behaviour is reduced to the level of etiquette, with members of the profession never understanding the fundamental principles on which they operate nor questioning the rationale behind their Guide to Professional Conduct (RCVS 2010), then veterinary leaders and educators have betrayed veterinary ethics in the same way as those occupying similar positions in the medical profession (Brody 2003; Hafferty & Castellani 2010).

The aim of this paper is to provide a principled exploration of this complex area for the veterinary profession. It:

- looks at the nature of the modern profession from the perspective of Thomas Hobbes' 'Social Contract';
- argues the case that veterinary professional ethics is more than etiquette;
- examines the effect of the societal context on the profession and its members;
- explores the implications for 'physician agency' and professional conduct towards clients;
- highlights the lessons for veterinary education in the twenty-first century; and
- discusses how the professional model for the organisation of human affairs remains as relevant as ever to society as a whole.

4.2 The Nature of the Modern Profession

At first sight, the work of Thomas Hobbes (1588–1679) may seem an unlikely starting point for a discussion about the modern veterinary profession. Hobbes' key concern was the legitimacy of political leadership and the powers associated with political office. He argued that an individual's normal state, in the absence of any organisation of our society, would be '*nasty, poor, solitary, brutish and short*' and that there were three main reasons for this: the scarcity of things human beings value, a passion for glory and a mistrust of others that leads to a perpetual state of war (Minogue 1995). Therefore, he concluded, at the same time recognising the individual loss of freedom that this entailed, that sovereignty had legitimacy in providing a structure for increased personal security, thus improving the human lot. In this sense, a 'social contract' existed between citizens and those in power that implied duties and responsibilities for both. In exchange for protection for families and goods, citizens should contribute to society and conform to its rules, and in exchange for the privilege of power, leaders should act in the interests of the whole of society (Hardin 1968; Scruton 1995).

In a little over 100 years, from the formation of the Royal College of Veterinary Surgeons (RCVS) in 1844 to the current UK Veterinary Surgeons Act (1966), the profession has advanced from acts of veterinary surgery that could be performed by anyone to procedures that are reserved exclusively for veterinarians. This sequential progress was achieved because the profession argued that its members alone had the knowledge and skills to promote and protect animal health and welfare, the interests of animal owners and keepers, and the interests and concerns of society (also see Paper 1). A Hobbesian social contract developed, like in medicine (Cohen 2006; Thistlethwaite & Spencer 2008), so that in exchange for the restriction of acts of veterinary surgery to the profession, veterinarians must act in the interests of society and its members. A part of 'the bargain' reached in the UK, in the Veterinary Surgeons Act 1881, in exchange for it being made illegal for anyone other than an individual on the RCVS Register to receive payment for veterinary work, was a requirement for the profession to deal with conduct that was disgraceful in a professional respect (Pattison 1984).

In a world where increasing distrust of experts and those in positions of power means that the model of external regulation has become a dominant paradigm, many see the concept of self-regulation by professions as both flawed and anachronistic. However, it emphasises the distinct difference between a craft or trade, where the outputs, and effectiveness in achieving these can be widely understood, and a profession, where the abilities of the practitioner and the quality of their work can only be fully comprehended by those in the profession (Edgar 2011). A balance is achieved by the profession taking its responsibility for regulation seriously, enforcing the high standards expected by the public from its members, and never protecting the interests of those members at the expense of society and its citizens. This has been well captured by Rollin (2006) in a societal warning to veterinarians: '*You regulate yourselves the way we would regulate you if we understood in detail what you do (which we don't), but if you violate this charge and trust we will know and hammer you with Draconian rules*'.

4.3 Veterinary Professional Ethics – More than Etiquette!

The concept of a social contract with clear responsibilities and duties for a profession at once elevates the behaviours of its members to more than etiquette. The conduct of a veterinarian should not result merely from the unthinking adoption of contemporary social, or even professional, behavioural norms, but should always start with a recognition of duties of service that the privilege of membership of the profession confer. A veterinarian's knowledge must be continuously updated and applied with a skill that avoids maleficence and maximises the likelihood of beneficence on the part of a patient. At the same time, the veterinarian must respect client autonomy for decisions over their animals and ensure that the principle of justice is applied to service delivery (Beauchamp & Childress 2001). This may come at a financial cost to veterinarians when, on occasion, they need to act in the interests of animal welfare, knowing that they have little chance of reward for their services or they need to turn down business after consideration of their professional limitations leads to the recognition that the work is outwith their range of competence. An understanding of the foundations for such decisions, and the ability to engage in ethical reasoning, to complement the more obvious clinical reasoning that is central to veterinary practice, will help ensure that individuals retain the respect of their clients and preserve the status and credibility of their profession (Rollin 2006; Mellor 2010).

4.4 The Effect of the Societal Context on the Profession and Its Members

The professional ethic, with its emphasis on a balance between privilege and responsibilities, represents a special case of the broader concept of citizenship, with its attendant duties, rights and privileges. Although many philosophers would see a correlation between natural or moral rights and duties, in practice, when these and other legal and constitutional rights are framed in law, there can be considerable difficulty in ensuring that one mirrors the other, and tensions can arise as a result of the expectations of different parties in any relationship (Donnelly 1982; Fieser 1992; Kobrin 2009). The asymmetry has also been enhanced in recent years by a political emphasis on rights, arguably, in part, to address a failure of various leaders to understand their responsibilities that combined with an unfortunate neglect of the discussion of duties. This has led to at least two consequences in the way in which citizens view their relationship with society. Whereas a duty of individuals to provide for the disadvantaged in society emphasises a collective relationship that recognises a balance in terms of what is possible, and engenders gratitude towards the donor, a right to be provided for emphasises recipient demands that may ultimately overwhelm the ability of society to provide, which will lead to resentment (Gillon 1985). In addition, when legislators confer rights on individuals, governments may be seen as primarily responsible for fulfilling the subsequent demands, allowing citizens to side-step what, in a different framework, may be seen as a collective duty of individuals to provide. The danger is that, progressively, the predominant thinking of all citizens relates to what they can get out of society – in some cases 'what they can get away with' – rather than what they have a duty to put in!

The emphasis on rights at an individual level has coincided, in the last 40 years, with an emphasis on the market at the level of society (Friedman 1970; O'Shaughnessy 1994; Steil 2009). This has led, in some quarters, to an instrumental view of corporate social responsibility and a view that wealth creation, and a contribution to society through taxes, is the sole responsibility of corporations (Garriga & Melé 2004). In the market, it makes sense to minimise the amount that needs to be paid to the state, so, at both corporate and individual levels, self-interest has been emphasised, with the model for control being based on external regulation rather than the self-regulation historically accorded to the professions.

Professions have not been immune to this overall shift in emphasis from responsibility to society to self-interest. Hafferty (2002) has recognised a sharp contrast between the attitudes of his general medical practitioner father and uncle and his medical students, with the latter group rejecting any sense of obligation and being clear that they would '*do good … on their own terms*', a perspective that May (1975) has described as '*the conceit of philanthropy*'. This next generation of medical practitioners emphasised the need 'to take care of oneself before one can take care of others' and 'to have "balance" in terms of their lives'. They framed the latter 'balance' in terms of personal and family needs.

There are sound ethical arguments and moral traditions that can be advanced to support the principle of work-related reward – like the ox, '*the labourer is worthy of his hire*' (Holy Bible, English Revised Version, 1 Timothy 5:18) – and a balanced approach to service and self-care. However, the tendency of free market thinking to emphasise excess is in sharp distinction to, for instance, Aristotle's doctrine of virtue as the mean between excess and deficiency (Brown 2009; Sellman 2011). Cohen (2006) has gone further and declared a profound incompatibility between capitalism and professionalism, neatly portrayed in the two mottoes: *caveat emptor* and *primum non nocere*. The whole meaning of a profession would be lost if it counselled wariness on the part of those it served. Therefore, it is predictable that the predominance of human capital theories focused on wealth (Gilead 2009), as well as attitudes expressed by some members of the professions, together with examples of unprofessional behaviours, has led to profound distrust on the part of economists and politicians of the professional model, even at a time when the alternative, of externally regulated expertise within a free market framework, has failed so spectacularly (Bragues 2010). This has meant that, in medicine, veterinary medicine and the law, each instance of behaviour 'disgraceful in a professional respect', and any perceived leniency toward a member being disciplined, notwithstanding the constraints that Human Rights legislation has placed on disciplinary bodies, is seen as a failure of the whole professional model, necessitating movement towards the preferred external regulatory framework.

4.5 Professionalism and Physician Agency

A pervasive political message, oft repeated since the 1970s, has been the concept that private and public life can be divorced, and that an individual whose personal morality is questionable can, at the same time, wield political power with honesty and integrity. Therefore, it should not be surprising that many politicians sincerely believe that external regulation can enforce professional behaviours, in the interests of society, whatever the natural inclination (which is assumed to be self-interest) of the individual. However, the requirement that, in the face of a vulnerable individual, a member of a profession acts altruistically in their client's interest, and does not take advantage, even in the absence of external scrutiny, is so important as to be central to the identity of the doctor (Martimianakis *et al.* 2009) and the veterinarian. It is clear that to perform at the highest professional level, there must be little or no dissonance between professional values and values in private life and that genuine values 'are not disposable, to be taken up with a white coat or uniform and set aside at the end of the working day' (Badcott 2011).

There have been various attempts in the professions to characterise the key professional value set, the enaction of which would constitute professionalism. In engineering, these have been suggested as a respect for nature, a commitment to the public good, an awareness of the social context of technology and a sensitivity to risk (Harris 2008), although, yet again, the requirement for 'benefitting humanity' has been challenged as violating an engineer's rights to seek happiness and '*act according to one's true self-interest*' (Stieb 2011). In medicine (Williams 2001), professionalism has also been viewed as an ethical concept, with three key features (easily identified in veterinary medicine as well) flowing from the social contract as duties for individual doctors: (1) altruism – leading to a strong commitment to others, respect for patients and respect for society; (2) competence – related to a body of knowledge and skills, reflective practice and teamworking and (3) integrity based on high moral standards and acceptance of accountability.

Once the foundations on which a profession operates and the values that flow from the social contract are understood, the important focus of veterinary ethics is the processes that allow rational and defensible decisions to be made. In the UK, the RCVS has drafted a revised declaration to be made by new members as they enter the profession that emphasises, in addition to animal welfare and working with integrity, the veterinarian's responsibilities to 'clients, the public, the profession and the RCVS', the statutory body in the UK, itself (RCVS 2011). Rollin (2006) has identified the same responsibilities in the form of four obligations to society, the profession, the animal(s) receiving attention and the client, and added a fifth obligation of the individual veterinarian to himself or herself.

As in medicine, particularly with infectious disease, a key issue may be balancing the interests of a group or population of animals with those of an individual in the group and the interests of society or a community with those of an individual animal owner. An important value in this dimension is reciprocity (Viens *et al.* 2009), and farmers have accepted the principle of slaughter with compensation for notifiable diseases. However, difficulties arise when there is distrust over the need for contiguous culls, particularly when these involve pet farm animals and seem to relate more to politics than scientific evidence (Vidal 2001; Michell 2005). The perceived imperative to prioritise the welfare of individual animals may also be in conflict with responsibilities to clients in the case of zoonoses such as tuberculosis or psittacosis.

A major difference between veterinary ethics and medical ethics is the expansion of the clinician–patient relationship to a triangular clinician–patient–client relationship. This is at the heart of the majority of veterinary ethical dilemmas facing the general veterinary practitioner on a day-to-day basis, and the way these dilemmas are resolved will depend on an additional element, the concept of the profession held by the individual clinician. Rollin (2006) has characterised the two extremes as 'the paediatrician' and 'the garage mechanic'. The paediatrician, analogous to their medical counterpart, may need to be an advocate for the patient who cannot speak for themselves and will tend always to prioritise their perception of the needs of the patient over the wishes of the client. In contrast, the garage mechanic is focused on the client and is much more likely to try to match their diagnostic and therapeutic approaches to the wishes of the client. There are gender differences in the balance between these two extremes. Although veterinary students and recent graduates are more paediatrician- than garage mechanic-orientated, males are more garage mechanic in their attitudes when they enter veterinary school and this difference increases as they move into their early years in practice (Ogden & May 2009, unpublished data).

The balancing of patient needs with the ethical principle of client autonomy is at the heart of ethical dilemmas around physician agency and informed consent. Agency theory is a branch of economics that relates to conflicts of interest between individuals who have different interests in an asset. A veterinarian may have different views on the treatment of a patient from a client for both worthy – a treatment is superior to an alternative – and less worthy – a treatment is more financially advantageous – reasons. Veterinarians have an 'Aesculapian authority' (Rollin 2006) that comes with their professional position and, particularly if they are adept communicators (Main 2011), this allows them to wield significant influence over the ultimate client decision. Physician agency deals with the power, motives and behaviours of clinicians as they deal with their patients (McGuire 2000), and difficult areas such as quality of service and physician-induced demand for services.

The danger of the abuse of power leading to consent of questionable value means that considerable thought needs to be given to shared decision making (Kon 2010). A naïve view of autonomy has led some young veterinarians to see their role as laying a mass of information and options before the client and leaving the decision up to them! Indeed, this may be the relationship that some clients demand, but for others it will represent an abdication of the responsibility to recognise their needs, in terms of help in understanding the options and dealing with the emotions that may cloud their ability to make a rational decision. A collaborative framework recognises this, with the clinician and the client resolving how much responsibility the client wants to take and how much they should take (Politi & Street 2010).

Further issues can arise in trying to work with difficult clients in the interests of their animals. Clients who have faith in homoeopathic remedies need to be persuaded of the necessity for the concurrent use of analgesic agents in animals that are in pain, together with disease-modifying therapies where appropriate, without the veterinarian giving the impression that they are endorsing the efficacy of homeopathy. Care also needs to be taken in the use of unproven therapies by veterinarians themselves and the provision of a diagnosis to a client wanting an answer in the absence of adequate evidence to support a conclusion. Such actions not only undermine the credibility of the individual but will also reflect badly on the profession of which they are a member and represent a breach of trust with the society that has given power to the medical and veterinary professions on the basis that they are 'scientifically and evidentially based' (Rollin 2006).

The resolution of the potential conflicts between all these separate issues and interested parties, at the same time as maintaining a focus on animal welfare, requires the balancing of multiple ethical principles, such as a deontological perspective that highlights the interests of the individual and a utilitarian perspective that maximises the benefit for all involved (Tannenbaum 1995; Rollin 2006). Alternatively, Sellman (2011) has found it helpful to approach professional values in nursing using a virtue ethics framework and the principle of the Aristotelian mean (Brown 2009). In dealing with limited resources for healthcare, the professional goal of excellence and the market's drive for efficiency might be seen as two extremes in a dimension called efficacy. The mean would be the point at which a good standard of care could be delivered at an affordable cost.

4.6 Lessons for Veterinary Education

In the same way as the focus on animal welfare has detracted from a broader and more balanced view of veterinary ethics, the focus in veterinary curricula on the organic disease aspect of the complex interaction between the patient and client has led to a relative neglect of business principles and theory, ethical reasoning (in contrast to clinical reasoning) and interpersonal, including verbal and non-verbal, skills (as opposed to written communication). As in medicine (Thistlethwaite & Spencer 2008), the deficiency has been recognised in a redefinition of day one skills (RCVS 2001, 2006); in the UK (May 2008) and elsewhere (Lane & Bogue 2010), curricula are being revised to include more substantial professional skills strands.

However, the transformation of veterinary education will require more than the revision of curricula. Educators, who currently do not see the broader professional development of their students as part of their role (Lane & Bogue 2010), will need to expand their skills in this area and recognise how their academic focus on technical skills, to the exclusion of other skills that make up the repertoire of the successful general practitioner, can lead to a 'hidden curriculum' (Hafferty & Franks 1994) that may undermine the necessary curriculum changes. It will be important that a similar emphasis on practical application of knowledge and skills, in the area of veterinary professional ethics, to that advocated and adopted in clinical education (Lucke 1991), is achieved.

4.7 Continued Relevance to Society of the Professional Model

Over the last 100 years, sociologists have held a variety of views on professions and professionalism, ranging from professionalism as a value system, emphasising altruism and subjecting individualism to the needs of society, to professionalism as a conspiracy of powerful occupational workers (Evetts 2003). The different accounts emphasise that however the professions are best understood, professionalism is about much more than a list of attitudes and behaviours (Martimianakis *et al.* 2009). A neglected theme has been the importance of the professions in the creation of modern capitalist order in the liberal democratic state, and the way in which professionalism represents a 'third logic' alongside consumerism – the market – and bureaucracy – government (Freidson 2001). The evidence in the professions of a workable, organisational model, based on self-regulation by individuals with standards and integrity, and value systems that emphasise the good of society, provides an important contrast with the amorality of market-driven behaviours and ever-increasing bureaucratic measures that try to defend the broader community interests. As the latter approach fails, there is even talk of the rediscovery of a social contract for banking (Wilson 2011). It is important that members of the professions, who understand the ethical framework of their value system, are able, and willing, to take up their broader social responsibility to ensure that this third logic, a key to social stability, with its ability to broker efficacy, as a balance between its ideal of excellence and the market's pressure for efficiency (Sellman 2011), is not drowned out by the voices of the market and governments!

4.8 Conclusion

The value systems that characterise the professions flow from the social contract that has created and maintained their existence. Veterinary ethics deals with the complex judgements that lead to the professionalism with which veterinarians discharge the responsibilities to their patients, their clients, the public, the profession and themselves. Continued excellence in service provision, through veterinarians acting with honesty and integrity, is essential to the health and sustainability of the professional model, and this will only be achieved if all members of the profession have a clear understanding of their professional *raison d'être* (Morrison *et al.* 2009).

Professionalism has been an important logic, alongside consumerism and bureaucracy, in the development of society as we know it, in the democracies of the western world, and provides an important contrast to the externally regulated marketplace in terms of an informed and balanced model of how communities can ensure that the needs of all their members are met.

References

Beauchamp, T.L. & Childress, J.F. (2001) *Principles of Biomedical Ethics*, 5th edn. Oxford University Press, Oxford.

Badcott, D. (2011) Professional values: Introduction to the theme. *Medicine, Health Care and Philosophy*, **14**, 185–186.

Brody, H. (2003) Professionalism, ethics or both? Does it matter? *Medical Humanities Report*, **24**, 1–4.

Brown, L. (2009) Introduction. In: *Aristotle: The Nicomachean Ethics* [Translated by W.D. Ross] (ed. L. Brown), pp. vii–xxix. Oxford University Press, Oxford.

Bragues, G. (2010) Leverage and liberal democracy. In: *Lessons from the Financial Crisis: Causes, Consequences, and our Economic Future* (ed. R.W. Kolb), pp. 3–8. John Wiley & Sons, Hoboken, New Jersey.

Cohen, J.J. (2006) Professionalism in medical education, an American perspective: From evidence to accountability. *Medical Education*, **40**, 607–617.

Donnelly, J. (1982) How are rights and duties correlative? *Journal of Value Inquiry*, **16**, 287–294.

Edgar, A. (2011) Professional values, aesthetic values, and the ends of trade. *Medicine, Health Care and Philosophy*, **14**, 195–201.

Evetts, J. (2003) The sociological analysis of professionalism: Occupational change in the modern world. *International Sociology*, **18**, 395–415.

Felipedia, (2011) Veterinary ethics. Available at: http://www.felipedia.org/~felipedi/wiki/index.php?title=Veterinary_Ethics (accessed on 11 July 2011).

Fieser, J. (1992) The correlativity of duties and rights. *International Journal of Applied Philosophy*, **7**, 2.

Free Dictionary (2011) Veterinary ethics. Available at: http://medical-dictionary.thefree dictionary.com/veterinary+ethics (accessed 11 July 2011).

Freidson, D. (2001) *Professionalism: The Third Logic*. University of Chicago Press, Chicago.

Friedman, M. (1970) The social responsibility of business is to increase its profits. *The New York Times Magazine*, September 13, 1970.

Garriga, E. & Melé, D. (2004) Corporate social responsibility theories: Mapping the territory. *Journal of Business Ethics*, **53**, 51–71.

Gilead, T. (2009) Human capital, education and the promotion of social cooperation: A philosophical critique. *Studies in Philosophy and Education*, **28**, 555–567.

Gillon, R. (1985) Rights. *British Medical Journal*, **290**, 1890–1891.

Hafferty, F.W. (2002) What medical students know about professionalism. *The Mount Sinai Journal of Medicine*, **69**, 385–397.

Hafferty, F.W. & Castellani, B. (2010) The increasing complexities of professionalism. *Academic Medicine*, **85**, 288–301.

Hafferty, F.W. & Franks, R. (1994) The hidden curriculum, ethics teaching, and the structure of medical education. *Academic Medicine*, **69**, 861–871.

Hardin, G. (1968) The tragedy of the commons. *Science*, **162**, 1243–1248.

Harris, C.E. (2008) The good engineer: Giving virtue its due in engineering ethics. *Science and Engineering Ethics*, **14**, 153–164.

Kobrin, S.J. (2009) Private political authority and public responsibility: Transnational politics, transnational firms and human rights. *Business Ethics Quarterly*, **19**, 349–374.

Kon, A.A. (2010) The shared decision-making continuum. *Journal of the American Medical Association*, **304**, 903–904.

Lane, I.F. & Bogue, E.G. (2010) Perceptions of veterinary faculty members regarding their responsibility and preparation to teach non-technical competencies. *Journal of Veterinary Medical Education*, **37**, 238–247.

Legood, G. (2000) *Veterinary Ethics: An Introduction*. Continuum, London.

Lucke, J. (1991) *Report of the Working Party on Veterinary Undergraduate Education*. Royal College of Veterinary Surgeons, London.

Main, D.C.J. (2011) Influencing clients. *Veterinary Record*, **168**, 383–384.

Main, D.C.J., Thornton, P. & Kerr, K. (2005) Teaching animal welfare science, ethics and law to veterinary students in the United Kingdom. *Journal of Veterinary Medical Education*, **32**, 505–508.

Martimianakis, M.A., Maniate, J.M. & Hodges, B.D. (2009) Sociological interpretations of professionalism. *Medical Education*, **43**, 829–837.

May, W.F. (1975) Code, covenant, contract or philanthropy. *Hastings Center Report*, **5**, 29–38.

May, S.A. (2008) Modern veterinary graduates are outstanding – But can they get better? *Journal of Veterinary Medical Education*, **35**,573–580.

McGuire, T.G. (2000) Physician agency. In: *Handbook of Health Economics*, Vol. 1 (eds A.J. Culyer & J.P. Newhouse), pp. 461–536, Chapter 9. Elsevier Science, Amsterdam, the Netherlands.

Mellor, D.J. (2010) Ethics, expectations and excellence in veterinary professionalism. *VetScript*, December 2010, pp. 6–8.

Michell, B. (2005) FMD and the contiguous cull. *Veterinary Record*, **156**, 847–848.

Minogue, K. (1995) *Politics: A Very Short Introduction*. Oxford University Press, Oxford.

Morrison, J., Dowie, A., Cotton, P. & Goldie, J. (2009) A medical education view on sociological perspectives on professionalism. *Medical Education*, **43**, 824–825.

Ogden, U. & May, S.A. (2009) Veterinary attitudes to euthanasia, death and coping. Royal Veterinary College undergraduate research project: London.

O'Shaughnessy, T. (1994) Economic Policy. In: *A Conservative Revolution?: The Thatcher-Reagan Decade in Perspective* (eds A. Adonis & T. Hames), pp.89–113, Chapter 5. Manchester University Press, New York.

Pattison, I. (1984) *The British Veterinary Profession 1791–1948*. J. A. Allen, London.

Politi, M.C. & Street, R.L. (2010) The importance of communication in collaborative decision making: Facilitating shared mind and the management of uncertainty. *Journal of Evaluation in Clinical Practice*, 1–6. doi: 10.1111/j.1365–2753.2010.01549.x.

Rollin, B.E. (2006) *An Introduction to Veterinary Medical Ethics*, 2nd Ed. Blackwell Publishing, Ames, Iowa.

Royal College of Veterinary Surgeons (RCVS) (2001) *Veterinary Education and Training: A Framework for 2010 and Beyond*. Royal College of Veterinary Surgeons, London.

Royal College of Veterinary Surgeons (RCVS) (2006) Day One Essential Competences as at April 2006. Available at: http://www.rcvs.org.uk/search/?keywords=day+one+skills (accessed on 11 July 2011).

Royal College of Veterinary Surgeons (RCVS) (2010) *Guide to Professional Conduct*. Royal College of Veterinary Surgeons, London.

Royal College of Veterinary Surgeons (RCVS) (2011) Available at: http://www.rcvs.org.uk/about-us/consultations/our-consultations/draft-code-of-professional-conduct-for-veterinary-surgeons/ (accessed on 11 July 2011).

Schneider, B.J. (2002) Veterinary ethics: An introduction. *Canadian Veterinary Journal*, **43**, 770–771.

Scruton, R. (1995) *A Short History of Modern Philosophy*. Routledge, London.

Sellman, D. (2011) Professional values and nursing. *Medicine, Health Care and Philosophy*, **14**, 203–208.

Steil, B. (2009) *Lessons of the Financial Crisis*. Council on Foreign Relations, New York. Special Report No. 45.

Stieb, J.A. (2011) Understanding engineering professionalism: A reflection on the rights of engineers. *Science and Engineering Ethics*, **17**, 149–169.

Tannenbaum, J. (1995) *Veterinary Ethics*, 2nd edn. Mosby, Missouri.

Thistlethwaite, J. & Spencer, J. (2008) Personal development and self-care. In: *Professionalism in Medicine*, pp. 117–133, Chapter 8. Radcliffe Publishing, Oxford.

Thornton, P., Morton, D., Main, D., Kirkwood, J. & Wright, B. (2001) Veterinary ethics: Filling a gap in undergraduate education. *Veterinary Record*, **148**, 214–216.

Tulgan, B. (2001) *Winning the Talent Wars*. Nicholas Brealey, London.

Viens, A.M., Bensimon, C.M. & Upshur, R.E.G. (2009) Your liberty or your life: Reciprocity in the use of restrictive measures in contexts of contagion. *Bioethical Inquiry*, **6**, 207–217.

Vidal, J. (2001) Confusion rises over cull policy after Phoenix. Available at: http://www.guardian.co.uk/uk/2001/apr/27/footandmouth5 (accessed on 11 July 2011).

Wikipedia (2011) Veterinary ethics. Available at: http://en.wikipedia.org/wiki/Veterinary_ethics.

Williams, J.R. (2001) Professionalism in Medicine. CMA Series of Health Care Discussion Papers, pp. 1–24. Canadian Medical Association, Ottawa.

Wilson, H. (2011) Banks need new 'social contract' says Bank of England's Tucker. *Daily Telegraph*, Print Version: Business, June 2011, B2.

Questions and Answers

Q: I was interested to hear you talk about the need to move away from professional and personal circumstances. The veterinary profession has, to some extent, been saddled by the declaration that veterinarians make when they qualify to look after the best interests or welfare of animals committed to their care. This has, in some circumstances, allowed individuals, and perhaps the veterinary profession as a whole, to conveniently push to one side the best interests of animals that are not committed to their care. Does the balance need to shift in order to make sure that veterinarians don't end up simply looking after animals that they are paid to look after?

A: No individual or group can fight all the battles in the world on every front. Animals in a veterinarian's care are the obvious ones that they have to deal with, but part of my argument is that the veterinary profession has a responsibility that relates to the veterinarian's specific knowledge and skills, which clearly allows veterinarians to take proactive roles in areas such as animal welfare more generally. One of the reasons why veterinarians have come under challenge is that they have often been reactive; indeed, latterly, they've perhaps forgotten that they only have a legitimacy because of their contribution to society. Their monopoly is not something that it is likely that twenty-first century politicians would create. It developed historically because it was in society's interests, even though at times it was something for which individuals were arguing to pursue their own interests. The only legitimacy in the twenty-first century is in relation to what veterinarians contribute to society. The veterinary profession should contribute to the broader debate about animals, both those within and outwith the veterinarian's care.

Q: I agree that introducing animal ethics into the curriculum is important: introducing new elements on ethics and increasing the understanding of the profession should help change behaviour. However, I would like you to comment further on the role of continuous professional development (CPD); you mentioned that animal ethics was only recently introduced in the curriculum.

A: The, at times, controversial RCVS Certificate in Advanced Veterinary Practice was introduced by the RCVS, as a result of a move within the profession, particularly by the Society for Practising Veterinary Surgeons. It includes a Professional Skills Module, which deals with many elements that are now part of the undergraduate course. In relation to CPD that is centred on this Certificate, ethics and professionalism play a big part. As someone who marks essays from colleagues in practice who are engaged in studying the CertAVP, I have been humbled, moved and felt very privileged to hear their reflections on what they are trying to achieve.

   We have seen magnificent examples, for example individual farm animal practitioners, who recognise that the way to improve animal welfare is to make things better for the farmer. If veterinarians obtain economic benefits for farmers, that's great and is one way that they can get onto farms and improve animal welfare. Veterinarians see themselves as having a dual role when they get onto farms; they recount areas in which they feel they have made real advances on individual farms for groups of animals at the same time as addressing agricultural economics and the needs of the business. This does not happen on every farm, but is at the core of the way these individuals practice their professional science and art.

Q: I appreciated the way you took a different perspective on the veterinary profession and touched on political philosophy, history and sociological issues. We've heard this morning about the need for social science. Is it enough to introduce ethics, business and communication into the veterinary curriculum or do we need veterinary humanities – in the same way that medical schools now teach medical humanities – that deal with the fundamental questions about what it means to be a veterinary professional in today's society?

A: Professional skills are relevant in the veterinary curriculum but in a different way from that conceived in the past. In the 1990s, we introduced the Professional Skills Module – we already had animal ethics in the first year of the programme – but they were very much 'bolt in' extras. One of the real issues has been how we integrate these themes effectively with the 'organic disease aspects' of the course that every 18-year-old expects to study at vet school. We weren't, historically, very successful, in part perhaps because the individuals teaching professional studies were seen, at times, as a separate group and clinicians don't seem to have seen professional skills as part of their responsibilities, namely, clinical reasoning about diagnosis and treatment. Nowadays, there are more clinicians, who integrate these themes. There's more to do, but it's all about getting case-based reasoning to integrate ethical and economic aspects alongside the purely clinical.

There's also the affective domain that needs to be considered. There are some issues around the ideal treatment for the animal (which the owner may even be able to afford) that mean that its adoption may not be in the best interests of the animal. The animal's treatment has to be of a type that the owner can administer and with which they can cope emotionally. The animal may be able to be re-homed to receive the ideal treatment, but this would have to be considered carefully and discussed very sensitively with an owner. Veterinary students have never engaged in that sort of thinking during their undergraduate courses.

Q: I teach ethics to veterinary and other students. I would draw attention to the way a previous speaker pictured ethicists as showing different options that promote good ethical reasoning. You can start here or there, and can end here or there, but it's all good ethics if you argue well. That's what ethicists are supposed to do. On the other hand, we need veterinarians who have an idea of the 'veterinarian view', for example 'We, veterinarians, think "this and that" regarding slaughter, regarding humane killing, etc.'. However, it's important that we make it clear that there are different ways of reasoning well and making good points. I have a picture that you think there is only one way of doing it and one way that should be transferred to the new students. What is the situation in Britain?

A: When a veterinarian is presented with an individual case, there isn't necessarily just one way of treating it. There are situations where he or she may euthanase an animal and others where the animal may be treated: there may be alternative treatments that are partly based on the animal's and the owner's circumstances. This is the sort of decision making that veterinarians have to make on a day-to-day basis. I become concerned if people say that there's one way of dealing with a case that has a particular diagnosis; that is not my experience of practice.

Q: You mentioned the veterinarian's responsibility to patients, clients and profession. Increasingly, many veterinarians are responsible to their employers, who are very often not veterinarians. This is addressed in the Guide to Professional Conduct,

Annex F. What are the veterinarian's responsibilities to an employer when these conflict with professional responsibilities?
A: It's a difficult balance but I would argue that professional responsibilities come first. When I was in private practice, even though I had a veterinary employer, there were times when I felt that there were things that needed doing that my employer didn't always think necessary. I reflected on what I was going to do, and, if it was right, carried on and did it, because it was part of my professional role. There can be a conflict, at times, between the market and professional responsibility. Although the veterinary surgeon is – like the ox – worthy of his hire and is paid reasonably well for a good job, he or she should not take advantage of the client. The market gets as much as it can, and tries to get away with what it can, in relation to the law. It has a different philosophy from the veterinary profession: the two need to be reconciled. If the market and the profession work together and with government, then that is the best balance. However, there is an issue when the market becomes dominant.

Justifying Ends – The Morality of Animal Use

JUDY MACARTHUR CLARK

Home Office

The presentations shared a common theme in that each offered a challenge to the ways in which we might make decisions within an ethical framework. In my introduction to the session, I outlined an ethical model used in the field of animal research to achieve a balance between animal welfare and a concern to ensure delivery of the scientific advances needed. This is illustrated in Figure 1.

In an ethical regulatory system, it is essential to ensure that bureaucracy does not become so burdensome as to inhibit scientists from developing high quality proposals, which address important scientific questions. However, it is also important to ensure that animals do not suffer unnecessarily. There needs to be an ethical balance between the needs of science and those of animals. Furthermore, there is strong evidence to show that good animal welfare leads to good scientific outcomes.

This balance between science and welfare provides the public with confidence that a regulatory system is working on its behalf. The public not only wants to benefit from new scientific advances but also wants to be reassured that animals are not suffering unnecessarily. The nature of this balance differs between countries, taking into consideration their diverse cultural, economic, religious and social factors. However, the guiding principles provide a tool to be applied universally when making decisions to determine the right approach to regulation of animal use in research.

Veterinary & Animal Ethics: Proceedings of the First International Conference on Veterinary and Animal Ethics, September 2011, First Edition. Edited by Christopher M. Wathes, Sandra A. Corr, Stephen A. May, Steven P. McCulloch and Martin C. Whiting.
© 2013 Universities Federation for Animal Welfare. Published 2013 by Blackwell Publishing Ltd.

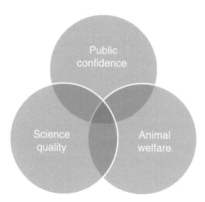

Figure 1   A decision support tool for achieving balance when considering the use of animals in research. Source: MacArthur Clark (2011).

This session sought to provide a number of other decision-making tools which veterinarians, and others concerned about animal welfare, can readily apply in their ethical frameworks. Hence, the tools need to be both appropriate and accessible. In both regards, the session succeeded well and the various presenters are to be congratulated.

Martin Whiting carefully analysed how we make decisions whether to provide veterinary treatment to animals and compared this with the delivery of medical treatment. Some of his assumptions were challenging, particularly in relation to medical delivery in countries without free health provision. Of relevance is the work of medical policy makers such as Paul Farmer (2003), who coined the term 'structural violence' when considering human healthcare provision as a key factor in the failure to deliver social justice. It is clear that comparisons between medical and veterinary healthcare provision are far from simple but nevertheless are worthy of careful consideration.

Bernie Rollins' recognition of *telos* as a significant factor in ethical consideration was illuminating. When deciding standards of welfare, he invited us to understand the factors which matter most to the particular species and which create pleasure and happiness as opposed to mere absence of pain. He reminded us that the conditions in which we hold animals in domestication have the potential to contribute greater violence than any specific procedures we impose upon them.

Steven McCulloch challenged the food policy of sustainable intensification from the perspective of environmental sustainability and animal welfare. His decision to promote instead 'radical naturalism' has many attractions but is premised on a confidence that the human race will decide to behave well. But as Winston Churchill astutely noted, an optimist finds the opportunity in every difficulty, compared with the pessimist who finds difficulty in every opportunity. Steven's optimism is shared by prominent animal welfare organisations such as Compassion in World Farming (Philip Lymbery, personal communication). Indeed, if this optimism is combined with intellectual rigour as well as political will from national and international bodies, perhaps we may yet make the right decisions to save our world.

Kate Millar proposed a tool for ethical decision-making involving a matrix approach. Her modified ethical matrix, which considered well-being, autonomy and fairness, was a compelling tool. I found her approach particularly inspiring as a means to generate new ideas about what may seem to be old concepts. However, I would join with those in the discussion who advocated an approach with some focus on outcomes. This would fit well with Bernie Rollins' view of *telos* and should provide suitable outcome measures which can be used as a basis for future decisions.

Finally, James Yeates took us on a journey through 'animal enhancement' and persuaded us that even defining the term is a significant challenge. Nevertheless, we should ponder the benefits (or lack of them) of developing 'intelligent sheep' or 'dumb chickens' for our moral decision-making. Do these enhancements provide benefits for the animals themselves, or is their *telos* simply adjusted to suit the way in which man chooses to keep these animals? This is clearly an area for ongoing debate in choosing which future interventions should be implemented and what will be their impact, as perceived by the affected animals.

In conclusion, I believe this session stimulated the audience to consider ethical and moral decision-making from a number of different, but related, perspectives. It provided some tangible frameworks which paved the way for practical considerations in Sessions III and IV. All speakers fulfilled their roles admirably: they presented often complex concepts in a readily digestible fashion which was particularly appropriate to the mixed, but also enthusiastic, audience at the conference.

References

Farmer, P.E. (2003) *Pathologies of Power: Health, Human Rights, and the New War on the Poor*. University of California Press, Berkeley, California.

MacArthur Clark, J.A. (2011) *International developments relating to the use of animals in science*. Proceedings of the Fifth Pan-Commonwealth Veterinary Conference. Accra, Ghana.

Justice of Animal Use in the Veterinary Profession

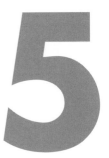

MARTIN C. WHITING

Royal Veterinary College

Abstract: One foundation of medical justice for physicians and their patients is that each patient has equality in their access to healthcare. Human patients should not be denied, or granted, treatment based upon clinically irrelevant data. Veterinary medicine is an allied profession with many similar requirements to medical 'principlism' and is able to offer many of the advanced treatments and interventions of human medicine. Yet, veterinary medicine differs on this fundamental point: treatments are offered, and patient end-points decided, with consideration of non-clinical data such as the utility of the animal to mankind. This has been justified by claims of decreased moral status for animals in relation to people, and the property status of animals, but has been rejected by those who claim animals have a right to absolute liberty. While human patients receive treatment independent of their 'purpose', animal treatment is dependent upon it. Treatments choices maybe dependent upon what the animal can give to people in return, notwithstanding other confounding factors (e.g. financial constraints).

This paper considers the concept of medical justice, some of the differences between humans and animals, and the absence of medical justice in the veterinary sphere. The concept of medical justice may be inappropriate in veterinary medicine, appropriate but not applied or appropriate if in a modified form.

Keywords: animal use, dog, healthcare, justice, medicine, moral status, patient, pig, property, rights, treatment, utility, veterinary ethics

Veterinary & Animal Ethics: Proceedings of the First International Conference on Veterinary and Animal Ethics, September 2011, First Edition. Edited by Christopher M. Wathes, Sandra A. Corr, Stephen A. May, Steven P. McCulloch and Martin C. Whiting.
© 2013 Universities Federation for Animal Welfare. Published 2013 by Blackwell Publishing Ltd.

5.1 Societal Relationships with Animals

Most societies have a formal policy or social agreement upon how they consider the moral worth of animals. The dominant view in the Western world, and of the three monotheistic religions that have formed our societal norms and laws today, was an instrumental view of animals; animals were seen as things to be used by man (Spinoza 1960, p. 215). Aristotle proposed that animals did not need to be considered in the realm of justice, nor should they be afforded any moral worth due to a lack of rationality (Aristotle 1998, p. 1161). To Kant (1997, p. 212), irrational animals could be, at most, a means for a human end and not an end on their own. Plato considered the 'ideal condition' where humans do not consume meat due to the consequence for human health. This view of animal use was instrumental only; animals themselves received no explicit moral consideration, their use was in service to mankind (Cochrane 2010, p. 13). The moral status of animals has been questioned for centuries, from Descartes' claim that they are mere automatons to Voltaire's response 'has Nature arranged all the springs of feeling in this animal to the end that he might not feel?' (Voltaire 1764, p. 23). Bentham claimed that animals require consideration if they are beings that can suffer (Bentham 1789, p. 283); Regan (2004) presents a case for animal rights and Singer (1990) argued for equal consideration of interest. The resolution of the moral status of animals has not been achieved.

Today, animals are ubiquitous within society. They are considered companions, livestock, vermin, laboratory tools and wildlife, and animal products are found within medicines, food and clothing. These divergent uses of animals have been associated with different levels of care and protection, but their socially accepted moral status is not absent. As Beauchamp and Childress (2009, p. 66) expressed '*an outright denial of moral status is implausible in light of the fact that virtually every nation and major scientific association has guidelines to alleviate, diminish, or otherwise limit what can be done to animals …*'. The presence of legal protections for these animals prohibits the conclusion that they have no moral status. Importantly, the law protects animals for their intrinsic value, not an instrumental value. The moral status that animals have is a socially accepted and legal one, but cannot be considered universal or absolute, and the increasingly protective legislation is reflective of our continuing adaptation of culturally accepted norms for their increasing moral status.

5.2 The Different Uses of Animals and Their Moral Status

Veterinarians engage with animals through many different forms of animal use in society. Animals may be owned as companions; utilised as a form of 'tool' such as on the farm or in the laboratory, working as traction or draft animals, or they may be wild (owned or not) where the veterinary involvement may be protection (conservation/preservation) or they are killed as pests. Animals in each category have different legislative protections or permitted harms, appearing to have different levels of moral worth. This variation of views of the moral status of animals involved in each of these types of uses was described by Arluke and Sanders (1996, chp 7) as the socio-zoological scale. They describe animals as being given a moral worth dependent upon two aspects: first, species membership dictates one layer of moral status, then the usefulness or harmfulness of that species to humans denotes a second layer. A pet cat, for example, may exist high on the scale, receiving high moral consideration being both a regarded species and one which is integrated within family life, while a vermin rat may be lower on the scale. This is described as attributing a moral status to an animal based upon both an intrinsic and extrinsic value (Collins *et al.* 2010) and explains why debate surrounding some species or issues are highly emotive, while others, such as fish farming, evoke very little emotion due to the low nature of fish on the scale (Sandøe *et al.* 2009).

The varying levels of moral concern and protection are exemplified in legislation about the killing of rats. As vermin, rats may be killed by non-specific anticoagulant use that is known to produce prolonged harm prior to death (Littin *et al.* 2000), while the laboratory rat is protected to some extent from this. In the UK, a Home Office Project License would be required to kill a rat by this method; the standard method of killing should induce instantaneous death (Animal (Scientific Procedures) Act 1986, Schedule 1, Table A) and cervical dislocation is commonplace. Pet rats are further protected, as legislation does not permit these rats to be killed by anticoagulants or any method that would cause avoidable harm (Animal Welfare Act 2006, S4). Pet rats would normally be killed by a veterinary surgeon and public perception of a 'happy death' would prohibit the use of cervical dislocation. Typically anesthetic overdoses would be used to kill these rats; in terms of animal welfare, this is the preferred method (AVMA 2007; RCVS 2008, para 9). Consideration of a cat in these three situations would involve administration of anesthetic overdose in all cases. Animals are considered and protected under UK laws in a manner that supports the socio-zoological scale.

5.3 The Separation of Animals from Humans

While the dominant view is that animals have a lower intrinsic worth than humans, it is unclear if animal conspecifics have an intrinsic moral status that is equally relative to each other within that species. To paraphrase Ingrid Newkirk (Spacter 2003), it would be uncontroversial to say 'a dog is not a pig is not a boy'; however, it is difficult to conclude other than 'a dog is a dog'. There is no morally relevant information to separate the intrinsic moral status of one dog from another: in the same way, we cannot separate one boy from another. All the traits that query the separation of moral status between humans and higher animals, such as pain perception, preservation of life, various shared desires, their own rationality, intelligence, etc., cannot be used as a way to separate individual members from a species group.

When determining the intrinsic moral status of a single species (to differentiate between species), status may hinge on a trait or a collection of traits. The example from the human sphere, however, is that intrinsic value of conspecifics must remain the same. All humans are to be considered equal in terms of moral status; the very nature of being part of the human category gives them equal consideration. Is it then possible to have logical cause not to apply the same reasoning between all conspecifics? Historically, extrinsic values have been used to rebut equality between all humans. Traits such as gender or race are normally considered determinant in removing full moral status from some humans, this is from the extrinsic value placed on those traits. Consequently, '[t]hose without moral status have been regarded as having no moral rights (e.g., historically, slaves in many, and almost certainly most, societies). Those with a lower moral status have fewer or weaker rights (e.g., historically, women in many, and probably most, societies)' (Beauchamp & Childress 2009, p. 64). The application of classes or categories of humans without full moral status have been met with refutation. It seems that without the need to broach the human–animal boundary, we may be able to consider all those conspecifics with equal intrinsic worth (whatever that worth may be), while the application of extrinsic values, as happens within the socio-zoological scale, may present an unjust approach to variation in moral worth.

5.3.1 Property, rights and liberty

There are important differences to note when considering the role of veterinarians and their relationship with animals when compared with that of doctors and their patients. Firstly, animals are property (with the exception of wildlife), while human patients are un-owned. Secondly, almost all the common animals dealt with by veterinarians have an instrumental interest in liberty accompanied by preference autonomy, not an intrinsic interest in liberty with full Kantian autonomy as do the majority of human patients. Both conditions could affect the concept of justice to be applied to animals, which may not allow direct comparison with physicians.

A companion or tool animal is owned and has been considered standard property, usable as the owner wishes. Ownership of an object in this instance conveys an absolute right to complete and exclusive control over it. While this may be an accurate explanation of ownership of certain objects, for example a pebble, it is not an accurate reflection of the concept of ownership that should be applied to an animal. In this instance, ownership '*signals … a certain set of relations with regards to a particular thing*' (Cochrane 2009b). Ownership does not always permit the owner absolute power over the object. For example, the owner of an area of land is not permitted to build what they want, to prevent access to anyone else nor to have '*sole and despotic dominion over it*' (Cochrane 2009b); there are limitations to ownership in this instance. Owners of property are limited in different ways and to different extents depending on the type of property that is being considered. It is not possible to claim *a priori* that because an animal is owned, the owner has dominion over it. Being owned or being a property is not necessarily detrimental to animals, as we may say it is for the case of humans. To be harmed by being property, one must be aware of the concepts of property and ownership and the social stigma associated with it (e.g., connotations of slavery or instrumentalisation), which is a human social construct. Animals can only suffer from being owned if they have an intrinsic interest in their own liberty. Cochrane (2009a) argues as Dworkin (1988) did, that animals do not '*possess the ability to frame, revise and pursue their own conceptions of good*'. While autonomous humans have an intrinsic value in being unconstrained, self-governing and not dominated by others, sentient animals only have an interest in liberty that permits them to achieve their preferences, an instrumental interest. This view is consistent with Rollin's idea of *telos* as the '*wants, needs and desires*' are intrinsic, their interest in being free to achieve them in necessarily instrumental (Rollin 1981). Restricting the complete liberty of animals is not against the principle of justice as it would be in human medicine, nor does being owned give absolute control to the owner.

Property itself can possess meaningful rights, independent of the owner. For example, corporations are not only property but they also possess legal rights, obligations and duties (Cochrane 2009b). It is possible for an item of property to have meaningful rights, and this too is reflected in the animal welfare laws giving certain animals in certain conditions the right to be free from cruelty (Animal Welfare Act 2006, S4). Despite an animal being a chattel and owned by a person, it can still have meaningful rights. However, these rights are attached to the ownership category (companion, farm, laboratory use, etc.) and not attached to the moral status, sentience level or species of animal (between a certain species threshold). Thus, different rights apply to the same species of animal in different situations. The rights mentioned here may not be direct rights of the animal but rather duties of care for them as explained in medical ethics by Gillon (1985) '*[rights are] justified claims that require action or restraint from others – that is, impose positive or negative duties on others*'.

This does not mean there are absolute rights for animals as there are for people (cf. human rights). Cochrane (2009b) suggests that geese have an absolute right not to undergo the farming practices required to produce *foie gras*. He argues that this absolute right of geese has overruled the interests of humans (consumers, chefs and farmers). However, the Animal (Scientific Procedures) Act (1986) allows for licensed people to overrule this right of geese if the benefits of research can justify it. Within the UK legal system, animals do not have absolute protected rights, they are always dependent on the purpose of the animal, the nature of the ownership and/or when un-owned, the nature of harm intended. Wolff describes this condition for animals as a 'near right' (Wolff 2011, p. 26). Francione proposes that human interests are always considered more important than animal interests (Francione 1995, p. 4), and the Animal Welfare Act (2006) protects owned animals' legal rights to their five welfare needs (S9(2)(a)–(e)), to a certain extent, over that of their owners preferences. Yet when there is a conflict of interests, the owners can opt for euthanasia of the animal, indicating that Francione's assessment that *'animals almost never prevail, irrespective of what may be a trivial human interest at stake and the relative weighty animal interest'* is correct. Whenever an animal 'right' becomes too burdensome on an owner, the animal may lawfully be killed, reinforcing Wolff's *'near right'* idea. Animals have a claim on our duty of care if we own them, but that is not absolute and currently does not extend to preservation of life if the cost is too great for owners.

To conclude this section on ownership, property and liberty, I have shown, using the arguments of Cochrane and others, that in respect to animals being treated with justice, owning an animal does not limit the concept of justice we can apply. Animals as property can be subject to limitations of interference and can have their own direct rights and duties that do not always permit dominion. Ownership of an animal resulting in restriction of its 'absolute' liberty is not necessarily contrary to animals that only have an instrumental interest in liberty in order to satisfy preferences. Claims of absolute animal liberation are not fully validated if ownership and liberty infringements are agreed to not cause harm. These claims are made from a mix of moral and legal premises. Yet they separate out animals from humans in a substantial and morally relevant way when we consider justice.

5.4 Justice as Understood by the Medical Profession

A commentary on justice within medical ethics (Campbell *et al.* 2005, pp. 14–15) suggests that treating two people with equal and telling needs differently due to non-medical criteria is an unjust discrimination. Justice within human healthcare does not require a compulsory, uniform standard of care for everyone, but an appropriate standard of care should be delivered to all irrespective of non-medical criteria of individual patients. Examples of 'non-medical criteria' such as *'gender, race, IQ, linguistic accent, ethnicity, national origin and social status'* should not contribute to decisions of healthcare provision allocation (Beauchamp & Childress 2009, p. 248). Diseases and predispositions may occur depending on some of these factors but they are not to be used as exclusion criteria for access to treatments. This is not always clear-cut. Hope *et al.* (2008, p. 5) use an example of doctors confusing age as a discriminatory trait in an 82-year-old patient in need of cardiac surgery. The surgeon describes the sole life-saving treatment as *'not clinically indicated'*, demonstrating the fine line between interventional requirements and ethical decision-making using non-clinically relevant data. Other examples of non-clinically relevant information used in clinical decision-making are seen at the extremes of healthcare choices and resource allocation such as organ allocation in transplant surgery. The limited availability of livers for transplant may mean that they are given in priority to patients, who do not remain alcohol dependent, although Glannon (1998) disagrees with this citing Morreim's (1995) argument that *'it is generally wrong to deny medical care because of a patient's lifestyle'*. The basis of the objection to using non-clinically relevant data in decision-making is that all humans are equal to each other in respect to being human. Although medical justice contains many other concepts, it is the basis of elimination of non-clinical data and equality, where appropriate, that is the questionable transferable idea to veterinary medicine.

5.5 Veterinarians and Animal Justice

The veterinary profession is embroiled in meeting many conflicting duties. It is dominated by a triad of duties between the veterinarian and the animal, the owner and society (or back to the profession itself). The profession is regulated by self-imposed codes of conduct (authorised under the Veterinary Surgeons Act 1966), with additional minor powers through other Acts. There is a stark difference in terms of justice when considering how veterinarians approach an animal, when compared with how physicians approach a patient. The veterinary profession relies heavily on non-medical patient data when determining what level of intervention should be given or even if that intervention is positive or negative. The non-medical data are predominately the animal's purpose. A person's purpose (which we often interpret as their job) is not a criterion used to determine the distribution of health-care resources.

The relationship between veterinarians and animals represents a similar scenario to that of doctors when dealing with people without mental capacity (e.g. very young children) (Morgan 2007). However, such a view of surrogate decision-making does not accurately capture the veterinary current relationship. The decision-making process that is involved in mentally incapacitated patients revolves around their best interests (previously expressed wishes and life plans) and those that support prolonged life, in general, in the case of children (Mental Capacity Act 2005, S4). It would be disingenuous to assert that decision-making in the treatment of laboratory, farmed or vermin animals be characterised as surrogate decision-making under the auspices of 'best interests'. Surrogate decision-making in relation to pet animals is limited by restraints of personal time, finance and inconvenience as well as what the owner of the animal perceives to be an acceptable quality of life. In general, companion animals are considered to be an 'end' in their own right and are rarely treated as a 'means' (exceptions to this may include fighting or status dogs, which are a 'means'; these would more appropriately be categorised as tools).

Tool animals are considered as a means not an end; decision-making regarding their treatment has a different prioritisation than 'best interest' surrogate decisions. The primary factor in the decision-making process is the purpose of the animal or the usefulness of the animal to the owner. This purpose is to exist within the experiment or farm, to produce data for research or generate a product for others. It does not necessarily matter if the outcome of either of these is for animal or human benefit (e.g. veterinary therapeutics or pet food). The purpose of keeping these animals is to fulfill their task within their environment; their treatment and their moral worth are linked to their ability to meet that task. For example, the cost of treating a dairy cow with mastitis is calculated against the likely chance of successful recovery to continue producing high volumes of saleable milk; if the treatment was unrelated to its purpose and the cow was considered an end, then the consideration would relate only to the financial cost and welfare of the cow during and after the treatment (with disregard to its milk product). Costs associated with improving welfare of tool animals are promoted through instrumental reasons rather than as a result of them being intrinsically beneficial to the animal's interest. Examples are found in the animal research dictum '*good welfare results in good science*' (Gilbert & Wolfensohn this volume) or in farming when subscribing to the RSPCA's Freedom Food scheme, '*Many shoppers are prepared to pay more for higher welfare, and this growing trend has increased the demand for Freedom Food labeled products, which could increase your profits*' (RSPCA, unspecified date).[1]

Vermin animals rarely involve veterinarians except through policy making. The interaction is associated with prioritising the interests of one species against another, either directly, for example removal of foxes from around chicken farms, or indirectly, for example removal of badgers to prevent the spread of *Mycoplasma bovis* to cattle, which may cause disease or financial harm to humans (Anon 2007; Torgerson 2008). Badgers are not culled for the sole benefit of cows.

In the UK, veterinarians should have the welfare of animals under their care as their constant endeavor (RCVS 2008, S1A (2)) and they should '*treat all patients, of whatever species, humanely, [and] with respect*' (RCVS 2010, S1C (1a)). This requires them to take into consideration the species being treated when making decisions, including welfare, and their actions must be humane (assumed to mean compassionate and benevolent) and respectful to the animal. The code of conduct does not specify that all animals of the same species should be considered equally, nor does it require that all animals with a similar purpose should be treated equally. Both money and the owner's wishes are determinate in the choice of treatments for animals unless the decision is contrary to welfare (and here euthanasia is not considered contrary to welfare). The RCVS does not acknowledge a difference in moral status connected to species or purpose. There appears to be a disconnection between the foundations of justice in medical ethics and that in veterinary ethics. Treatment options available for the same condition within the same species vary according to the purpose of the animal. The treatments and considerations of a rat under the different statuses of vermin, laboratory tool and companion, represent value placed upon extrinsic factors used to separate out individuals of equal intrinsic moral worth.

Currently, it is not possible for veterinarians to treat all conspecifics equally, irrespective of their purpose. 'Purpose' remains a deciding factor for the owner as to what treatment may be given; when animals become too costly for purpose euthanasia can be elected.

---

[1] Although the authors' intent is unknown.

5.6 Conclusion

The debate surrounding public policy and animals does not hinge upon whether animals have rights or equality with humans, but rather it is about what the morally relevant traits of the animals are that need to be protected or that induce duties (Wolff 2011, p. 36).

A claim that animals have an equal moral status to humans is contentious, but claims that their moral status is limited due to their status as property are unjustified. Infringing liberty is not necessarily harmful so long as the animal can achieve its goals. People have a duty of care to animals, which may or may not be a claim right of the animal, but more accurately, it is a 'near right'. Animals do not have absolute rights in law. Many factors separate out humans and animals in a morally relevant and substantial way, but there seems to be no morally relevant trait that separates out conspecifics in a meaningful way. In veterinary medicine, the purpose of the animal is a non-clinical data point that decides the treatment an animal will receive.

In human healthcare, Weale (1998) and Butler (1999) described an 'inconsistent triad' in healthcare balancing: (1) high quality care, (2) equality in access and (3) affordability. The RCVS is responsible for maintaining the first point, and the third point should be regulated by the profession itself. The second point is the crux of this paper; equality in access to healthcare, that is equality of access to similar levels of care (treatments, efficacy and protections) as appropriate to the species, not according to the purpose of the animal, equality is not attached to the extrinsic factors. While it seems that those of equal intrinsic moral worth should be treated equally as a fundamental principle of medical ethics, it may be considered in veterinary medicine that it is the owners who are considered equally. This is not the approach applied in substituted judgments in the human sphere where the patient is paramount. It seems commonplace in veterinary medicine, as well as animals at large in society, that this principle is not adhered to. The role and importance of justice when treating animals remains unclear, which may mean that either (i) justice does not apply in the veterinary sphere; (ii) our understanding of justice needs to be refined when considering animal use; or (iii) a radical reformation of veterinary policy on treating animals is required. The key question for this debate will be 'is the purpose or use of an animal a morally relevant trait?'

Acknowledgements

I would like to thank Pat Walsh, Nadia Shihab, Lorna Treanor, Rachel Warren, Stephen Barrett and Rowena Packer for their generous help, contribution and detailed reading of the manuscript.

References

Animal (Scientific Procedures) Act. (1986) HMSO, London.

Animal Welfare Act. (2006) HMSO, London.

Anon. (2007) In for the cull. *Nature*, **450**(7166), 1–2.

Aristotle. (1998) *The Nicomachean Ethics*. Oxford University Press, Oxford.

Arluke, A. & Sanders, C. (1996) *Regarding Animals*. Temple University Press, Philadelphia.

AVMA. (2007) AVMA Guidelines on Euthanasia [Online]. American Veterinary Medical Association. Available at: http://www.avma.org/issues/animal_welfare/euthanasia.pdf (accessed 20 May 2011).

Beauchamp, T.L. & Childress, J.F. (2009) *Principles of Biomedical Ethics*, 6th edn. Oxford University Press, New York.

Bentham, J. (1789) Introduction to the principles of morals and legislation. In: *The Collected Works of Jeremy Betham 1996* (eds J.H. Burns & H.L.A. Hart). Oxford University Press, Oxford, U.K.

Butler, J. (1999) *The Ethics of Health Care Rationing*. Cassell, London.

Campbell, A., Gillet, G. & Jones, G. (2005) *Medical Ethics*, 4th edn. Oxford University Press, Oxford, U.K.

Cochrane, A. (2009a) Do animals have an interest in liberty? *Political Studies*, **57**, 660–679.

Cochrane, A. (2009b) Ownership and justice for animals. *Utilitas*, **21**(4), 424–442.

Cochrane, A. (2010) *An Introduction to Animals and Political Theory*, 1st edn. Palgrave Macmillan, London.

Collins, J.A., Hanlon, A., More, S.J., Wall, P.G., Kennedy, J. & Duggan, V. (2010) Evaluation of current equine welfare issues in Ireland: Causes, desirability, feasibility and means of raising standards. *Equine Veterinary Journal*, **42**(2), 105–113.

Dworkin, G. (1988) *The Theory and Practice of Autonomy*, 1st edn. Cambridge University Press, Cambridge, U.K.

Francione, G.L. (1995) *Animals, Property, and the Law*. Temple University Press, Philadelphia, Pennsylvania.

Gilbert, C. & Wolfensohn, S. (2011) This proceedings. Chapter 11.

Gillon, R. (1985) Philosophical medical ethics. *Rights. British Medical Journal*, **290**, 1890–1891.

Glannon, W. (1998) Responsibility, alcoholism, and liver transplantation. *Journal of Medicine and Philosophy*, **23**, 31–49.

Hope, T., Savulescu, J. & Hendrick, J. (2008) *Medical Ethics and Law. The Core Curriculum*, 2nd edn. Churchill Livingston, Elsevier Health Sciences, Edinburgh, U.K.

Kant, I. (1997) *Lectures on Ethics*. (trans P. Heath). Cambridge University Press, New York.

Littin, K., Connor, C.O. & Easton, C. (2000) Comparative effects of brodifacoum on rats and possums. *New Zealand Plant Protection Society*, **53**, 310–315.

Morgan, C. (2007) Autonomy and paternalism in quality of life determinations. *Animal Welfare*, **16**(s), 143–147.

Morreim, E. (1995) Lifestyles of the risky and infamous: from managed care to managed lives. *The Hastings Center Report*, **25**, 5–13.

RCVS (2008) Advice Note 17: Euthanasia [Online]. Royal College of Veterinary Surgeon. Available at: www.rcvs.org.uk/document-library/an17-euthanasia/Advicenote17.pdf (accessed 20 May 2011).

RCVS (2010) *Guide to Professional Conduct*. Royal College of Veterinary Surgeons, London.

Regan, T. (2004) *The Case for Animal Rights*, 2nd edn. University of California Press, Berkeley, CA.

Rollin, B. (1981) *Animal Rights and Human Morality*. Prometheus Books, New York.

RSPCA (unspecified date) Join Freedom Food: What are the benefits? [Online]. Available at: http://www.rspca.org.uk/freedomfood/producers/join/benefits (accessed 1 June 2011).

Sandøe, P., Gamborg, C., Kadri, S. & Millar, K. (2009) Balancing the needs and preferences of humans against concerns for fishes: How to handle the emerging ethical discussions regarding capture fisheries? *Journal of Fish Biology*, 75(10), 2868–2871.

Singer, P. (1990) *Animal Liberation*, 2nd edn. Jonathan Cape, London.

Spacter, M. (2003) The Extremist: The woman behind the most successful radical group in America. *The New Yorker*, 4 April.

Spinoza, B. (1960) *Ethics and the Improvement of the Understanding* (ed. J. Gutmann), Part 4, prop 37, note 1. Hafner Publishing Company, New York.

Torgerson, P. (2008) Does risk to humans justify high cost of fighting bovine TB? *Nature*, 455(23), 1029.

Veterinary Surgeons Act (1966) HMSO, London.

Voltaire, F.M.A. (1764) *Voltaire's Philosophical Dictionary*. Bibliobazaar.

Weale, A. (1998) *Rationing health care. British Medical Journal*, **316**(7129), 410.

Wolff, J. (2011) *Ethics and Public Policy. A Philosophical Inquiry*. Routledge, Abingdon, U.K.

Questions and Answers

Q: You pointed out that rights correspond with corresponding duties. Do duties differ between people? Similarly, when you said that two boys are the same, this may be true for the doctor treating them; but my boy is not the same as your boy and therefore my duties in relation to them differ. My duties in relation to two animals are similarly different. This perhaps puts even more onus on a veterinarian to be an animal's advocate, that is to discount those differences which the owner or others may put on animals from their point of view. Additionally, religions may well have regarded the animal as instrumental but they also talk about the duties people have towards careful stewardship.

A: With regards to rights and duties relationship, I refer to legal rights, that is what is written into legislation and the duties that the legislation imposes upon us. It becomes unnecessarily complex if we start talking about moral rights and their related duties. The socio-zoological scale in its original form is interesting when we look at the status of animals because we can bypass the moral status question and jump straight to where legislation starts. Moral distance is of no importance to the veterinary surgeon dealing with an animal. The purpose of the veterinary surgeon is to be the advocate for an animal, undertaking interventions to ensure their welfare is maximised until their death. The onus is on the veterinarian to treat justly, focusing on their welfare, this is independent to who the client is, but to work with the client within their means.

It might be a historical disservice to exclude the dominant view that several religions have prioritised the instrumental view of animals and the substantial influence this has had on our legislation. Recently, people have interpreted these differently, but the historical influence has been strongly associated with statute formation and it is to the statute that I am referring in this paper.

Q: UK medics have a relation to UK citizens. What does the British Medical Association think about British medics' duties to citizens in Africa or India, for example?

A: One of the dangers in the veterinary sphere is looking at how medics deal with similar issues and then transposing their solutions and viewpoints into the veterinary world. Beauchamp and Childress' four ethical principles are the underlying ones to be taught. Although beneficence and non-maleficence are straightforward to transfer to veterinarians, autonomy and justice are troublesome. If we restrict justice to a doctor's interactions with his/her patients on an individual daily basis on a single ward, then perhaps the concept of medical justice can be transferred. But we must remember that the relationship is part of the UK legal system and the NHS structure while empowerment of veterinarians is largely through the social contract.

Q: In the UK, we have an unusual view of the doctor–patient relationship because of the NHS. What is the relationship in the USA where the patient has to pay?

A: Finances and the status of animals as property are a major rebuttal to this argument. Finances are difficult to understand, especially when the argument is transferred from the medical to the veterinary side. We have to look at the basic level of healthcare. In the UK, it is high for humans, as it is in the veterinary sphere. I'm not proposing that every dog in the world should be vaccinated but the basic level should be even more primitive, such as non-interference or alleviation of suffering.

Q: I am intrigued by your concept of justice and its limitations to the animal and the veterinarian. You haven't considered much about society. In human medicine, there is the risk of the patient to society, for example the patient who infects others. Similarly, in veterinary medicine if animals are of great risk to society, like cattle or pigs with foot-and-mouth disease, then we treat them differently. An ethical framework has to account for the consequences for society.

Your perspective is that of the UK, but elsewhere in Europe, for example the Balkans, legislation states that animals should not be euthanised merely because they're not wanted any more. Where is the justice in that practice?

A: Foot-and-mouth disease is not a good example as it does not affect the health of people; rabies is better. An animal with rabies is normally considered to be harmful to the society and is dealt with accordingly. However, this is not the concept of harmfulness which I consider. I do not mean for harm to be calculated on an individual level in the theory. The 'vermin rat group' is harmed because society does not want it. The theory highlights legislation prejudging a group of animals because of a perceived harm or use rather than an actual physical harm. When Arluke and Sanders talk about harm, they don't mean causing disease but usually an indirect problem. This paper focuses on UK Legislation, the concept contained within it may be transferrable internationally but it would need to be applied to the local legislation.

Telos

BERNARD E. ROLLIN

Colorado State University

Abstract: The foundation of animal ethics in the English-speaking world has historically been the ability of animals to experience pleasure and pain. But pleasure and pain are not the only things that *matter* to animals. Following Aristotle, my work in animal ethics recognises the *telos* or nature of an animal, the set of interests constitutive of its unique form of life – the 'pigness' of the pig, the 'dogness' of the dog. Thus, an adequate morality towards animals should address not only pleasure and pain, but the full range of possible 'matterings' following from animals' natures. When we evaluate, for example, gestation crates for sows, we must compare them to what a sow does in nature when she actualises her *telos* – covering a mile a day rooting and foraging, nest building, all of which behaviours are impossible to perform in a crate. Violation of *telos* may be more significant to an animal than physical pain. Full satisfaction of *telos* creates happiness. When *telos* is added to Plato's point about the most successful method for expanding people's ethical concerns being reminding rather than teaching, one can create a robust and comprehensive ethic for animals based on what people already believe.

Keywords: animal ethics, animal happiness, concern, dog, 'mattering', pleasure and pain, recollection, telos

6.1

Thanks to a series of British 'commonsensical' thinkers, animal ethics, at least in the English-speaking world, has focused overwhelmingly on pleasure and pain.

Veterinary & Animal Ethics: Proceedings of the First International Conference on Veterinary and Animal Ethics, September 2011, First Edition. Edited by Christopher M. Wathes, Sandra A. Corr, Stephen A. May, Steven P. McCulloch and Martin C. Whiting.
© 2013 Universities Federation for Animal Welfare. Published 2013 by Blackwell Publishing Ltd.

These thinkers generally worked in the Utilitarian tradition, and included Bentham, Mill, Sidgewick, Salt, Singer, as well as related philosophers like Hume. Being empiricists, the desire on the part of all organisms to seek pleasure and avoid pain seemed to them to be an observable and obvious basis for ethics that lent itself well to quantification. This focus enabled British moral thought to escape from continental European, rationalistic skepticism about more complex animal thought to exclude animals from the realm of moral concern, as articulated by Descartes, Spinoza and Kant. Animal ethics could thus be grounded in common sense awareness that animals experienced pleasure and pain even as we did; that pleasure and pain *matter* to animals.

But an adequate account of animal ethics must transcend exclusive concern with pleasure and pain, though such a view may be simple and attractive. An adequate morality towards animals must recognise the full range of possible 'matterings' unique to different sorts of animals. To accomplish this, we must look to Aristotle, the greatest common sense philosopher of the ancient world, specifically to his concept of *telos* or animal nature, a root notion of his functional, teleological biology. Whereas modern biology focuses on reductionist, molecular and mechanistic explanations, Aristotle's biology emphasises the unique set of traits and powers that make the animal what it is – the 'pigness' of the pig, the 'dogness' of the dog.

Aristotle recognised that different animals evidenced different ways of fulfilling the fundamental nature of living things, for example nutrition, locomotion, sensation, cognition and reproduction. Biology studies these functions in different sorts of animals, and it is the set of these functions that constitutes an animal's nature. Secondary school biology is still studied in this Aristotelian way. There is nothing mystical about *telos*; it is simply what common sense recognises as 'fish gotta swim, birds gotta fly'. The only departure that must be made from Aristotle today is to see *teloi* not as fixed and immutable but as slices or snapshots of a dynamic process of evolution, genetically encoded and environmentally expressed.

Thus, an adequate morality towards animals should address not only pleasure and pain, but the full range of possible 'matterings' following from animals' natures. When we evaluate, for example gestation crates for sows, we must compare them to what a sow does in nature when she actualises her *telos*, covering a mile a day rooting and foraging, nest building, all of which behaviours are impossible to perform in a crate. In fact, given the *telos* template, it is evident that we regularly violate fundamental interests of animals determined by their natures; we prevent their moving; we stop them from eating what they are naturally built to consume by not letting them graze, hunt or forage; we lessen their ability to cope with weather change; and we do not allow them to exercise. Denying these natural activities harms the animals in many ways, impeding their exercise of powers they possess to survive.

A non-obvious example of violating animal nature may be found in a story recounted by Hal Markowitz. He recounts that the Portland, Oregon zoo built a showpiece exhibit for servals, even importing sand and plants from the Kalahari (Markowitz & Line 1990). The exhibit was a dud; the servals lay around in obvious depression, even refusing to eat. When Markowitz visited their native habitat, he found that the bulk of these animals' time was spent predating low-flying birds, their main source of food. He told the zoo that instead of feeding horsemeat in chunks, the keepers should grind the rations into meatballs, which were then to be shot randomly across the exhibit enclosure by a compressed air cannon. The animals' behaviour changed overnight; they became excited and active, clearly exercising the predating aspect of their *telos*. Despite the power of the food drive, it was trumped here by failing to accommodate *how* they had evolved to eat. Similar strategies provide for *telos* accommodation for many animals in captivity.

An example from coyote behaviour strikingly illustrates how *telos* needs can trump even major physical pain. It has been recounted for years that coyotes, caught in a leg-hold trap, will chew their legs off, enduring terrible pain, rather than submit to immobility. (This is also true for other animals, such as raccoons.) This is understandable given the coyote's *telos* as a free ranging predator (or, on occasion, prey). It is not plausible to suggest that the animal chews its leg off to avoid death, since it is not possible that a non-linguistic being *has* a concept of death, though it clearly understands the inability to escape. Clearly the animal is not chewing the leg in order to escape the pain, as any attempt to chew the leg off will greatly *increase* the pain.

Other animals, wild and domestic, will endure pain and injury to escape close confinement. Though confinement agriculturalists in the United States claim that all needs of confined sows, for example food, water, protection from the elements and protection from predators, are met in confinement, these animals escape when they can, with no reports of any ever trying to return. Chickens will trade *ad libitum* feeding in confinement for sporadic access to food outdoors. Chickens will also work for food in confinement when given a choice of doing so (Duncan & Hughes 1972). Monkeys and other animals will self-mutilate in deprived, impoverished environments, the pain presumably providing some stimulation, as a counter to boredom (Berkson 1967; Ridley & Baker 1982; Chamove *et al.* 1984).

Kilgour (1978) cites evidence showing that cattle being exposed to a new herd show a physiological response for 30 days. In animals, the initial exposure to the experimental setting (i.e. major novelty) evoked the largest elevations in plasma cortisol (Mason *et al.* 1957; Hennessy & Levine 1979). This is not surprising, since cattle are herd animals who come to know their conspecifics as individuals and hence do not know how new animals will behave. Novelty of any sort evokes stress in most if not all animal *teloi*. Even in human experiments, the introduction to the experimental situation for the first time was often more effective in increasing steroid level than anything else the experimenter could devise, including electric shock (Michalski 1998).

Researchers know that animals can be trained by reward to willingly accept some physically painful experimental procedures. In one instance, my friend was drawing blood from dogs daily for a vaccine study. She would enter the facility, play with each dog, draw the blood and give the dog a treat after the draw. On one

occasion, one of the dogs set up such a howl as she was leaving that she raced back
to see if his paw was caught in the cage door. It turned out she had forgotten to
draw blood from that dog and he had missed his play and his treat, which bothered
him more than the blood draw. Separation of a newborn calf can cause mooing on
the part of the mother cow, bespeaking distress for over a week and even longer if
the cow can see the calf (Flower & Weary 2001). This is no surprise, as calves in
more natural situations will suckle and remain with the mother for up to 9 months
or more.

All of these examples illustrate three major points:

1. Pain, as a physical phenomenon, does not begin to capture all the ways that
   what we do to animals matters to them.
2. Other things we do to animals can be worse for them than physical pain.
   Unfortunately, we have no words for many of the myriad ways we can harm
   or cause animals to suffer, for example not allowing the pig to forage, separating
   a newborn animal baby from its mother at birth or stopping a chicken from
   nest building. For others, of course, we do have words, for example creating
   boredom, social deprivation and fear.
3. In general, interfering with or impeding actualisation of *telos* creates a negative
   experiential state for an animal.

Further, there is no simple word to express the many ways we can hurt animals
besides creating physical pain; the ways are as countless as the multiplicity of *teloi*
and the interests that flow from them. So I will introduce a barbarous neologism
to express this concept, 'negative mattering'. 'Negative mattering' means all
actions or events that harm animals or create misery, for example frightening an
animal, removing its young unnaturally early, keeping it so it is unable to socialise,
maternal deprivation, social separation that can not only cause distress but also
lead to physical illness and causing grief. Physical pain is perhaps the paradig-
matic case of 'negative mattering' but only constitutes a small part of what the
concept covers. 'Positive mattering' would, of course, encompass all states that are
positive for the animal, for example freedom of movement, pleasure, a sense of
security, companionship, play, exposure of young boars to allomimesis (i.e.
learning from older boars by imitation), to model and teach reproductive behaviour and so on.

If this analysis is correct, it is morally obligatory to expand the scope of veterinary
medicine and/or animal welfare science to study all of the ways things can matter
negatively as well as positively to animals, as society grows ever more concerned
about animal treatment. In addition, it is necessary to attempt to understand which
forms of 'negative mattering' are most problematic from an animal's perspective.
Obviously the challenge is to study these without hurting the animal subjects.

In sum, then, using *telos* as the core concept in animal ethics, rather than pleasure
and pain, has numerous advantages. It helps us to understand our obligation to

animals in higher resolution. It stops us from classifying insults as diverse as a blow, sickness, grief and loneliness on a continuum of only one axis, that is pain. (The same holds, of course, for various states of pleasure.) It comports well with Darwin's realisation that if physiological and morphological traits are phylogenetically continuous, so too are mental and psychological ones, a point I have stressed since 1980 to counter ideological skepticism about animal consciousness among scientists. It accords better with common sense, which has little problem attributing mental states to animals based on *telos* fulfilment or violation. (*Vide* the common sense insight expressed in the song 'fish gotta swim, birds gotta fly'.) And, equally importantly, as concern for animal welfare continues to evolve in society, it makes perfect sense attributing happiness to animals, that is satisfaction of most (or all) of an animal's needs arising from its *telos*.

6.2

It is becoming increasingly clear to society that ethical obligations to animals are not restricted to a set of admonitions designed to curtail pain, other noxious states or even physical harm to them. Merely being able to affirm that one has not harmed an animal does not entail that one has behaved morally towards that animal, particularly regarding domestic animals. One could perhaps argue cogently that our only obligation towards wild animals is to leave them alone and perhaps not to destroy their environment (see Chapter 10). That is an issue beyond the scope of our discussion. But few would argue that that is our only obligation to domestic animals, that is those whom we have made dependent on us, be they farm, zoo, research or companion animals. In the case of all domestic animals, one can mount the argument that we are responsible not only for shielding them from harm but also for assuring that we create a context in which they can flourish. We certainly act morally towards our horses when we provide them with food, water, shelter and shade, so that their lives are not negative. But, I believe, we are also morally required to make their lives positive, that is happy. Anyone who has kept horses is aware that there are positive resources we can provide these animals, for example when we give them access to a pasture where they can eat, play and run freely. No one, except perhaps the most extreme skeptic, can deny that equine behaviour displayed under such conditions evidences that these animals are experiencing happiness.

The more that a person makes it his or her business to learn about an animal's *telos* and the individual differences that may be found among different animals of that kind, as when some dogs like to horse-play with humans and others do not, the more we can be assured that we are not only not harming our animals but providing them with opportunities for positive pleasure and happiness.

In sum, I have argued that the concept of *telos* provides a very sound basis for animal ethics. First, it avoids the oversimplification error of assimilating all the ways in which animals can be made to suffer to the single rubric of 'pain'. Secondly, it activates ethical recollection rather than requiring assimilation of an unfamiliar ethical category. Thirdly, it allows and even directs us towards not only the avoidance of negative experiences for the animals we care for but also enjoins us in the direction of maximising positive experiences emerging from the animals' biological and psychological natures. In other words, acknowledging *telos* as the basis for animal ethics is the most likely way to assure that we respect animals' intrinsic value.

Perhaps the most poignant example of the efficacy of the ethic I developed occurred in 1980, when, having finally published the ethic, I did a full day seminar on animal ethics for representatives from every Canadian Federal Ministry that dealt with animal issues. In the course of the discussion, they reasoned that the best way to make progress in legislation derived from animal ethics was to create a Bill of Rights for animals. In attendance at the seminar was a high official from the Ministry of Fisheries and Oceans. Some years later, I received an anonymous copy of a memo from someone at this ministry. The memo had been sent to the director of the Vancouver aquarium, who had requested permission to take two killer whales from Canadian waters for an exhibit at the aquarium. The Minister responded that such permission would be granted only when the aquarium had demonstrated that the exhibit was designed to respect and accommodate animals' *teloi*.

References

Berkson, G. (1967) Abnormal stereotyped motor acts. In: *Comparative Psychopathology: Animal and Human* (eds J. Zubin & H.F. Hunt), pp. 71–87. Grune and Stratton, New York.

Chamove, A.S., Anderson, J.R. & Nash, V.J. (1984) Social and environmental influences on self-aggression in monkeys. *Primates*, **25**, 319–325.

Duncan, I.J.H. & Hughes, B.O. (1972) Free and operant feeding in domestic fowls. *Animal Behaviour*, **20**, 775–777.

Flower, F.C. & Weary, D.M. (2001) Effects of early separation on the dairy cow and calf: 2. Separation at 1 day and 2 weeks after birth. *Applied Animal Behavioural Science*, **70**, 275–284.

Hennessy, J.W. & Levine, S. (1979) Stress, arousal and the pituitary-adrenal system: A psychoendocrine hypothesis. In: *Progress in Psychobiology and Physiological Psychology*, Vol. 8 (eds J.M. Sprague & A.N. Epstein), pp. 821–865. Academic Press, New York.

Kilgour, R. (1978) The application of animal behaviour and the humane care of farm animals. *Journal of Animal Science*, **46**, 1478–1476.

Markowitz, H. & Line, S.W. (1990) The need for responsive environments. In: *The Experimental Animal in Biomedical Research*, Vol. I (eds B.E. Rollin & M.L. Kesel), pp.152–172. CRC Press, Boca Raton, Florida.

Mason, J.W., Harwood, C.T. & Rosenthal, N.R. (1957) Influence of some environmental factors on plasma and urinary 17-hydroxy-corticosteroid levels in the rhesus monkey. *American Journal of Physiology*, **190**, 429–433.

Michalski, A. (1998) Novel environment as a stress-inducing factor. An event-related potentials study. *Acta Neurobiologiae Experimentalis*, **58**, 199–205.

Ridley, R.M. & Baker, H.V. (1982) Stereotypy in monkeys and humans. *Psychological Medicine*, **12**, 61–72.

Questions and Answers

Q: *Telos* definitely passes the common sense test and it's great for communication to talk about the 'piggyness' of the pig, 'doggyness' of the dog. It encourages you to think about the animal. But why present it as a conflict with pleasures and pains? With the example of servals fed by 'flying' meat, where's the *telos*? That's pleasure.

A: Actualisation of *telos* in a successful way is going to be pleasurable; but in a situation where you can't let servals predate but create an approximation thereof, it's certainly pleasure but it's more than pleasure. Mere pleasure would be creating a situation so that every time servals ate, they felt a little thrill of pleasure. But that would not necessarily be in accord with the predating capacities that servals have evolved.

Q: But surely they're deriving pleasure from chasing the meat?

A: Yes, but that doesn't mean it's nothing but pleasure. It's pleasure that arises from eating the way servals were made to eat.

Q: Is there not a distinction between animal welfare and ethical decisions, in the sense that *telos* is very important to welfare and should be considered? It also makes us more aware that animals should be allowed to behave, so to speak, or behave in accordance with their natures. But when you come to decisions where there are ethical dilemmas, A versus B, it becomes more difficult. Should the animal welfare issues not come before ethical decision makings, for example, the use of animals in experiments where they're perceived as being of benefit to humans versus the disadvantage for animals?

A: Good results don't lead to good welfare, necessarily.

Q: Not necessarily, but it's something that should happen anyway. But the ethical decision of whether or not to experiment on animals is almost separate. Animals should experience good welfare. The scientific results should be good, but the ethical dilemma of whether or not you should actually experiment on that particular animal is further down the line.

Q: Should we experiment on animals? The decision has been made that we will experiment on animals. No society has risen up and said, 'We demand its abolition', with the possible exception of Switzerland.

A: It is clear that some people believe that every research protocol is painful. The most extreme estimate is that 15–20% of research protocols involve significant pain. On the other hand, 100% of research animals are kept under conditions which are violative of how they are built to live. There is absolutely no excuse to impose that degree of suffering because that is not required for human benefit. In fact, in the last 20 years, when we started to create environments for these animals that do approximate their natural living environment, all our baseline data were shown to be wrong because the baseline data were derived from stressed animals.

Q: In order to identify *telos* you need to do empirical research. And there are certain things, for example, where reducing stress might actually be adverse for the animal. Hans Selye used to make his point about new stress and good stress; it can make a very big difference to one's life to have a bit of stress. It's an empirical question.
A: It's very much an empirical question. A putative place to start in identifying *telos* is with people who know animals well, for example herdsmen. There was a wonderful response that David Morton once gave when somebody asked him *'How do we define pain?'* He said, *'Our job is not to define it, it's to control it'*.

Q: In traditional ethology, there is a distinction between function and mechanism. *Telos* corresponds to function, but for every function there are various ways of solving that problem for the animal. Wallowing in mud is a natural behaviour for pigs. It might be said that it's part of their *telos*, but you can solve the possible heat stress in other ways, which don't require the animal to wallow. Why should wallowing be included as a behavioural need?
A: It's a preference. Temple Grandin took a fiftieth generation Landrace pig that had been raised for generations in the University of Illinois confinement barn and turned it loose. It immediately went to wallow.

Q: If it's not hot, if it's cold, the pig won't wallow. Wallowing is a response to the heat.
A: Your account is too mechanistic. You're treating the animal as if it's a robotic mechanism that when the temperature goes up, it mechanically moves to wallow. An animal is more than a robot. The pig is not indifferent to how it cools down.

Q: I want to ask about relativity in terms of *telos*. In India, China and Africa with a working horse, for example, you're trying to explain to horse-keepers or veterinarians about *telos* and the importance of matterings to that animal. Would you comment on the relativity of matterings? Are the things that matter to a working horse covered in harness sores, dragging heavy weights, etc., likely to be different to the things that matter to a performance horse, for example?
A: There are certainly levels of mattering. Contrary to popular belief, Amish working horses are in terrible condition, their tack doesn't fit and they've got sores. Common sense would dictate that before you could create an actualisation of its desire to work, you'd get some tack that fitted and didn't cause physical lesions. It's not a matter of relatively but priority.

Q: I'm wondering about using *telos* in a society that is concerning itself with naturalness. It's much harder where you haven't seen horses doing the fart of happiness on the streets of Mexico, for example.
A: What can I do about people in societies where there's no animal ethics?

Author's Commentary

By introducing the concept of *telos* to animal ethics, I hope to provide a more comprehensive and rational theoretical basis for our moral obligations to other sentient beings than has traditionally been found in approaches based in pleasure and pain. Many of the wrongs we perpetrate on animals do not easily lend themselves to categorisation along a pleasure/pain axis. After all, such negative modalities as fear, loneliness, boredom, social isolation and anxiety do not in ordinary language and common sense categorisation lend themselves well to being subsumed under the rubric of pain. Certain things are more important to animals than physical pain, as when animals will endure physical pain to escape captivity.

Historically, the only societal consensus ethic, that is law regarding animals, was that embodied in the anti-cruelty laws, which laws mainly restrict themselves to the deliberate, sadistic and purposeless infliction of physical pain, identifiable by evidence of physical trauma or outrageous neglect, such as failing to provide adequate food and water to an animal. Yet, it is common sense that this does not cover the full spectrum of animal abuse. Animals suffer if they are tied on a short lead continuously, if they are not permitted to run or play, if they are bullied or threatened or frightened constantly, if they are not allowed interactions with others of their own kind, if they receive no exercise or stimulation and even if there are no pleasant surprises in their lives. Thus, basing our obligations to animals on their physical, social, psychological and behavioural interests accords well with pre-reflective intuitions. Similarly, equating happiness in animals with allowing them to actualise the full range of the interests dictated by their biological and psychological natures is plausible to common sense.

Using *telos* as a basis for formulating what counts as animal abuse – be it sadistic, thoughtless or arising out of human convenience – provides us with a much more comprehensive theory of harm to animals as well as positive obligations to them, by giving us a baseline of non-negotiable needs and interests inherent in an animal's unique form of life. Focusing on *telos* also explains the discomfort many of us feel when seeing an animal or a bird in a small cage, a killer whale confined in a pool, a horse alone in a small paddock or a dog kept on a short lead.

The anti-cruelty laws would be greatly rationalised and augmented if the traditional sole emphasis on physical pain were to be replaced by respect for animals' natures. It is also possible that if respect for *telos* became a widespread concept governing our view of animals, people would think twice before developing agricultural confinement systems such as battery cages, veal crates and sow stalls. Most importantly, our sense of moral obligation to the animals we use would be significantly sharpened, given a heightened awareness of the many ways we harm them beyond the infliction of physical pain.

Agriculture, Animal Welfare and Climate Change

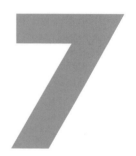

STEVEN P. McCULLOCH

Royal Veterinary College

Abstract: In the second half of the twentieth century, agricultural production in the UK intensified, first for food security and then for economic reasons. Since the 1960s and 1970s, both animal welfare and environmental advocates have criticised intensive systems of agriculture. Intensive livestock farming methods translate to confinement, high stocking densities and rapid growth rates, which can cause poor welfare. Campaigning organisations have successfully lobbied the government for improved animal protection legislation. Also, British society increasingly demonstrates preference for food from animals reared compassionately in a sustainable way. Agriculture may contribute up to 30% of global greenhouse gas (GHG) emissions and it is the largest contributor by industrial sector. GHG emissions contribute to global warming, which may cause droughts, flooding, lower agricultural yields and the extinction of species. Further, the human population is set to reach 9 billion by 2050, meaning a greater demand for food, water and energy. In response to John Beddington's perfect storm scenario, 'sustainable intensification' has been recommended. However, livestock intensification can be detrimental to animal welfare, which is ethically unacceptable. In contrast, this paper defends 'radical naturalism', a position which argues for more fundamental changes in human activities. In particular, the growing human population and increasing and excessive meat consumption must be addressed. Philosophically, sustainable intensificationism and radical naturalism may be based on different conceptions of human nature. Sustainable intensifiers have faith in scientific progress, hold an anthropocentric worldview and see humankind as rightful master of the world. Radical naturalists are more sceptical about science and technology, have a biocentric worldview and see humankind as steward, and not master, of the natural world.

Veterinary & Animal Ethics: Proceedings of the First International Conference on Veterinary and Animal Ethics, September 2011, First Edition. Edited by Christopher M. Wathes, Sandra A. Corr, Stephen A. May, Steven P. McCulloch and Martin C. Whiting.
© 2013 Universities Federation for Animal Welfare. Published 2013 by Blackwell Publishing Ltd.

Keywords: agriculture, climate change, environment, ethics, farm animal welfare, intensive farming, legislation, livestock, production, protection, radical naturalism, sustainable intensification

7.1 Introduction

In 1964, the classic book *Animal Machines*, by Ruth Harrison, was published. Harrison had read Rachel Carson's *Silent Spring*, an *exposé* of pesticides and their effects on the environment (Carson 1962). *Animal Machines* was an *exposé* of modern industrial intensive farming, in particular the conditions in which pigs and chickens were kept (Harrison 1964). In response to widespread public concern after publication, the British Government appointed a committee to investigate intensive livestock farming. The *Report of the Technical Committee to Enquire into the Welfare of Animals kept under Intensive Livestock Husbandry Systems* was published in 1965 (Brambell 1965). The Brambell Report, as it is known, has had an enormous influence on farm animal welfare.

The same period witnessed a resurgence in writings of professional philosophers on the moral question of how we ought to treat animals. Singer argued that animals deserve equal consideration of interests (Singer 1975); Regan defended animal rights based on intrinsic worth as 'subjects of a life' (Regan 1983) and Rollin used the Aristotelian concept of *teleology* to argue that animals should be treated according to their species-specific natures (Rollin 1981; this proceedings). As well as intellectual discourse, there has been an increase in non-governmental organisation (NGO) activity, for example by the campaigning organisation Compassion in World Farming (CIWF).

Recently, developments in the sciences, to understand animal wellbeing and suffering, and in philosophy, to examine our moral relationship with animals, coupled with persistent and effective campaigning from NGOs, have helped to increase public concern about the plight of farm animals. Consumer behaviour has changed as a result of greater awareness and concern about farm animal welfare. Perhaps the most significant advance for the welfare of farm animals is the Treaty of Lisbon, which amends the founding Treaty of European Union (EU Treaty). The Treaty recognises animals as 'sentient beings' and mandates that Member States must pay 'full regard to the welfare requirements of animals' (Treaty of Lisbon 2009).

During the same period, there has been a parallel, but largely distinct, environmental movement, which comprises intellectual, campaigning, social, legislative and policy strands. For example, the Gaia hypothesis proposes that living organisms, together with the inorganic environment, form a single and self-regulating system on Earth (Lovelock 1979). Disturbances to this system will threaten the stability of environmental conditions, such as the Earth's surface temperature. The Kyoto Protocol to the United Nations Framework Convention on Climate Change is a legally binding agreement to reduce GHG emissions worldwide (UNFCC 2011).

However, it is notable that both movements, despite some exceptions (e.g. Benton 1993), have followed separate but parallel developments. Over the last decade or so, animal and environmental issues appear to be converging; Dale Jamieson in the USA (Jamieson 2002) and Kate Rawles in the UK (Rawles 2010) have both synthesised an ethic that combines concerns for animals and the environment. Further advances in climate science would rapidly bring these movements into much closer proximity.

7.2 The Link between Agriculture and Climate Change

The Intergovernmental Panel on Climate Change (IPCC 2007) concluded that there is now widespread agreement that the Earth's atmosphere is warming, and the cause is anthropogenic. In 2006, the UN's Food and Agricultural Organisation (FAO 2006) made clear the connection between agriculture and emissions causing climate change; the livestock sector is a major source, responsible for 18% of GHG emissions measured in CO_2 equivalent. This is a higher share than transport. Other reports have calculated that agriculture may contribute up to 30% of global GHG emissions (e.g. see discussion in Garnett 2010).

Greenhouse gases at moderate concentrations in the atmosphere create an environmental temperature that has enabled humans to thrive on Earth. As their concentrations rise, more solar radiation is trapped, raising surface temperature. Small increases in global temperatures have profound effects on water availability, ecosystems, food systems, coasts and human health. More specifically, likely effects include water stress, increased risk of extinction of plants and animals, reduced agricultural yield, more flooding and increased human disease (IPCC 2007). Concern about the effects of global warming has gathered pace. Beddington's 'perfect storm' of food, energy and water shortages will happen by 2030 (Beddington 2009). Global demand for food and energy will jump 50% by 2030 and for fresh water by 30%, as the population tops 8.3 billion; these problems will be exacerbated by climate change.

The UK's Climate Change Act 2008 mandates the reduction of GHG emissions by 80%, compared with 1990 levels, by 2050 (Climate Change Act 2008). The global human population is projected to increase from its current 7 billion, to stabilise at between 8 and 10 billion in 2050 (IPCC 2007). This will increase demand for food, water and land. Large populations in countries such as China and India are in the process of rapid, sustained economic growth. As people become more prosperous, they tend to consume a higher proportion of meat in their diets. This phenomenon has been called the 'nutrition transition' (Popkin 2003). This increase is not only a problem because of high GHG emissions from livestock farming. Compounding the growing demand is the issue of the inefficiency of conversion of vegetable protein to animal protein. Animals waste much energy as heat when they convert vegetable protein to animal protein as meat. Up to 9, 4 and

2 kg of non-pasture feed energy are needed to produce 1 kg of beef, pig and chicken meat, respectively (McMichael and Butler 2010). Hence, large areas of land are required to grow crops, which are required to feed animals for a growing human population with changing consumption habits. In a similar scenario, many farmed fish are themselves fed fish, which is again inefficient in terms of potential energy use by humankind.

If the *Livestock's long shadow* report (FAO 2006) documented the connection between agriculture and global warming, the next major UK scientific report on farming offered policy recommendations in response to this problem. The Foresight *Future of food and farming* report suggests 'sustainable intensification' as a major agricultural policy recommendation (Foresight 2011). To summarise so far, the problems are: first, a demand in developed countries for safe, higher welfare provenance food (Eurobarometer 2007), which is locally produced and environmentally friendly. There is also a growing health problem in non-communicable diseases such as cardiovascular disease, diabetes and obesity, which are associated with excessive consumption of saturated fats (WHO 2011). Second, the global human population is growing. In developing countries, there is a trend towards consumption of more animal protein as a proportion of the diet – the nutrition transition. Third, there is scientific consensus that agriculture is a significant contributor to anthropogenic climate change. Finally, if we continue as we are the extent of global warming will cause serious and irreversible changes across most of the globe.

In response to this perfect storm, there appear to be two different schools of thought. Of course, not all proponents fall neatly into one of the groups, and there is crossover. Nevertheless, two different groups emerge. The first I shall call 'Sustainable Intensifiers', after the Foresight report; the second group I call 'Radical Naturalists'.

7.3 Sustainable Intensification

In January 2011, the UK government-commissioned *Future of Food and Farming: Challenges and Choices for Global Sustainability* report was published. The authors are aware of the contribution of greenhouse gases from agriculture (Foresight 2011, p. 28). In response to the problem, a central policy recommendation is sustainable intensification in agriculture. This phrase refers to both crop and livestock agriculture and was used earlier in a Royal Society report on arable agriculture (Royal Society 2009). Sustainable intensification, or intensifying food production in a manner that is sustainable, is an intuitively appealing solution to the growing demand for food. Intensification, an economic concept, involves reducing inputs (costs), increasing productivity (growth rates and yields) and economies of scale (larger production units). Sustainability is described in the Foresight report (2011, p. 31) as:

> *'The principle of sustainability implies the use of resources at rates that do not exceed the capacity of the earth to replace them. Thus water is consumed in water basins at*

rates that can be replenished by inflows and rainfall, greenhouse gas emissions are balanced by carbon fixation and storage, soil degradation and biodiversity loss are halted, and pollutants do not accumulate in the environment.'

Despite being intuitively appealing, we need to analyse sustainable intensification further: first because of the grave consequences of getting policy wrong, and second because the concept of sustainable intensification has since been criticised. Tim Lang, Professor of Food Policy at City University, London, has argued: Is another round of technical intensification needed to raise productivity? That's what the UK's Foresight report argued a few months ago, calling for the oxymoronic 'sustainable intensification' (Lang, The Guardian 2011).

Is the concept of sustainable intensification an oxymoron? Consider the concept in a formal sense, that is without any content. Intensification is a *process*, specifically the process of making something more intense. Sustainability means capable of being sustained or continued. Conceived without reference to content, the sustainability of the intensification should not be bound by time, that is it should be (at least in principle) indefinite. As a strictly formal concept, sustainable intensification does appear to be contradictory: any *object* of intensification must surely reach a limit of intensity.

But does Foresight's policy recommendation of sustainable intensification entail or even imply that intensification should continue indefinitely? The recommendation of sustainable intensification is based on population growth that is projected to *plateau* between 2050 and 2100; *'For the first time, there is now a high likelihood that growth in the global population will cease, with the number of people levelling in the range of eight to ten billion towards the middle of the century or in the two decades that follow'* (Foresight 2011, p. 13).

Therefore, the policy recommendation holds as long as the population is growing or, more accurately, for as long as demand for animal protein increases (due to the nutrition transition associated with economic development). Hence, Lang's claim that Foresight's use of sustainable intensification is oxymoronic is ambiguous, since the phrase contains contradictory terms but is not in itself contradictory if limited in time. But despite upholding the conceptual coherence of a limited, that is temporary, sustainable intensification, the more important question is this: Is sustainable intensification a coherent policy, when applied in a real sense to agriculture? To answer this question, we should first examine what sort of sustainable intensification the authors of the report intend. Second, we should analyse whether the goals are realistically achievable with these methods. Third, we should examine whether such methods will be ethically acceptable from society's point of view. First, the report describes sustainable intensification as: *'Sustainable intensification means simultaneously raising yields, increasing the efficiency with which inputs are used and reducing the negative environmental effects of food production'* (Foresight 2011, p. 35).

Second, examples of how sustainable intensification might be achieved: *'Developments in science or technology can influence and increase the efficiency of interventions to reduce greenhouse gas emissions. For example, precision agriculture with reduced volume of fertiliser application, breeding for improved nitrogen use by plants, and breeding for reduced greenhouse gas emissions in beef and dairy cattle and via genetic improvements in their fodder*' (Foresight 2011, p. 29).

And in the developing world: '*Appropriate new technology has the potential to be very valuable for the poorest people in low-income countries. It is important to incorporate possible beneficiaries in decision-making at all stages of the development process*' (Foresight 2011, p. 11).

Third, Foresight acknowledges concerns that certain options may not be culturally acceptable; '*New technologies (such as the genetic modification of living organisms and the use of cloned livestock and nanotechnology) should not be excluded a priori on ethical or moral grounds, though there is a need to respect the views of people who take a contrary view*' (Foresight 2011, p. 11).

In fairness, the authors of the report certainly do not recommend sustainable intensification as the sole policy to create more food at lower environmental cost: '*The solution is not just to produce more food, or change diets, or eliminate waste. The potential threats are so great that they cannot be met by making changes piecemeal to parts of the food system. It is essential that policy-makers address all areas at the same time*' (Foresight 2011, p. 12).

However, when writing in more detail about the consumption of meat, the Foresight authors appear reticent: '*Policy-makers should recognise that more proactive measures affecting the demand and production of meat may be required should current trends in global consumption continue to rise*' (Foresight 2011, p. 22).

That '*proactive measures*' *may* be required '*should current trends in global consumption continue to rise*' implies that the authors are not currently recommending proactive measures now, but why the delay? The only plausible reason is the authors have confidence in sustainable intensification significantly contributing to an 80% reduction in greenhouse gas emissions by 2050 that is a legally binding requirement (Climate Change Act 2008).

7.4 Livestock Intensification and Animal Welfare Problems

After the risk to UK food security exposed during World War II, the agricultural policy of the British Government was to be self sufficient in food production. Soon after this, economics replaced security as the main driver of intensification. There are limits to intensification, one of which is the living animal. Increasing stocking densities, for example, increases stress and susceptibility to infectious disease. However, the routine use of antibiotics and advances in technology, such as mechanical ventilation, has allowed for the widespread development of industrial farming (Rollin 1981).

Tradinal battery cages for laying hens reveal the extent to which intensification has gone. The birds are often kept on sloping mesh floor, deprived of materials (economic inputs) to satisfy behaviours with strong natural urges such as dust bathing and nest building. In terms of space, the birds are unable to stretch their wings, each having about the size of an A4 piece of paper. This can lead to feather pecking and even cannibalism, which is controlled by beak trimming. In many parts of the world, pigs are confined in stalls not much bigger than themselves. They are unable to move around, that is they cannot perform the most basic normal behaviours. Broiler chickens have been bred to grow so rapidly that some of them become severely lame, some to such an extent that they are unable to reach food and water; some die of dehydration (FAWC 2009). Modern dairy cows have been selectively bred to have such high milk yields that they cannot be sustained on grass, their natural diet, because it does not provide sufficient energy. Webster (1994) has calculated that the dairy cow works, in a metabolic sense, harder than any other farm animal. The modern British high-yielding Holstein–Friesian cow works harder than the *Tour de France* endurance cyclist. Such productivity has its price; there is a high prevalence of lameness, mastitis and infertility in the UK herd (FAWC 2009). Broiler chicken breeders are kept chronically hungry throughout their lives, for their appetite is so great that they would become too obese to breed if they were allowed to satisfy their appetites (FAWC 1998).

The true picture is one of being already a long way along the road of livestock intensification. Living animals have natural limitations, and the above examples clearly demonstrate these, all related to intensification of farming: unnatural aggression, chronic hunger, painful lameness, mastitis and infertility. In addition to these so-called 'production diseases', farm animals can have stereotypies and other abnormal behaviours (Mason 1991). To counter with the assertion that we do not have knowledge of the mental states of animals is simply a relic of behaviourism. There is no justification for demanding a higher epistemic burden of proof for suffering in animals other than our own species. Such thinking simply reflects prejudice.

This raises the question of what precisely is meant by further intensification. The intentions of Foresight could be interpreted variously: first, to further intensify already intensive aspects of production; or second, to promote a similar level of intensification in those places that are currently extensive, to a perceived 'maximum' level of intensification. Here, we should remind ourselves that to maintain high levels of meat consumption, *step changes* in livestock intensification would be required, to substantially reduced GHG emissions.

7.5 The Ethics of Genetic Modification

The Foresight (2011) report states that genetic modification, nanotechnology and cloning should not be ruled out *a priori* as possible solutions. In Europe, there is a widespread public opinion against the use of bovine somatotrophin (bST) hormone injections in cows to produce higher milk yields. There are undoubtedly many reasons for this, and the use of bST in cattle has been shown to detrimentally affect the welfare of cows (Millar and Mepham 2001). There is also widespread rejection of the practice of cloning animals for meat production in the UK (*The Telegraph* 2008). This has been brought into sharp focus by media coverage of cloned animals illegally entering the UK food supply (e.g. BBC 2010). Cloning animals has also been heavily criticised by animal welfare organisations, partly due to the high proportion of cloned animals that die shortly after birth (RSPCA 2010). The independent government advisory body, FAWC, recently commented on genetic modification techniques (FAWC 2009, p. 3):

> 'Would it be right to produce, whether by conventional breeding or modern biotechnology, a pig unable to feel pain and unresponsive to other pigs? If that were possible, such a pig would not be able to suffer and its use might lead to significant productivity gains. Someone arguing that such a course of action would be wrong, would not be able to argue thus on the grounds of animal suffering. Other criteria would have to be invoked. It might be argued that such a course of action would be disrespectful to pigs, that it is not respecting their integrity (i.e. telos), or that it would involve treating them only as a means to a human end and not, even to a limited extent, as ends in themselves. While the application of science offers many opportunities to improve animal welfare, FAWC does not favour the use of animal breeding practices and technologies including genetic modifications, new or existing, that would decrease the sentience of farm animals, e.g. their ability to feel pain or experience distress.'

7.6 Radical Naturalism: An Alternative to Sustainable Intensification

The Foresight *Future of Food and Farming* report (2011) emphasises sustainable intensification as a central policy recommendation. Radical naturalism is an alternative position to one that relies on sustainable intensification. Rather than suggesting that human population growth and consumption patterns may need to be addressed in the future, radical naturalists believe that these are vital elements to influence now. Radical naturalism is so called because it seeks to change the basic causes of global warming. Sir David Attenborough recently gave a lecture on population, entitled 'People and Planet' (Attenborough 2011):

> 'We now realise that the disasters that continue increasingly to afflict the natural world have one element that connects them all – the unprecedented increase in the number of human beings on the planet.'

In terms of meat consumption and policy recommendation, the conservative tone of Foresight's words is highlighted by comparison with the more urgent recommendations of other reports. Oxfam's *4-a-week Changing food consumption in the UK to benefit people and planet* paper sets out '*four ways in which we can adapt our consumption to achieve both environmental and social sustainability and justice. These are: waste less; eat less meat and dairy; buy more Fairtrade products; and buy more produce from developing countries'* (Oxfam 2009).

Dr Rajendra Pachauri, chair of the United Nations Intergovernmental Panel on Climate Change, has publicly said that people should reduce their meat consumption (The Guardian 2008):

> *'In terms of immediacy of action and the feasibility of bringing about reductions in a short period of time, [reduced meat consumption] clearly is the most attractive opportunity…. Give up meat for one day [a week] initially, and decrease it from there.'*

There are also serious questions about the role of free market growth-based economics in the current crisis. In his book *Prosperity without Growth*, Tim Jackson, economics commissioner on the UK government's Sustainable Development Commission, asks the following:

> *'In a world of finite resources, constrained by strict environmental limits, still characterised by 'islands of prosperity' within 'oceans of poverty', are ever-increasing incomes for the already-rich really a legitimate focus for our continued hopes and expectations? Or is there perhaps some other path towards a more sustainable, a more equitable form of prosperity?'* (Jackson 2011)

7.7 Discussion

The current problem is to feed a growing human population without destroying the environment for future populations, that is sustainably. To begin with, there is no disagreement between sustainable intensifiers and radical naturalists about the nature of the problem. Rather, it is the emphasis on different aspects of the solution that are in dispute. The ethical stance that the following discussion assumes is an anthropocentric one. The problem is how to feed the world's population sustainably. An anthropocentric position allows moral consideration of sentient animals and the wider environment, but the interests of the human take priority. What follows is a suggested logical approach to the problem of sustainably feeding a growing population, from an anthropocentric perspective.

The first element to address is human population size. Demographic projections are best estimates and it is possible that the human population will *not* plateau as forecast. The optimal solution, all things considered, will account for all reasonable projections. Since GHG emissions are a function of population size, this is the first factor to address.

Second, an analysis of the problem should look at similar problems now and in the past. The central problem is how to feed an increasing number of people sustainably. Policy failure will result in either more hunger or increased climate change beyond manageable limits. What lessons can we learn from the problem of hunger today? Top of the United Nations Millennium Development Goals list is to halve the proportion of hungry people in the world (United Nations 2011). Although good progress was made in the 1980s and first half of the 1990s, hunger has been rising for the last decade (World Food Program 2011). The World Food Program (WFP) asks on their website:

> 'Food has never before existed in such abundance, so why are 925 million people in the world going hungry? In purely quantitative terms, there is enough food available to feed the entire global population of 6.7 billion people. And yet, one in nearly seven people is going hungry. One in three children is underweight. Why does hunger exist?' (World Food Program 2011)

The answer is divided into short sections on nature, war, poverty trap, agricultural infrastructure and over-exploitation of environment. The diagnosis of the WFP for the hunger problem is that *droughts* are the most common cause of food shortages and basic agricultural infrastructure would improve this. There is therefore a serious problem with water supply and basic infrastructure.

The developing world has food problems of hunger and malnutrition. In contrast, the developed world has health problems caused by excessive nutrition, including obesity, cardiovascular disease and type-2 diabetes (WHO 2011). This state of affairs suggests that the current food problem is one of inequitable distribution and *not* absolute deficiency.

Third, the conversion of vegetable to animal protein is inherently inefficient. The efficiency of conversion of energy ranges from 9:1 to 2:1. Intensively reared livestock are often fed cereals that could be used more efficiently to feed humans directly. Despite this, universal ethical veganism does not necessarily follow. Meat is a good source of essential nutrients, such as iron, zinc and vitamin B12, which are vital for human health. In many areas, it is much easier to access these nutrients through eating meat. Farm animals can convert energy not available to humans. Pigs and poultry are like scavengers and can convert poor quality/ unwanted/waste food to animal protein (Tudge 2010). Ruminants graze fibrous grasses to convert energy into edible meat and milk. Tara Garnett, in her Livestock and Climate Change, describes this approach as 'Livestock on Leftovers' (Garnett 2010). Other limitations in the future will be water availability and land. Livestock use far more water and land (via inefficiencies of conversion) compared with crop agriculture.

How does sustainable intensification measure against these facts? First, a large part of the problem is distribution and not absolute deficiency. Increasing quantity may help with distribution, but indirectly. It is more sensible to directly target the underlying problem of distribution. Second, inefficiencies of conversion mean that intensifying livestock agriculture can lead to further reductions in vegetable energy and protein available to the people of poorer nations. Third, intensive livestock agriculture is associated with deforestation and other land use change to grow cereals to feed the animals.

Since excessive meat consumption in developed nations is associated with non-communicable diseases, the most sensible solution is for developed nations to reduce meat consumption. The most rational policy is called contraction and convergence (McMichael and Butler 2010). This recommends a contraction in meat and dairy consumption in parts of the developed world, which currently consumes an excessive quantity, and an increase in parts of the developing world, ultimately leading to convergence of consumption at a sustainable level. This is consistent with feeding the world more equitably and achieving food justice. Finally, all of this is consistent with respecting the welfare of sentient farm animals because intensification has led to diminished animal welfare. This is consonant with society's current move towards concern for animal welfare. It also avoids the risk that agricultural intensification is at or close to the point of decreasing marginal returns.

Sustainable intensification does not in itself require structural societal and economic changes. It is simply the aim to produce a larger amount of food, in a sustainable way, through continued intensification. The above analysis has shown that there are serious problems with this view. A central argument of this paper is that further intensification is not likely to be sustainable, due to natural and physical constraints. Radical naturalism, as its name suggests, involves more fundamental changes. This includes changes in consumption patterns, more serious consideration of demographics, a re-examination of the economy and an appreciation of risk analysis.

7.8 Conceptions of Human Nature

The doctrine of sustainable intensification is premised on a confidence that science and technology can play a large role in preventing the impending perfect storm. The Foresight report is based on the belief that current scientific knowledge and technology, as well as future developments, can significantly contribute to the solution. Since science and technology are tools that are created and used by humans, this approach implies a confidence in the capacity of humans both to disseminate current technology and to use our creative abilities to produce more knowledge that can be put to good practical use. At a deeper level, the utilisation of science and technology to solve problems with the natural world implies an underlying conception of human nature. This is the outlook of the enlightenment, in which man dominates nature for his own purposes. Indeed, this analysis is entirely consistent with modern scientists being the grandchildren of the early scientists of that time. In contrast, radical naturalists are more sceptical about the human understanding of the natural world and believe that there are limits to the utility of technology. Rather than seeing the rightful place of humankind as above and in control of nature, radical naturalists see humans as a *part* of nature. If *Homo sapiens* are the dominant species, then our natural role is as stewards of a susceptible ecosystem rather than artificers of control. These characterisations of sustainable intensifiers and radical naturalists are but the modern rationalists and romantics, each with its own perspective on mankind's proper relation with nature.

7.9 Summary

Sustainable intensification is neither necessary nor sufficient to address the demographic and climate crises that the human family faces. To reduce emissions of greenhouse gases to levels that will enable a stable and hospitable climate, the growth in population must be checked and the habit of eating excessive meat and dairy products reversed. Indeed, intensification of livestock agriculture that leads to increased productivity and cheaper meat could increase demand for these products and fuel, on a global basis, the current level of excessive consumption in the developed world. Further intensification will also cause the suffering of sentient animals, which society has judged to be morally unacceptable. Succeeding in this difficult challenge may require unpopular social and economic policies and an unprecedented degree of global cooperation. The human race has lived unsustainably since some time after the industrial revolution and old habits die hard. But die they must, for nothing less than the future of the planet might well be at stake.

Acknowledgements

The author is grateful to Michael Reiss and Tara Garnett for valuable comments on earlier drafts of this paper.

References

Attenborough, D. (2011) People and planet lecture to the RSA, 10 March 2011. Available at: http://puttheworldright.com/population_people_and_planet.html (accessed on 16 June 2011).

BBC (2010) Meat of cloned cow offspring in UK food chain, FSA says. Available at: http://www.bbc.co.uk/news/uk-10859866 (accessed on 16 June 2011).

Beddington, J. (2009) *The Guardian*. Available at: http://www.guardian.co.uk/science/2009/mar/18/perfect-storm-john-beddington-energy-food-climate (accessed on 20 June 2011).

Benton, T. (1993) *Natural Relations?: Animal Rights, Human Rights and the Environment.* Verso Books, London.

Brambell, R. (1965) *Report of the Technical Committee to Enquire into the Welfare of Animals Kept under Intensive Livestock Husbandry Systems.* Her Majesty's Stationary Office, London.

Carson, R. (1962) *Silent Spring*, 40th edn. Houghton Mifflin (Trade) (23 October 2003).

Climate Change Act (2008) Available at: http://www.legislation.gov.uk/ukpga/2008/27/contents (accessed on 20th June 2011).

Eurobarometer (2007) Attitudes of EU citizens towards animal welfare. Eurobarometer, March 2007.

FAO (2006) *Livestock's Long Shadow*. Food and Agricultural Organisation of the United Nations, Rome, Italy.

FAWC (1998) *Report on the Welfare of Broiler Breeders*. Farm Animal Welfare Council, London.

FAWC (2009) *Farm Animal Welfare in Great Britain: Past, Present and Future*. Farm Animal Welfare Council, London.

Foresight (2011) *The Future of Food and Farming. Executive Summary*. The Government Office for Science, London.

Garnett, T. (2010) Livestock and climate change. In: *The Meat Crisis* (eds J. D'Silva & J. Webster), pp. 34–56. Earthscan 2010, London.

Harrison, R. (1964) *Animal Machines*. Vincent Stuart, London.

IPCC (2007) *Climate Change 2007: Synthesis Report. Contribution of Working Groups I, II and III to the Fourth Assessment Report of the Intergovernmental Panel on Climate Change* (eds Core Writing Team, R.K. Pachauri & A. Reisinger), 104 pp. IPCC, Geneva, Switzerland.

Jackson, T. (2011) *Prosperity without Growth*. Earthscan, London.

Jamieson, D. (2002) Animal liberation is an environmental ethic. In: *Morality's Progress: Essays on Humans, Other Animals, and the Rest of Nature* (ed. D. Jamieson), pp. 197–212. Clarendon Press, Oxford, U.K.

Mason, G. (1991) Stereotypies and suffering. *Behavioural Processes*, **25**(2–3), 103–115.

McMichael, A.J. & Butler, A.J. (2010) Environmentally sustainable and equitable meat consumption in a climate change world. In: *The Meat Crisis* (eds J. D'Silva & J. Webster), pp. 173–189. Earthscan 2010, London.

Millar, K. & Mepham, B. (2001) Bioethical analysis of biotechnologies: Lessons from automatic milking machines systems (AMS) and bovine somatotrophin (bST). In: *Occasional Publication*, number 28 (eds C.M. Wathes, A.R. Frost, F. Gordon & J.D. Woods), pp. 29–36. British Society of Animal Science, Edinburgh.

Oxfam (2009) *4-a-week, Oxfam GB Briefing Paper*, March 2009. pp. 2.

Popkin, B.M. (2003) The nutrition transition in the developing world. *Development Policy Review*, **21**, 581–597.

Rawles, K. (2010) Sustainable development and animal welfare: The neglected dimension. In: Animals, Ethics *and Trade: The Challenge of Animal Sentience* (eds J. Turner & J. D'Silva), pp. 208–216. Compassion in World Farming Trust, Surrey.

Regan, T. (1983) *The Case for Animal Rights*, revised edition (14 September 2004). University of California Press, Berkeley, California.

Rollin, B. (1981) *Animal Rights and Human Morality*. Prometheus Books, New York.

Royal Society (2009) *Reaping the Benefits: Science and the Sustainable Intensification of Global Agriculture*. The Royal Society, London.

RSPCA (2010) Concern over recent cloned animal claims. Available at: http://www.rspca.org.uk/media/news/story/-/article/EM_Cloning (accessed on 22 June 2011).

Singer, P. (1975) *Animal Liberation*, 4th revised edition (5 October 1995). Pimlico, London.

The Guardian (2008) Available at: http://www.guardian.co.uk/environment/2008/sep/07/food.foodanddrink (accessed on 22 June 2011).

The Guardian (2011) Available at: http://www.guardian.co.uk/commentisfree/2011/jun/01/food-prices-doubling (accessed on 22 June 2011).

The Telegraph (2008) Consumers reject food from cloned animals. Available at: http://www.telegraph.co.uk/earth/earthnews/3343589/Consumers-reject-food-from-cloned-animals.html (accessed on 16 June 2011).

Treaty of Lisbon (2009) Available at: http://ec.europa.eu/food/animal/welfare/references_en.htm (accessed on 17 June 2011).

Tudge, C. (2010) *How to Raise Livestock – and How Not To* In: *The Meat Crisis* (eds J. D'Silva J & J. Webster), pp. 9–21. Earthscan 2010, London.

United Nations (2011) Millennium development goals. Available at: http://www.un.org/millenniumgoals/bkgd.shtml (accessed on 22 June 2011).

UNFCC (2011) Kyoto protocol to the United Nations framework convention on climate change. Available at: http://unfccc.int/resource/docs/convkp/kpeng.html (accessed on 17 June 2011).

Webster, J. (1994) *Animal Welfare: A Cool Eye towards Eden*. Blackwell Publishing, Oxford, U.K.

WHO (2011) WHO/FAO release independent Expert Report on diet and chronic disease. Available at: http://www.who.int/mediacentre/news/releases/2003/pr20/en/ (accessed on 22 June 2011).

World Food Program (2011) Available at: http://www.wfp.org/hunger/causes (accessed on 22 June 2011).

Questions and Answers

Q: You've said that we need an unprecedented level of cooperation across the planet. We've not seen very positive moves in that direction with the likes of Copenhagen, for example. Is there any optimism for the political possibility of what you're saying is necessary?

A: There will be cooperation, but the question is whether it will be too little too late. James Lovelock and others are more pessimistic and believe that we need a few more natural disasters to hasten action. There is a middle ground with increasing levels of cooperation. For instance, international organisations, which are necessary to solve a global problem, are becoming more important and this trend will likely continue in the future.

Q: Inter-governmental organisations like the FAO are aware of the issues and take them very seriously. All these different aspects are now addressed at that level with the OIE, FAO, World Food Programme and so on. I want to pick up on our tendency to generalise and use averages. You talked about the contraction and convergence model and the different levels of consumption in developed countries versus developing countries. It's important to remember the diversity within those categories. The massive increase in animal product consumption in developing countries is primarily people of middle and higher income; it's not the poor and malnourished, who need those animal products. So policies are required that take account of protection of poor and malnourished people in developed and developing countries rather than simply looking at average intakes.

A: Yes, I entirely agree.

Q: The Pew Foundation is the Sun Oil Company, a $6 billion trust. It was the first to investigate confinement agriculture over a period of 2½ years. The phrase 'sustainable intensification' sounds like an oxymoron because the Pew Foundation uncovered structural reasons to believe that intensification is inherently non-sustainable in many ways.

C: The question is that there needs to be a route map to go better than sustainable intensification. Do you have any comments on that?

A: I have taken the phrase 'sustainable intensification' from the Foresight *Future of Food and Farming* report, which was published January 2011 and commissioned by the UK Government. In contrast, I have coined the term 'radial naturalism' to describe a different, broader position represented by, for example, David Attenborough and Tim Jackson. The paper is a critique of sustainable intensification for being insufficient to address the food issue and also for it being problematic ethically in terms of animal welfare. In this way, it is consistent with the findings of the Pew Commission. The point about it being oxymoronic has been made by Tim Lang of City University, London. In my paper, there is a philosophical analysis of whether this claim is justified. The concept is oxymoronic in a purely formal sense because you can't intensify something indefinitely. However, applied in a real sense to agriculture, and critically if it is based on a model where the population plateaus, it is not oxymoronic. This is because the idea is to intensify production to a certain level and then remain at that level. Presumably that is what sustainable intensifiers would argue, but of course this also reveals that the policy is crucially dependent on the population indeed stabilising.

Q: Do you know what is the environmental footprint of pet ownership? Many talks like yours focus on meat and dairy consumption; I'm concerned that we should look at other social things.

A: One of the next big issues in veterinary ethics may well be pet foods, both for environmental reasons and also welfare provenance; do the cows and pigs which produce the beef and pork for dogs and cats to consume live happy lives? It's an issue that hasn't been addressed and it should be.

Q: Unless we recognise that human greed and human growth are getting us into this problem, we are going to be dealing with palliative fixes instead of addressing the underlying problems. The feed conversion ratios are correct but we have to remember that for a lot of the world outwith Europe, there are huge tracts of land on which crops cannot be grown. The only way to use this land is by using ruminants which convert those products which are unavailable to humans, that is cellulose and hemi-cellulose, to something useful. Even though it is relatively inefficient for the people who live in those areas, it is very important.

A: Yes I entirely agree, hence why universal and ethical veganism doesn't follow from the radical naturalism position, even though in general consumption of animal products is less efficient than consumption of vegetable protein. The problem is, for example, de-forestation of the Amazon, which creates massive carbon emissions through land use change and with cereals and soya which are grown to feed cattle in intensive systems. These practices should stop: arguably, further intensification is likely to rely on such methods. Radical naturalism is consistent with using ruminants to graze land that is unsuitable for other purposes.

Q: Does the British Veterinary Association and other professional associations have policies that they would like to see their members abide by?
A: Increasingly more organisations will become involved. The target is 80% reduction in greenhouse gas emissions by 2050, relative to 1990 levels, which is mandated by the UK Climate Change Act (2008). The majority of people aren't aware of the scale of change needed. I hope that once this becomes better known, more people will change their behaviour.

Q: The Royal Society is currently engaged in a big project on people and the planet. The population issue is complicated because in many parts of the world where the population is declining, governments are actually encouraging people to have more children. This is an appalling thought, but one of the big issues, of course, is consumption. The difficulty is getting people to reduce their consumption, for example as a result of a disaster or a war. We, in the UK, adopted a rationing policy as a result of war which led to better health but it's going to be a real problem in the USA where people are very resistant to any kind of government action. While many people are optimistic, I'm a bit pessimistic about getting people to reduce their consumption.
A: Both demographics and food security are very complex issues. Various policy instruments and changes in society will be needed. But let us hope things do change before we get to the point of war. As you know, even now people are forecasting conflict over water stress, which is already occurring in some parts of the world. The WHO recommendation for meat consumption is about 80 g/day. But we eat on average over 200 g in the UK, and it's over 300 g in the USA. Many people simply don't realise that the international authority on health, the WTO, is advising that we eat too much meat. In Germany, there is a public education campaign to reduce meat consumption. There is politics involved in the issue, partly due to the strength of the agricultural lobby.

Ethics and Ethical Analysis in Veterinary Science: The Development and Application of the Ethical Matrix Method

KATE MILLAR

University of Nottingham

Abstract: Animal professionals, veterinarians and scientists working with animals deal with a unique and complex set of ethical dilemmas that arise out of the nature of clinical practice and animal use. This paper discusses the complexity of these ethical dilemmas and examines the development and use of ethical tools to support decision-making. The paper focuses on the development and use of the ethical matrix, originally presented by Ben Mepham in particular discussing how this method has been adapted for a number of different uses. Several recent applications of this approach are discussed. Finally, the need and opportunities for further development of these types of tools is explored.

Key words: ethical matrix, ethics, principles, reflexivity, veterinarian

Veterinary & Animal Ethics: Proceedings of the First International Conference on Veterinary and Animal Ethics, September 2011, First Edition. Edited by Christopher M. Wathes, Sandra A. Corr, Stephen A. May, Steven P. McCulloch and Martin C. Whiting.
© 2013 Universities Federation for Animal Welfare. Published 2013 by Blackwell Publishing Ltd.

8.1 Introduction

Ethical dilemmas can be observed in all professional settings, from design engineering through to the retail industry. A number of these are common to all professions, involving issues such as the protection of personal information, misappropriation of funds, etc. The drive to create a knowledge-based society, rapid technological innovation and ICT modernisation is challenging the way in which various professionals manage data and resources, interact with clients and define professional standards, to name but a few areas of decision-making. However, some groups appear to face distinctive challenges, that is veterinarians and scientists (hereafter termed 'animal professionals'), who are confronted with unique ethical issues when working with animals.

Embracing the assertion, which could be tested empirically, that animal professionals face a challenging and unique range of ethical issues, the question that then arises is: how should their ethical decision-making skills be developed and supported? This question has been taken up by a number of applied ethicists. A range of approaches are needed, from undergraduate training, through the embedding of institutional mechanisms that encourage and support reflexivity, to state-of-the-art, good practice guidance (Magalhães-Sant'Ana et al. 2009; Rogers & Ballantyne 2010). Decision-support methods can assist professionals when considering ethical issues; these are often referred to as ethical tools (Mepham & Millar 2001; Beekman & Brom 2007). One such 'tool' is the ethical matrix (EM), originally proposed by Mepham (1996, 2000).

This paper briefly discusses the complexity of animal-centred ethical dilemmas, before examining in more depth the nature and use of ethical frameworks to support decision-making, specifically focusing on the use of the EM and its development over the past decade. Finally, the recent application of the EM as a decision-support tool, the potential value of the tool for animal professionals, and the need for its further development are examined.

8.2 Professional Ethics and Animals

Although veterinarians and scientists working with animals deal with a number of challenging issues that are faced by others (e.g. fair employment, equal opportunity, etc.), they deal with unique and complex ethical dilemmas that arise out of the nature of veterinary practice and animal use. It is important to understand the nature of these ethical issues and how animal professionals approach them on a day-to-day basis as this knowledge will have an impact, not only on how they might be supported through training and decision-support services but also on their overall well-being through greater awareness and insight of the challenges that they face, which may in turn lead to greater empowerment.

Focusing on the experiences of veterinarians, it is increasingly acknowledged that they face difficult ethical decisions in their daily work; for example Bartram and Baldwin (2008; 2010) have attempted to deconstruct the issues that contribute to a high suicide rate amongst veterinarians, with access to lethal pharmaceuticals believed to have a significant impact on annual figures. Among other factors, routine euthanasia is believed to be stressful and, through contextual effects, may contribute to a high suicide rate, as noted by Bartram and Baldwin (2010) *'Veterinary surgeons may experience uncomfortable tensions between their desire to preserve life and an inability to treat a case effectively'.*

Although veterinary consultations that directly involve decisions about euthanasia present prominent ethical dilemmas, other issues may also be characterised as value-based conflicts. These may often represent complex ethical dilemmas as they are either opaque or involve numerous value conflicts embedded within one case. In addition, they may not be traditionally identified as key ethical dilemmas, which may make them more stressful, as there are limited opportunities to discuss these issues openly. Examples of common ethical dilemmas include some orthopaedic surgeries in companion animals, castration in farm animals, the use of animals in toxicity tests and the use of various reproductive technologies in dogs. For these and many other issues, the practices may seem embedded and are rarely questioned due to economic 'realities'.

In terms of the nature of the issues and how they 'play out' in practice, veterinarians and others often encounter complex relationships. At times not all parties with responsibility for a patient may agree on that patient's ethical standing: this relationship is often expressed through sentiments such as 'it's only a dog' or '… but it is my baby'. These simple caricatures highlight that conflicting 'voices' may be underpinned by different, although not consciously expressed, ethical beliefs. Being able to identify different ethical positions, facilitate discussion between individuals within complex multi-actor relationships (e.g. patient, two owners, associated animals to consider, etc.) and balance this against a clinician's individual ethical position is a significant challenge. Add into this mix notable financial constraints (as there is no National Health Service for animals in the UK) and operating commercially within a regulatory framework (e.g. AWA 2006; VSA 1966, A[SP]A 1986, etc.), then it is not hard to imagine the day-to-day challenges. In addition, technological innovation now allows greater and more significant intervention in an animal's life. The development and application of biotechnologies such as animal cloning, stem cell techniques and transgenics raise complex, potentially unique ethical questions.

Are the ethical challenges that animal professionals face significantly underestimated and is the profession under supported as they deal with these issues? This is an empirical question which cannot be fully answered here. However, the above discussion implies at the very least that the ethical challenges are notable and finding ways to support these professionals is important. This leads on to a normative question in itself, what ought to be done, or more specifically, how can bioethics support professionals working with animals?

When addressing what is needed, the responses to the problem could be characterised under four themes: (i) insight: the need to better understand the nature of the ethical dilemmas that are presented, through interdisciplinary research that combines social science, ethics and clinical expertise; (ii) transparency: the need for greater acknowledgement of the complexity of the issues faced by professionals working with animals and the ethical dimensions of these issues; (iii) reflexivity: identification of new ways to encourage ethical reflexivity as well as providing spaces and time where this can happen; and (iv) empowerment: development of new training approaches that can empower professionals so they feel increasingly confident and secure in the ethical position they develop and the value decisions they make, as well as being willing to discuss and reflect upon these positions.

In order to empower animal professionals, create insight and transparency as well as encouraging reflexivity, three practical approaches may be needed, for example skills training, provision of ethics tools and conducive institutional arrangements. Practically this should involve some form of ethics training, development of decision-support tools and institutional support allowing individuals to invest time and resources in these activities.

Before discussing tools, it is important to note the role of ethics training, particularly in relation to an individual's ability to respond and be prepared for significant ethical challenges, that is 'the art of anticipation'. The role of ethical theory in the work of animal professionals can seem abstract and obscure; however, the value of ethics knowledge and skills has been clearly presented by leading authorities, such as Sandøe and Christiansen (2008) and Rollin (2006). That said, this need is highlighted by applying Guston's metaphor (2008) to ethical issues:

> 'Anticipation ... denotes building the capacity to respond to unpredicted and unpredictable risks. Many of us frequent gyms to lift weights. But we do not predict that our lives will depend on our ability to perform a 'lat pull' (lat pulldown exercise) or ... to bench-press our weight. Instead, we rightly believe that these exercises will build in our bodies a capacity to withstand whatever physical and emotional stresses we might confront .... We must exercise the various intellectual and imaginative capacities that will prepare us for the challenges.'

Beyond ethics training, the development and application of ethical tools may be one of the most effective ways of responding to "the challenges" under these four themes. The next section examines the role of ethical tools and focuses on the EM as a means to help support decision making.

8.3 Ethical Tools: The Role of the Ethical Matrix

Both animal professionals and ethicists have been interested for a number of years in the development of tools that can aid ethical analysis and reflection. When discussing ethical tools, it is useful to present a general definition: here, tools are considered as methods that are used to structure an ethical assessment by providing a broad set of values and to encourage reflection on the outcomes of an action or policy on a wide range of stakeholders that have ethical standing. They are intended to function amongst a plurality of concerns with the aim of assisting policy makers (within both public and private organisations) to examine key ethical dilemmas or the issues raised by the prospective use of a new technology or innovation. Beekman and Brom (2007) have further discussed the role and diversity of ethical tools, such as the EM.

Millar *et al.* (2007) have discussed ethics within research and technology development (RTD) programmes, identifying four forms of ethics, which are equally applicable when considering research or clinical work with animals. These are: (i) regulation, which is a formally required decision-making process conducted by an external committee (e.g. RCVS or ERP Committees); (ii) engagement, which requires a value-based discourse with external stakeholders, who may be directly or indirectly affected by an action (e.g. veterinary consultation) or the RTD process; (iii) analysis of a programme or practice that is conducted (usually externally) by an individual, committee or consultative group but a final judgement is not necessarily required; and (iv) reflection, which is an informal review process, facilitated through internal reflection and value-based discourse. These forms can be conducted on an individual basis or as part of an on-going project in which clinicians or researchers reflect on key ethical issues. In an extension of Millar *et al.* (2007), a further category is proposed, that is scoping, which is exploratory and explicitly assesses the ethical dimensions of future strategies or policies which are pertinent to policy options.

Defining the nature of an ethical tool and presenting a view on the different forms of ethics is important. An individual tool may operate in different ways in order to fulfil each of the roles listed above. One tool may not be suitable for use across all forms. That said, although the EM was essentially developed to facilitate ethical analysis, it has subsequently been developed and applied in a number of additional ways.

8.4 Original Development and Application of the Ethical Matrix

The EM was proposed by Mepham (1996) as a way of analysing ethical issues raised by new biotechnologies. It was first applied to food and dairy technologies (Mepham 2000; Millar 2000; Millar and Mepham 2001). In its original form, Mepham described it as a *'form of checklist'* that, at its simplest, could be used to map key issues. He hoped that it could also be used to conduct ethical analysis and that it could be used by those with little training or background in applied ethics. Subsequently, it has been developed at Nottingham and elsewhere across Europe; new uses include a participatory approach and a tool to encourage reflexivity as part of upstream research planning and management.

Table 8.1   Generic ethical matrix.

Generic ethical matrix (Translation of principles for the corresponding generic interest groups)

	Well-being	**Autonomy**	**Justice**
Treated organism	Welfare of the animal	Behavioural freedom	Intrinsic value
Producer (e.g. farmer)	Adequate income and working conditions	Freedom to adopt or not adopt	Fair treatment in trade and law
Consumer	Availability of safe food, acceptability	Consumer choice	Affordability of food
Biota	Protection of biota	Biodiversity of biotic populations	Sustainability of the biotic populations

Source: Mepham (2000). Copyright © The Nutrition Society 2000, published by Cambridge University Press, reproduced with permission.

The EM is constructed using a set of *prima facie* principles, derived from those proposed by Beauchamp and Childress (2001), that is respect for well-being (combining the original non-maleficence and beneficence), autonomy and justice. These principles encapsulate western ethical traditions by representing deontological and utilitarian theories as well as Rawlsian notions of justice as fairness. The principles are then applied to interest groups that may be affected by a proposed action or practice, for example the use of a new biotechnology in the dairy industry. Its early use was to assess animal biotechnologies; the interest groups were treated animals, producers, consumers and the biota (Table 8.1). This form has been subsequently described as the generic ethical matrix.

Each individual cell of the EM is a translation of the principle for the specified interest group. Many of the 'translations' represented in the cells are familiar terms (e.g. animal welfare considerations), that is they represent assessment criteria that are used commonly. However, when analysing other cells, such as the principle of justice translated as 'intrinsic value' for the treated organism, these aspects may not be traditionally 'assessed' when determining the implications of the use of a new technology in an animal production system. As Millar and Morton (2009) proposed, it is important to find ways to incorporate discussions of concepts such as integrity or intrinsic value in an overall analysis of how human actions affect animals, as such *'respect for animal integrity plays a significant role in determining what society defines as acceptable human-animal interactions, expressed either implicitly or explicitly through legislation and codes of practice'*. The EM may be one way of doing this by incorporating a broad range of scientific and philosophical concepts into one tool. This may, in turn, encourage individuals to engage in a broad and more transparent ethical discourse (and an ethical analysis process) and assessment.

The inclusion of data or more specifically evidence within the EM is another important aspect. As set out in an instruction manual for the matrix. (Mepham *et al.* 2006)

'... *ethical deliberation entails an appeal to several forms of evidence. Evidence is defined here as anything that provides material or information on which a conclusion or proof is based. Such forms of evidence include, for example: (a) scientific and economic data; (b) assessments of the consequences of risk and uncertainty; (c) assessments of the intrinsic value of different forms of life (which may reflect peoples' differing world views); (d) tacit, folk or practical knowledge.*'

The original formulation of the EM involves the selection of interest groups. Their choice was originally influenced by the focal use of the EM, that is agricultural and food-related issues, but ultimately selection is determined by the activity that is being analysed. In the original use of the EM, Mepham attempted to limit the number of interest groups to four (see Table 8.1). There are practical and substantive reasons for adopting this approach as the interest groups represent those that are deemed to have ethical standing and who may be notably affected by the activity. The number of interest groups could be subdivided and extended *ad nauseam*, but the EM is intended to be a comprehensive tool, representing a common morality amongst the primary groups that may be affected by or have key concerns about the specified action. One of the original aims was to encourage users to put themselves in the 'shoes of others', including interest groups that are unable to express their concerns, such as the treated organism. This is hopefully achieved through the specification of interest groups.

Finally, the overarching aim of this approach is to present a useful tool that is constructed on ethical principles yet is still user-friendly and applicable as a tool for those who have little or no training in theoretical ethics. The approach is also an attempt to open the 'black box' of ethical deliberation, highlighting how data (and other forms of evidence) and values are brought together to form a position or to map ethical issues.

8.5 Further Development of the Ethical Matrix

Following its initial proposal by Mepham in the late 1990s, the EM has been further developed by a core group of researchers at Nottingham (Mepham *et al.* 2006) and in Norway (Kaiser & Forsberg 2001). Millar *et al.* have attempted to develop the EM as a form of participatory tool that can be used by a variety of groups to explore the ethical implications of RTD programmes, agriculture and food policy, or determine strategic policies. Beyond this, further collaborations between the Nottingham and Norwegian researchers have also resulted in the use of the tool to build capacity and encourage ethical reflection, without the need to engage with external stakeholders, within large research consortiums conducting work on the genetic basis of animal disease.

The increasing use of the EM as a tool or reference point for ethical analysis is highlighted by a recent research literature analysis (conducted in 2011) that identified 60 peer-reviewed papers that either applied the EM, referred to it as framework of value, or noted the potential utility of the EM. These papers have been published in an array of journals (e.g. *Journal of Environmental Radioactivity, Journal of Pharmacological and Toxicological Methods* and *In Practice*) highlighting what many of the authors believe to be the wide applicability of the EM. The topics that have been analysed using the EM range from the use of animals in experimentation, management of contaminated agricultural ecosystems, through to the use of AI in dogs, etc. (Howard 2005; England & Millar 2008; Webster *et al.* 2010). Others groups and individuals have proposed the value of using this approach in the future to assess precision livestock farming and inform euthanasia practice (Wathes *et al.* 2008; Yeates 2010). In addition, over 65 further book chapters, conference papers, articles and reports have also referred to or applied the EM, ranging from reports by the UK Food Ethics Council, to education briefing documents (e.g. HEA, UK Centre for Bioscience), to direct application of the EM by an FAO Committee (analysing ethical issues in fisheries), thorough to working papers produced by legal specialists examining biotechnology policy in Zimbabwe (Mohamed-Katerere 2003; FAO 2005; FEC 2006).

Several researchers have examined the foundational basis of the matrix in the hope of improving the method and developing further applications. Schroeder and Palmer (2003) have pointed out some of the limitations in the individual articulation of one of the principles, proposing that the principle of solidarity should substitute the principle of justice. A response has been made by Mepham (2010), where he reiterates the value of the three principles, well-being, autonomy and justice. Crooney and Anthony (2010) have examined the EM comparing it with the use of a framework proposed by Campbell and Hare (1997), referred to as an ethics assessment process, claiming that both these approaches present '*models to combine socio-ethical concerns with relevant factual information, thereby facilitating decision making that is ethically responsible and that offers viable solutions … [these tools provide] ways of examining ethics that offer real solutions to conflicts of interests and not merely "one size fits all" answers*'. Forsberg (2007a, b) has claimed that the use of the EM can result in better decision making and has explored the use of decision support tools in expert ethics committees. She argues that '*societies are characterized by respect for value pluralism*' and, as such, '*even if the ethical matrix process does not determine an answer, its function is so comprehensive that it would be misleading to call it simply a checklist*' (Forsberg 2007b, p. 466). Forsberg finally goes on to state '*I will tentatively conclude that a pragmatist ethical matrix method may yield justified conclusions on concrete cases while still being compatible with principled pluralism and value pluralism*' (Forsberg 2007b).

Thus, Forsberg claims, albeit tentatively, that the use of the EM *per se* can result in better decision-making. This in itself raises opportunities as well as threats for the matrix. It has long been claimed by Mepham and Millar that one of its strengths is that it is not prescriptive. If the tool does steer the user in a direction, this may undermine the value of EM in any mapping or reflection. In addition, any sense of steer may also shut down dialogue, rather than opening it up, as is intended by the EM and other ethical tools. Further work is needed in this area of ethical regulation, i.e. using the EM and other tools in ethics committees.

8.6 Development of the Ethical Matrix and Its Use in Veterinary Practice

The above analysis shows that the EM has been applied across many sectors and the tool itself has developed substantially over the last decade. It has now been used in all five forms of ethics applicable to animal professionals: (i) regulation (e.g. Forsberg 2007a); (ii) engagement (e.g. Kaiser & Forsberg 2001); (iii) analysis (e.g. Mepham 2000; Millar & Tomkins 2007); (iv) reflection (e.g. Millar *et al.* 2007; Jensen *et al.* 2010) and (v) scoping (England and Millar 2008; Mepham 2010). The EM has developed from a tool that was used originally to assess animal biotechnology, licensing and research programmes into more general uses such as supporting committee based ethical decision-makings.

However, although the EM has previously been used by veterinary and animal research groups and is currently being used by groups conducting research in canine genomics and highly infectious zoonotic diseases, it has rarely been applied to ethical dilemmas in veterinary practice. This application may not be suitable for individual consultation in real-time, but it may still be useful as a reflective or scoping tool. Reviewing two examples of the use of the EM may be helpful.

Clinicians could either use the EM to reflect retrospectively on complex cases, as proposed by Yeates (2010) for euthanasia cases. Yeates and Main (2011) imply that principle-based approaches are unsuitable for the complexity of veterinary decision-making. However, Yeates' reference (2010) to the EM and some of its previous uses indicates that principlism, as an approach, can support veterinary clinicians as they weave through the ethical dilemmas that they face week-by-week. Yeates and Main (2011) indicate that there is a need for ethics training at the undergraduate level. In addition, more research is needed to identify the most applicable uses of the EM for the veterinary profession. England and Millar (2008) applied the EM to the use of surgical AI in dogs. This highlights how the EM could be adapted in order to analyse the issues raised by a surgical intervention or a veterinary practice (see Table 8.2).

This application involved the mapping of issues for this surgical intervention, an analysis of the options and a number of policy options. It showed how the EM may be used as a tool to support the development of personal or institutional guidelines or policies for professional governing bodies.

As the veterinary profession seeks to find ways to support ethical deliberation and reflection across the research and clinical communities, a recent discussion within the medical community highlights that embedding of ethics through reflection, scoping and engagement can at times be preferable to formal regulatory

Table 8.2 Example of a modified ethical matrix.

Modified ethical matrix (Translation of the ethical principles for the corresponding interest group)

	Well-being	**Autonomy**	**Fairness**
Dogs	Welfare	Behavioural freedom	Intrinsic value
Breeders	Satisfactory income and working conditions	Managerial freedom	Fair regulations and trade
Owners	Safety and quality of life	Choice	Affordability of products
Veterinarians	Satisfactory income and working conditions	Professional freedom	Equitable standards of practice
Society	Safety and social harmony	Democratic choice	Fair resource allocation

Source: England and Millar (2008).

ethical processes. Sokol (2009) points out that large formal ethics committees may not help clinicians, as they deal with ethical dilemmas in everyday practice. He highlights the omnipresent nature of ethics and the presence of ethical dilemmas within the day-to-day activities of an average clinician and the distant hence potentially unhelpful approach (applied through formal ethical review) of ethics committees when attempting to address day-to-day cases. This observation appears as applicable to veterinarians as it does to physicians. Sokol claims that new ways of encouraging ethical reflection and supporting physicians as they tackle 'live' issues are needed. This, in turn, implies that we need to develop not only new tools but should also examine the process of reflection and interaction with colleagues as well as enlisting ethicists. Rather than focusing on more formal ethical review, embedding ethical reflection in Mortality and Morbidity (M&Ms) sessions in veterinary hospitals and large practices may be valuable. For smaller practices, short sessions that involve explicit application of an ethical tool may provide a much needed discussion of ethical dilemmas. There may be a role for tools such as the EM in these processes. However, more research within a clinical setting is needed. The use of the EM should be assessed alongside the current suite of informal and formal veterinary decision-support processes that are currently available.

References

Bartram, D.J. & Baldwin, D.S. (2010) Veterinary surgeons and suicide: A structured review of possible influences on increased risk. *Veterinary Record*, **166**, 388–397.

Beekman, V. & Brom, F. (2007) Ethical tools to support systematic public deliberations about the ethical aspects of agricultural biotechnologies. *Journal of Agricultural and Environmental Ethics*, **20**, 3–12.

Campbell, C. & Hare, J. (1997) Ethical literacy in gerontology programs. *Gerontology and Geriatrics Education*, **17**, 3–16.

Crooney, C.C. & Anthony, R. (2010) Engaging science in a climate of values: Tools for animal scientists tasked with addressing ethical problems. *Journal of Animal Science*, **88**, 75–81.

England, G. & Millar, K. (2008) The ethics and role of AI with fresh and frozen semen in dogs. *Reproduction in Domestic Animals*, **43**, 165–171.

FAO (2005) Ethical issues in fisheries. FAO Ethics Series No 4. FAO, Rome.

Forsberg, E.-M. (2007a) A Deliberative ethical matrix method – Justification of moral advice on genetic engineering in food production, Dr Art. Dissertation, Oslo: Unpublished/

Forsberg, E.-M. (2007b) Pluralism, the ethical matrix, and coming to conclusions. *Journal of Agricultural and Environmental Ethics*, **20**, 455–468.

Guston, D.H. (2008) Innovation policy: Not just a jumbo shrimp. *Nature*, **454**(21), 940–941.

Howard, B.J., Beresford, N.A., Nisbet, A., *et al.* (2005) The STRATEGY project: Decision tools to aid sustainable restoration and long-term management of contaminated agricultural ecosystems. *Journal of Environmental Radioactivity*, **83**, 275–295.

Jensen, K.K., Forsberg, E., Gamborg, C., Millar, K. & Sandøe, P. (2010) Facilitating ethical reflection among scientists using the ethical matrix. *Science and Engineering Ethics*. DOI: 10.1007/s11948-010-9218-2 (accessed on-line 22 May, 2011).

Kaiser, M. & Forsberg, E.-M. (2001) Assessing fisheries – Using an ethical matrix in a participatory process. *Journal Agricultural Environment Ethics*, **14**, 191–200.

Magalhães-Sant'Ana, M., Baptista, C.S., Olsson, I.A.S., Millar, K. & Sandøe, P. (2009) Teaching animal ethics to veterinary students in Europe: Examining aims and methods. In: *Ethical Futures: Bioscience and Food Horizons* (eds K. Millar, P. Hobson-West & B. Nerlich), pp. 354–359. Wageningen Academic Publishers, Wageningen, The Netherlands.

Mepham, B. (1996) Ethical analysis of food biotechnologies: An evaluative framework. In: *Food Ethics* (ed. B. Mepham), pp. 101–119, Routledge, London. Reproduced in: Chadwick, R. & Schroeder, D. (eds) (2002) *Applied Ethics: Critical Concepts in Philosophy*, pp. 343–359. Routledge, London.

Mepham, B. (2000) The role of food ethics in food policy. *Proceedings Nutrition Society*, **59**, 609–618.

Mepham, B. (2010) The ethical matrix as a tool in policy interventions: The obesity crisis. In: *Food Ethics* (eds F.-T. Gottwald, H.W. Ingensiep & M. Meinhardt). Springer, New York.

Mepham, B. & Millar, K. (2001) The ethical matrix in practice: Application to the case of bovine somatotrophin. In: *Food Safety, Food Quality, Food Ethics, Preprints of 3rd EURSAFE Congress* (ed. M. Pasquali), pp. 317–319. A&Q, University of Milan, Florence.

Mepham, B., Kaiser, M., Thorstensen, E., Tomkins, S. & Millar, K. (2006) *Ethical Matrix: Manual*. Agricultural Economics Research Institute (LEI), The Hague, the Netherlands.

Millar, K. (2000) The role of bioethical analysis in assessing automatic milking systems (AMS): Examples of animal issues. In: Robotic Milking (eds H. Hogeveen & A. Meijering), pp. 248–258. Wageningen Pers, Wageningen, the Netherlands.

Millar, K., Gamborg, C. & Sandoe, P. (2007) Using participatory methods to explore the social and ethical issues raised by bioscience research programmes: The case of animal genomics research. In: *Sustainable Food Production and Ethics* (eds W. Zollitisch, C. Winckler, S. Waiblinger & A. Haslberger), pp. 354–359. Wageningen Academic Publishers, Wageningen, the Netherlands.

Millar, K. & Mepham, B. (2001). Bioethical Analysis of Biotechnologies: Lessons from Automatic Milking Systems (AMS) and Bovine Somatotrophin (bST) In: *Occasional*

Publication Number 28, BSAS (eds C.M. Wathes, A.R. Frost, F. Gordon, & J.D. Wood), pp. 29–36. British Society of Animal Science, Edinburgh.

Millar, K. & Morton, D.M. (2009) Animal integrity in modern farming. In: *Ethics, Law and Society VI* (eds J. Gunning, S. Holm & I. Kenway), pp. 19–31. Ashgate Publishing, Surrey.

Millar, K. & Tomkins, S. (2007) Ethical analysis of the use of GM fish: Emerging issues for aquaculture. *Journal of Agricultural and Environmental Ethics*, **20**, 437–453.

Mohamed-Katerere, J.C. (2003) Rights and risk: Challenging biotechnology policy in Zimbabwe. *Institute of Development Studies (IDS) Working Paper 204*. IDS, Brighton.

Rogers, W. & Ballantyne, A. (2010) Towards a practical definition of professional behaviour. *Journal of Medical Ethics*, **36**, 250–254.

Rollin, B. (2006) *Science and Ethics*. Cambridge University Press, Cambridge.

Sandøe, P. & Christiansen, S. (2008) *Ethics and Animal Use*. Blackwell, London.

Schroeder, D. & Palmer, C. (2003) Technology assessment and the 'ethical matrix'. *Poiesis Prax*, **1**, 295–300.

Sokol, S.K. (2009) Ethics man: The unpalatable truth about ethics committees. *British Medical Journal*, **339**, 891.

Wathes, C.M., Kristensen, H.H., Aerts, J.-M. & Berckmans, D. (2008) Is precision livestock farming an engineer's daydream or nightmare, an animal's friend or foe, and a farmer's panacea or pitfall? *Computers and Electronics in Agriculture*, **64**, 2–10.

Webster, J., Bollen, P., Grimm, H. & Jennings, M. (2010) Ethical implications of using the minipig in regulatory toxicology studies. *Journal of Pharmacological and Toxicological Methods*, **62**, 160–166.

Yeates, J. (2010) Ethical aspects of euthanasia of owned animals. *In Practice*, **32**, 70–73.

Yeates, J. & Main, D.C. (2011) Veterinary opinions on the refusing euthanasia: Justifications and philosophical frameworks. *The Veterinary Record*, **168**, 263.

Questions and Answers

Q: I'm keen on the Ethical Matrix (EM). In an evaluation of whether we're doing the right thing, we're increasingly going from input measurements to output measures of outcomes in order to discover whether or not, whatever our motivation, we're getting it right. I had difficulty jamming fairness and justice in as a principle. Might it be helpful to re-evaluate justice or fairness as an outcome measurement?

A: The principle of justice needs exploring further in terms of its application in the EM. There is no short answer. One challenge is to assess outcomes for all issues when we wish to make a single decision. The value of the EM is that it collates all issues so that assessment of outcome and weighing is clearer. You could set a series of goals/outcomes, including one relating to justice and then analyse these using the EM. Instead of applying the EM and then looking at the impact, you could actually see if you reach, by a certain set of actions, a particular goal.

Q: How do you put a weighting in the EM?

A: Some individuals have tried to put a value on each cell, for example numerical scores. For others, this can be unacceptable, i.e. using a scoring system. A user can determine the significance of each cell through dialogue. Another option is to combine this approach with ranking methods, multi-criteria mapping, for example. Early attempts have created a form of 'visual volume' in relation to each cell, where volume indicates significance. Personally, I'm slightly nervous about this. There is benefit in looking at aspects like multi-criteria mapping as a way of further operationalising aspects of the matrix. It depends on the setting and the use of the EM. These are important considerations for all such tools.

Q: A starting point for empowering and engaging veterinary professionals in ethical decision-making would be to ensure that veterinary students thought about the use of animals as part of their education. In some veterinary schools, fewer animals are used in traditional physiology experiments and so on and more replacements have been sourced. We are informing veterinary undergraduates from the first year onwards of the animal audit that encourages lecturers to think about numbers involved and purposes of animal use in education. It would be good to engage students in this process to get them thinking about the ethical decision-making as they move forward in their veterinary career. What is your view?
A: This is an important issue that should be discussed within veterinary schools and an important issue generally. At Nottingham, ethical analysis sessions are embedded alongside clinical sessions; ethics teaching is split across the curriculum with a larger amount of the teaching in the second year, although there is some in the first year. Sessions pose challenging questions that relate to an individual's future within the profession and the type of policies within institutions. This issue could be discussed in sessions combining classical skills teaching with the exploration of notable ethical issues, for example the use of animals in teaching.

Q: We are trying to develop ethical training of veterinary students. It is quite important to demonstrate that ethical consideration does not necessarily have to result in a right or wrong decision because this causes immense pressure, that is students are supposed to know in every situation what is right and what is wrong, for example about companion animals. My feeling is that it's more important to show them that it might be adding value to identify the dilemma and demonstrate directions based on different presuppositions but not the final conclusion. What is your view?
A: I feel that skills-based teaching should be applied. We encourage an approach that introduces cases that make students think across the whole spectrum of ethical decision-making, allowing them to see how they might respond as an individual, learning from each other and seeing how and why they might differ from each other. Peter Sandøe is a Special Professor who applies this approach, presenting cases and getting students to explore them. We also ask students to think about the interactions between personal, professional and social ethics. Part of the approach involves setting out positions that are put forward by either individual clinicians or institutions and getting students to explore them. We also need to explore our own positions as institutions and be willing to discuss them. We should create a safe environment that enables students to deal comfortably with difficult ethical issues, especially early in their career.

The Ethics of Animal Enhancement

JAMES YEATES

RSPCA

Abstract: The issue of animal 'enhancement' is a good example that requires analysis on applied, abstract normative and meta-ethical levels. It draws in ontological, linguistic, semantic and ethical concepts. It also requires an understanding of scientific and medical elements, as well as cultural and societal concepts. Indeed the very concept of enhancement is vague, ambiguous and contested, and attempts to define it have methodological and ethical implications. Nevertheless, the issue has received limited discussion in the bioethical literature.

This paper tries to sketch some salient approaches to the analysis of animal enhancement. The issue of its definition is discussed. Some key ethical aspects are then discussed, some of which are related to definitional aspects while others introduce novel terminology. These approaches are described under the headings pertaining to animals' capacities and interests; effects on other animals, including humans; the concept of what is normal; 'yuk factor' ideas and moral repugnances; and potential ethical implications of altering animals' moral status.

These allow some ideas as to how the future debate may progress and some appreciation of what effect this debate – and what and how enhancing interventions are conducted in the future – will have for the animals themselves.

Keywords: animal welfare, conduct, debate, doping, enablement, enhancement, enrichment, moral discussions, moral status

Veterinary & Animal Ethics: Proceedings of the First International Conference on Veterinary and Animal Ethics, September 2011, First Edition. Edited by Christopher M. Wathes, Sandra A. Corr, Stephen A. May, Steven P. McCulloch and Martin C. Whiting.
© 2013 Universities Federation for Animal Welfare. Published 2013 by Blackwell Publishing Ltd.

9.1 Introduction

Modern developments in biotechnology, animal breeding and animal husbandry are providing new opportunities to 'enhance' animals. Now, or in the foreseeable future, animals may be altered by technological means such as surgery, genetic engineering, chimerification and pharmaceutical 'doping' to make them faster, happier, more productive, lower their 'carbon hoof-print' or just make them better looking.

The possibility of similar enhancements of human animals has spawned a wealth of opinion within the bioethics literature. But relatively little work (so far) has been done on the bioethical concerns surrounding animal enhancement (Caplan 2009). This paper reviews insights from the literature on human enhancement and considers issues specific to the enhancement of animals. As I shall describe, 'enhancement' covers a whole range of different interventions, so it is impossible for one paper to conclude what is mandatory, acceptable or impermissible. But it is possible to identify and introduce some terms of reference for the animal enhancement debate.

9.2 What Is Enhancement?

Enhancement is unavoidably a socially constructed term (Wolpe 2002) and is used in many ways. Often authors choose a definition that helps their moral argument, which, in a debate that is a plagued with futuristic and conservative rhetoric (Coenen *et al.* 2009), can be dangerous. Some have suggested that the term is so ambiguous and open to abuse that it should be avoided or used only in a general way (Parens 1998).

Consequently, I avoid defining enhancement, employing the term only as placeholder for a general concept. Instead of fixing on a single narrow definition, different types of intervention are characterised, all of which might be included within the general idea. Some of these classifications are purely fact-based, in that interventions are categorised depending only on the normative description of the cases. Others are more value laden, in that interventions are classified in terms of some ethical concept. In some cases, an apparently fact-based distinction is actually more value laden than it first appears. Some of the more value-laden categories are considered in detail later, but several apparently fact-based distinctions can be sketched now.

One fact-based categorisation is in terms of who or what is being enhanced: a normal adult human; a fetus; a mental health patient; an ape; a primate; a vertebrate or an invertebrate animal etc. Another useful distinction is between the body-systems affected (Table 9.1). One can also distinguish between enhancing an individual animal versus the enhancement of a species or strain.

Another fact-based classification is in terms of the method of enhancement (Table 9.2). Some interventions alter the animal internally (e.g. its anatomy or genes), others are external add-ons (e.g. animal–computer interfaces or limb prostheses). One can also characterise interventions as 'conventional' or 'traditional'

Table 9.1 Classes of enhancement by substrate.

System affected	Enablement	Enrichment	Moral enhancements
Immune system	Ability to avoid disease	Health	Exploitability
Neural, musculoskeletal and cardiovascular systems	Physical abilities	Achievement of physical goals	Responsibility, dependency
Peripheral nervous and sensory systems	Sensory abilities, reactions	Sensations	Sensitivity
Central nervous system	Cognitive abilities	Increased knowledge, understanding, etc.	Agency, self-determination
	Emotional abilities	Mood and feelings	Sentience (± higher pleasures)
General	Liveability	Lifespan	Increased value of life
Skeletal and integumental systems	Ability to inspire beauty	Beauty	Aesthetic value

Table 9.2 Classes of enhancement by method.

Class		Examples
Internal	Nutritional	Mineral supplementation (e.g. calcium, iron)
	Pharmacological	Pancreatic enzymes, thyroxine
	Surgical	Palate cauterisation, tie-backs
	Cyto-surgical	Chimerification (e.g. by nuclear transfer)
	Genetic	Breeding, genetic modifications
	Developmental	Training, habituation, socialisation
External	Interface technologies	Limb prostheses (Cyborg technologies)
	Symbiotic technologies	Probiotics

versus 'novel', or as 'medical' versus 'non-medical', and some have used these to try to differentiate non-enhancing versus enhancing technologies (e.g. Englehardt 1990; Pellegrino 2004; Ljungqvist 2005).

Enhancement–non-enhancement differentiation can also be attempted though classifications based on the outcome of the intervention (Table 9.3). For example, one may distinguish self-limited changes (e.g. somatic changes) from uncontainable changes (e.g. germ-line changes which can be passed onto an animal's progeny) (Juengst & Walters 1999). One can also differentiate outcomes in terms of the states that the intervention is meant to change. An obvious example is distinguishing interventions that treat disease (which may not be considered 'enhancement') from those that go beyond it and make the patient 'better than well' (Juengst 1998;

Table 9.3 Classes of enhancement by 'outcome' (and potential differentiations between non-enhancing and enhancing interventions).

Less extreme outcome of intervention, which could be argued to mean that the intervention is not enhancement	More extreme outcome of enhancing intervention, which might usually be thought to imply enhancement
Restorative or preventative treatment of disease	'Better than well'
Natural	Unnaturalness
Normal	Subnormal/supernormal
Intra-specific	Extra-specific
Resolution of absolute harms	Resolution of relative harms
Fulfilment of basic needs	Added value/'luxury'
Reversible	Irreversible
Self-limited	Uncontainable
Substantive change	Accidental change
Type change	Token change
Beneficial	Harmful
Fair	Unfair

Sandel 2004). Another distinction can be made between changes that increase a quality that an animal already possesses, such as a horse's speed, versus changes that give an animal a quality that it previously lacked, such as to fly unaided. Another difference is between 'extra-specific' enhancements that go beyond what is normal for the animal's species and 'intra-specific' enhancements that alter it within the normal range for the species.

9.2.1 Capacities and interests

An important issue is whether an intervention is in the interests of the animal, that is whether it is beneficial or harmful (Table 9.3). Within different types of enhancement, many interventions are aimed at helping the animal. Analgesia can decrease pain and suffering. Disabilities can be remedied by surgeries such as cataract surgery and external interfaces such as 'doggy carts'. Genetic modification can also alter animals, for example by altering apparent memory (Tang *et al.* 1999; Routtenberg *et al.* 2000; Wang *et al.* 2004) or pain experiences (Yeates 2010a). A more imminent possibility for species enhancement is through breeding manipulations, such as screening potential parents, calculating welfare-focused estimated breeding values (EBVs) or perhaps pre-implantation genetic diagnosis.

There is a debate about whether restorative and preventative interventions constitute 'enhancements'. On the one hand, they do make animals better and some have classified them as a type of enhancement, including the European Parliament STOA (Coenen *et al.* 2009). On the other hand, some have tried to define more conventional medical treatments as not being enhancement, partly in order to focus the debate and partly in order to ontologically distinguish morally separable categories. This, as with other 'lines in the sand' approaches to bioethics has its difficulties, not least that it is not easy to differentiate prevention and enhancement (Juengst 1997), at least without recourse to additional argumentation (e.g. based on 'conventional' or 'medical', but these then need defence, as discussed below).

In the human enhancement debate, several (utilitarian) authors have tried to *define* the term 'enhancement', as they use it, to include (only) interventions that are beneficial. This has the advantage of simplifying the debate about whether enhancement is acceptable by letting us tautologically decide that enhancements are by definition good for the animal. This firstly creates a requirement for a convincing account of what is 'good'. For animals, we have some recourse to animal welfare, although this has tended to avoid accounts of benefit and opportunity (Yeates & Main 2008). Secondly, we then have the problem of working out what interventions are beneficial, so this tactic simply defers normative assessment. In addition, such slight-of-hands create a danger that non-beneficial interventions are automatically considered better, without reflection, because they have been described as enhancement.

Another useful distinction cited in Table 9.1 is between 'enablements' and 'enrichments'. *Enablements* are interventions that increase an animal's capacities, for example its abilities to perform certain physical or cognitive tasks, its ability to experience feelings and so on. An example is making animals stronger, for example through genetic modification (Lee 2004), myostatin blockers (Lee & McPherron 2001) or bovine somatotropin. Enablements may also increase an animal's ability *not* to achieve certain outcomes, such as the ability to avoid disease or pain. Some authors have defined enhancement in this way (e.g. Pellegrino 2004).

Enrichments are interventions that increase the animal's 'quality' in some way, such as its aesthetic value, its pleasure and its integrity. In some cases, whereas enablements increase an animal's *abilities* to achieve X, enrichments increase their *predisposition* to achieving X. For example, on a hedonic account of value, an intervention that made an animal *more likely* to feel pleasure (see Yeates 2010a), would be an enrichment. Some authors have defined enhancement in this way (e.g. Savulescu *et al.* 2011).

An intervention may be both enabling and enriching. An increased ability to resist disease avoids the adverse experiences associated with pathologies. In general, an increased ability to perform a function may lead to greater achievement of an animal's goals. The reciprocal is also true – enrichments can have additional effects of enabling animals. For example, environmental enrichment has long been recognised as being able to promote resilience to neurological stress and neurotoxins (Schneider *et al.* 2001) and improve cognitive abilities (Walsh *et al.* 1969; Greenoug & Volkmar 1973; Diamond *et al.* 1975; Nilsson *et al.* 1999).

Nevertheless, enablements and enrichments are different types of enhancement: an animal is not necessarily or directly happier for being stronger (or even cleverer). Indeed, some enablements may in fact impoverish an animal, for example an enablement that made an animal able to feel grief might worsen its life. Conversely, an animal's well-being may actually be enriched by a 'disablement', for example decreasing an animal's ability to get pregnant by contraception. It follows that enablements are not necessarily beneficial. Indeed, it is an obviously fallacy to equate 'making an animal better at doing X' with 'making an animal better'.

In fact, even enrichments are not necessarily beneficial. Some interventions have harmful indirect effects. For example, the genetic change that can lead to an increased memory may come with an apparent increased sensitivity to pain (Wei *et al.* 2001) and loss of previous learning (Falls *et al.* 1992). Other such trade-offs may also exist, for example there may be an inverse correlation between increased intelligence and longevity (Gottfredson 2004) or intelligence and happiness (Gow *et al.* 2005). This should not make us conclude that evolution has created perfect animals whose lives we cannot enrich (Powell & Buchanan 2011), but it does suggest that we should be careful. In addition, some enrichments may perpetuate problems. For example making an animal impervious to pain could lead to increased injuries, as is the case with mice (and humans) that are congenitally insensitive to pain (Yeates 2010a). This means that, *at most*, we can only ever say that any given intervention is beneficial 'all else being equal'.

9.2.2 Other animals (and humans)

Sometimes interventions that deal with anthropogenic problems can have indirect effects on other animals. These may be beneficial, for example enhancing mothering ability or tolerance may decrease perinatal losses or aggression. But indirect effects may also be harmful. Treatments may allow genetic problems to be passed onto an animal's progeny, or mean imperfect husbandry conditions can be perpetuated. Genetic modification and chimerification may increase disease risks. Enablements may allow an enhanced animal to outcompete other animals for resources, effectively making unenhanced animals into 'relative runts'. Alternations may also alter animals' environmental impact (e.g. the Enviropig) (see Paper 7).

Humans may be similarly benefitted or harmed. Many enhancements are intended to make the animal more instrumentally beneficial to humans. Cosmetic 'enhancements', such as ear cropping and testicular prostheses, make the animal more aesthetically pleasing. Performance enhancement, such as tie-forwards, palate cauterisation and 'doping' using erythropoietin or simply pre-race intravenous fluids, may help the trainer and owner to win prizes and money (see Paper 14). Productivity enhancements, such as breeding programmes, mutilations and growth promoters, help farmers to make more money more efficiently. Some alterations, such as an increased 'ability' to contract HIV or cancer, make animals into better laboratory models. Others make humans' lives easier, such as pharmaceuticals that improve animal's resistance to disease.

Humans may also be harmed by indirect effects such as increased zoonotic disease risks. They may also experience relative harms. For example, an enhancement that makes one horse win a race means another trainer's unenhanced horse comes second (or, as more people enhance their horses, third, fourth or last). This scenario may also occur in farming, where the introduction of a new strain or method such as BST makes other farmers commercially disadvantaged.

For the human owners, one could leave the decision to the owner's choice. Much of the human enhancement debate centres on personal liberty, sometimes related to individual authenticity (e.g. Just 2011). This concept has been extended to ideas of 'reproductive autonomy' and, in general terms, animal owners are also thought to have a similar – and usually more extensive – right of 'property autonomy' (Yeates & Main 2010).

However, while providing requested enhancements may respect the autonomy of the particular individual, it can decrease the liberty of other humans (Jennings 2003). For example, farmers whose competitors use bovine somatotropin are faced with the choice of following suit or risking their business. Similarly, if most horse-trainers dope their horses, other trainers are left with a choice between losing or doping, and lose the option of competing 'fairly'.

The concept of fairness is covered elsewhere (e.g. Chapter 5), but it is worth noting several approaches that might be useful. Utilitarian approaches would consider enrichments to be good 'all else being equal' and enablements good insofar as they have utility. Concepts similar to enablements are included in Sen's capability approach (Sen 1985) and Nussbaum's capacities-based approach to animal ethics (Nussbaum 2004). Rawls's justice as fairness approach, which has been applied to nonhuman animals (VandeVeer 1979; Rowlands 1998), considers the fair distribution of 'primary goods', which represent all-purpose capacities to achieve each individual's aims, that is which could include enablements. Some approaches could include both enablements and enrichments. Rawls's approach might be extended to include enrichments, for example treatments that avoid suffering (Yeates 2010b). Parker and Yeates's list of opportunities could also include both enablements and enrichments (Parker & Yeates, 2011). These approaches may suggest that some enhancements are unfair (Elliot 2004), although obviously they provide arguments only against those enhancements that are unfair (Caplan 2004).

It is also worth noting that many enhancements that are beneficial 'all else being equal' do not actually provide any overall benefit since all else is far from equal. Many interventions simply rearrange the distribution of benefits and harms. For example, the reordering of race form from performance enhancement does not provide any overall benefit: it is what games theorists might call a 'zero sum' change. On Rawls's terms (under his difference principle), such changes are fair only insofar as the horse or trainer who benefits is the one who was the worst off. In utilitarian terms, they are fair only if the horse and trainer that win are benefitted more than the others are harmed. (These seem hard to calculate, and would be even harder to enshrine into Jockey Club rules.) Furthermore, potential harms such as drug reactions, however slight they may be, mean that there may be an overall loss of utility, since the opportunity for enhancement effectively creates a Prisoner's Dilemma scenario – in that it would be best for all if no animals were enhanced, but for each individual trainer it is rational to enhance, if one cannot trust others not to do so.

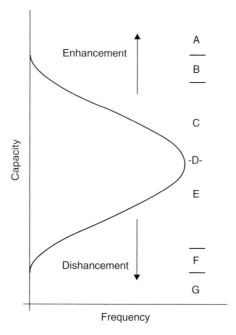

Figure 9.1 Normalising and super-normalising enhancements. Super-specific states (A); overall intra-specific range (B–F); extreme super-normality (B); normal range (C–E); normal average (D); extreme subnormality (F); sub-specific states (G).

9.3 Normalcy

Tacit concerns for fairness may underlie many of the proposed categorisations of enhancements in terms of extent relative to normalcy. Figure 9.1 shows how this idea may be applied to attributes that are normally distributed in the original population (for binary attributes or those that are not present at all in the original population, similar ideas can be used on a simplified model – that is with only categories of normal and supranormal). Some 'normalising' interventions bring an animal into what is normal for its species (or breed or strain). In contrast, 'super-normalising' enhancements go beyond that normal range.

As for naturalness, it is not clear what 'normal' means. Where no members of a species ever possess a capacity (e.g. horses and unaided flying), an intervention that provides this capacity constitutes an extra-specific change. But it is not clear what should constitute a 'normal' level of a capacity that is already normally distributed in a population (Figure 9.2). One option is to consider 'normal' as the overall range of the capacity within the species, and differentiate intra-specific enhancements that are within this range (e.g. from C to E in Figure 9.1), to extra-specific enhancements that go beyond it (i.e. from B to A). However, it is impossible to authoritatively judge what the overall range for a species is because of the bell shape of the Normal distribution.

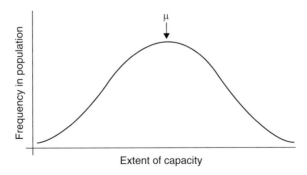

Figure 9.2 Average normally distributed capacity in a population (e.g. species); μ = average.

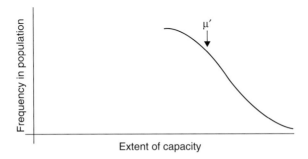

Figure 9.3 Altered average of a capacity after normalising enhancement; μ′ = new average.

An alternative approach is to use a statistical concept of normalcy (Sabin & Daniels 1994). One could use a narrower 'normal range', for example as within two standard deviations from mean (Savulescu *et al.* 2011), or in the inter-quartile range, and differentiate interventions that raise animals from the extreme subnormality to the normal range (i.e. from F to E). Or one could define normal as a statistical average point, such as the mean or the median, and distinguish interventions that raise an animal up to that point (i.e. from F/E to D) from those that go beyond. While all of these would fit a normalising–super-normalising distinction, they may have very different implications, the analysis of which will have to be left to another discussion.

Two other problems with the normalcy account are worth noting, because they relate to the contingency of what is normal. The first is the question of what to do with widespread problems. If all animals of a certain type have a condition (e.g. femoral head necrosis, brachycephalic syndrome or excessive skin folds), then correcting these conditions is super-normalising, while surely being acceptable. The second is that, as animals are treated at the lower end, this produces new statistical norms, for example a new median and mean (Figure 9.3). This means that performing only normalising enhancements would eventually have the same effect as super-normalising enhancements (Figures 9.2–9.4).

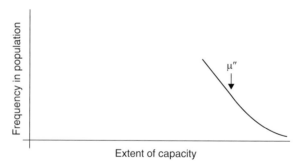

Figure 9.4 Further altered average of a capacity after normalising enhancement; μ″ = further new average.

9.3.1 Yukkiness

Arguments against enhancement often stem from ideas that what already exists should be left alone (what Parens [2005] calls a gratitude-based position). This idea can come from environmentalist concerns, who consider that 'nature' has a value; from natural law theorists, who consider animals to have an essence that should be respected; and from pre-reflective 'yuk factor' responses to the prospect of radical interventions.

Respect for naturalness could underpin arguments (a) against enhancements by unnatural methods (although this kind of argument might also rule out most of veterinary medicine!), (b) against enhancements that achieve unnatural outcomes outside the intra-specific range (e.g. hyper-intelligent 'superchimps') and (c) *for* enhancements that increase naturalness. This last possibility sounds counter-intuitive, but animals might be 'naturalised' by interventions such as pre-release training of captive-born wild animals or breeding and surgical methods that correct anthropogenic breed-related conditions.

Essentialist positions include those that consider animals have an essential quality that should be respected. In the human enhancement debate, several authors suggest that human nature is intrinsically good (Habermas 2001/2003; Fukuyama 2002; Kass 2003; Fenton 2006), and one lawyer, George Annas, has proposed a need for a UN Convention on the Preservation of the Human Species (Annas *et al.* 2002). The related concept of authenticity is also fundamental to the human enhancement debate (Christman 1988), although human ethics often talks of individual authenticity as well as being an authentic member of one's species (Taylor 1992). In animal ethics, one could consider that an animal's authentic nature – what we often term its *telos* – is similarly worth respect (Rollin 1981; also Chapter 6).

There are problems of what 'naturalness' and 'integrity' mean, since nature has many definitions (Collingwood 1945/1965). In addition, one might consider sanctity of nature arguments to be irrelevant for domesticated animals, which are already not insignificantly unnatural. Such arguments can lead people to dismissing naturalistic arguments as obfuscating (Nielsen 2011), and there have been several critiques of essentialism about human nature (e.g. Buchanan et al. 2002; Bayertz 2003). But the fact that nature-based concepts are ill-defined does not mean they are morally irrelevant (Nielsen 2011) and they may be useful in some cases, even if not all (Kaebnick 2007). Firstly, respect for nature need not be taken as an absolute value (Kaebnick 2000), and could be used for the more extreme cases, without necessarily implying any moral beliefs about less extreme cases (Nielsen 2011). Secondly, given the role of emotions in moral reasoning (Mameli 2004), it may be that emotional 'yuk' responses are an unavoidable part of ethical reasoning (Midgley 2000) and perhaps constitute a useful 'wisdom of repugnance' (Kaebnick 2008).

9.3.2 Altered moral status

The above moral issues largely assume that animals have a moral status that can be respected or disrespected. Some interventions go further and alter an animal's interests. An animal with increased immunity may have less need for antibiosis or vaccination. Physical and cognitive enhancements may decrease an animal's dependency on its carers. Conversely, other enhancements, for example cosmetic improvements, may increase carers' abilities to relate to the animals. Similarly, the genetic modification of an animal may mean it has a new integrity, which should then be respected. Such changes still leave the animal in roughly the same place in the overall moral (and ontological) landscape because they do not change the type of thing that the animal is (what scholastic philosophy would call an 'accidental change').

But there is another, deeper issue, where enhancements might go even further and alter an animal's moral status, by actually making the animal into something else (a 'substantive' change). One example would be an enhancement that made an animal into another species, either through the genetic creation of a new species or through sufficient chimerification that meant that the animal had changed species. Humans might be 'bestialised' by enhancements, such as genetic introduction of fluorescence genes (or, more everyday, the use of musk odours in perfumes). Animals might also be 'humanised' by the introduction of human tissues, such as the introduction of differentiated human embryonic stem cells (Darsalia *et al.* 2007). If these changes went far enough, the nonhuman animal could be said to have changed species.

Such substantive changes evoke a yuk factor and may cause welfare issues. They might also alter the animal's moral status. Many ethical theories attribute higher moral status to beings with certain properties such as being human, personhood, rationality or having a preference for life. For example, Peter Singer described a two-tier system in which all sentient animals have a moral status of their interests being worthy of consideration, alongside a higher level of respect for 'persons', which are defined as having various mental capacities including self-awareness or a preference for life (Singer 1992). A cognitive enhancement that made an animal (sufficiently) self-aware would elevate it into the higher moral status. This may be especially likely for changes to more neurophysiologically complex animals like great apes (DeGrazia 2007).

One could conclude that such substantive changes should be avoided, especially if we cannot guarantee that this new moral status will be respected (DeGrazia 2007). But this argument would appear to suggest that we should avoid whatever change it is that creates a human being's moral status. So a parallel of this argument would suggest that we should also prevent the change of human moral status being created by other means, such as fertilisation, neural crest formation, birth, development of speech or whatever change we consider makes humans have their moral status. In addition, separate agents may be responsible for the substantive enhancement and the later disrespect, so it is impossible to guarantee that an animal's moral status would be respected (just as one cannot guarantee that one's child's status will always be respected), which leaves it unclear as to where moral responsibility would lie.

As a final note, it is worth remembering that having a higher moral status may be *contrary* to an animal's interests – effectively through it having harmful indirect effects. For example, if higher status means absolute right to life, which would disallow active euthanasia, then this higher status would be contrary to the animal's interests if it later was in a state of terminal suffering. Indeed, in such cases a disablement that caused an animal to have a lower moral status may constitute an enrichment (e.g. rendering an animal in a painful experiment insentient). This brings me back to other determinants/approaches to moral status such as integrity. These may be useful concepts, but there may be situations where animals might sometimes be better off without them being applied – a chicken in an intensive system may thank you politely for your concern for its integrity, but if its suffering is reduced by technological means, then perhaps you should either prevent the more basic breaches of factory farming or please keep quiet.

9.4 Terms of Reference for the Future Debate on Animal Enhancement

With this variety of enhancements, multitude of ethical concerns and vagueness of the very term, it is impossible to conclude categorically on the morality of animal enhancement. A fuller debate is needed. The modest aim of these conclusions is to suggest some ways in which the future discussion of animal enhancement might avoid some of the problems that have befallen discussion on human enhancement.

The first is simply to ensure that the questions being asked are well described. Different work is needed to analyse different types of enhancements in different contexts, such as veterinary practice, laboratory experiments and agricultural contexts.

Secondly, practical decisions can draw upon a number of different approaches. Here I have sketched only a few, but this issue of animal enhancement draws on many ethical concepts. While animal welfare assessments are useful, ethical approaches based on naturalness or yuk-factors may also provide useful approaches.

Even from a welfare perspective they may prove to be good 'iceberg ethics indicators' that highlight cases that need further investigation.

Thirdly, it should be immediately recognised that these different ethical approaches may often share common ground. The underlying concepts may share common themes (Parens 2005; 2009). In addition, different ethical approaches may reach similar conclusions (Juengst 2009). Finding such commonalities can generate heuristics that suggest practical rules that are more widely acceptable (Bostrom & Sandberg 2009; Powell & Buchanan 2011). For example, one might suggest rules that limit enhancements only to certain methods (e.g. permitting nutritional advances but prohibiting human–animal chimerification) or outcomes (e.g. permitting only changes that are reversible, that affect traits with shallower ontological depths, or that are within the normal intra-specific range). In addition, certain conditions may be imposed (e.g. that medico-surgical enhancements are carried out only by regulated veterinary surgeons).

Fourthly, while finding common ground can be useful to forward debate, common ground is not the same as full consensus and should not end the discussion. Sometimes finding common terminology simply results in people using the same words to mean different things, albeit with a superficial appearance of consensus. Sometimes it may be better to continue a polarised debate than for stakeholders to erroneously think they understand each others' perspectives. It is also important that the debates are not reflected simply as pro-enhancement (or 'futurist') versus anti-enhancement (or 'conservative') viewpoints, as this can stifle debate and prevent a middle-ground position being reached. In addition, there can be a risk that the existence of a common ground reflects a lowest common denominator (as one might suggest the 3Rs do). As ethics and science move on, such consensus positions should be revisited.

Finally, given the variety of types of enhancement, and the risks of a misleading definition, I would suggest not using 'enhancement' except in general terms (e.g. in presentation titles). Instead, I would suggest a number of 'rules' by which terms should be responsibly employed within public debates on enhancement. These include:

a. Retaining the term 'enhancement' as a useful 'placeholder'
b. Producing an operational definition for particular projects
c. Using other terms where possible, for example enablement and enrichment
d. Not leaving terms unexplained in papers and reports
e. Not using the definition of enhancement to exclude or include any interventions or cases *a priori*
f. Identifying and clarifying how other discussants are using the term
g. Using the term transparently
h. Avoiding fallacies of ambiguity
i. Being consistent in how terms are used throughout a given document
j. Not drawing any normative arguments from the definition, directly or indirectly.

9.5 Animal Welfare Implications

Animal enhancements have great scope to alter animals' welfare, for example by increasing their ability to cope. Enrichments can improve their experiences. Some changes may even increase naturalness. In addition, such enhancements may also help owners, consumers, other animals or the environment. This can make enhancement seem like a win–win solution.

However, care must be taken to consider the side effects of any change, especially where enhancements that are beneficial 'all else being equal' can perpetuate welfare compromises, for example by allowing animals to survive in suboptimal environments, achieve zero sum effects or create Prisoner's Dilemma scenarios. Careful examination of each and every opportunity for enhancement is therefore warranted using both ethical and welfare science methods.

References

Annas, A., Andrews, L. & Isasi, R. (2002). Protecting the endangered human: Toward an international treaty prohibiting cloning and inheritable alterations. *American Journal of Law and Medicine*, **28**: 151–178.

Bayertz, K. (2003) Human nature: How normative might it be? *Journal of Medicine and Philosophy*, **28**, 131–150.

Bostrom, N. & Sandberg, A. (2009) The wisdom of nature: An evolutionary heuristic for human enhancement. In: *Human Enhancement* (eds J. Savulescu & N. Bostrom), pp. 375–416. Oxford University Press, Oxford.

Buchanan, A., Brock, D., Daniels, N. & Wikler, D. (2002) *From Chance to Choice*. Cambridge University Press, New York.

Caplan, A.L. (2004) Nobody is perfect – But why not try to be better? *PLOS Medicine*, **1**, 52–54.

Caplan, A.L. (2009) Good, better or best? In: *Human Enhancement* (eds J. Savulescu & N. Bostrom), pp. 199–209. Oxford University Press, Oxford.

Christman, J. (1988) Constructing the inner citadel: Recent work on the concept of autonomy. *Ethics*, **99**, 109–124.

Coenen, C., Schuijff, M., Smits, M., Klaasen, P., Hennen, L., Rader, M. & Wolbring, G. (2009) *Human Enhancement, IP/A/STOA/FWC/2005-28/SC35, 41 & 45*. European Parliament, Brussels.

Collingwood, R. (1965) *The Idea of Nature*. Oxford Paperbacks, Oxford.

Darsalia, V., Kallur, T. & Kokaia, Z. (2007) Survival, migration and neuronal differentiation of human fetal striatal and cortical neural stem cells grafted in stroke-damaged rat striatum. *European Journal of Neuroscience*, **26**, 605–614.

DeGrazia, D. (2007) Human-animal chimeras: Human dignity, moral status and species prejudice. *Metaphilosophy*, **38**, 309–329.

Diamond, M.C., Johnson, R.E. & Ingham, C.A. (1975) Morphological changes in young, adult and aging rat cerebral-cortex, hippocampus, and diencephalon. *Behavioral Biology*, **14**, 163–174.

Elliot, C. (2004) Pharma's gain may be our loss. *PLOS Medicine*, **1**, 52–53.

Englehardt, H. (1990) Human nature technologically revisited. *Social Policy and Philosophy*, **8**, 180–191.

Falls, W.A., Miserendino, M.J.D. & Davis, M. (1992) Extinction of fear-potentiated startle – Blockade by infusion of an NMDA antagonist into the amygdala. *Journal of Neuroscience*, **12**, 854–863.

Fenton, E. (2006). Liberal eugenics and human nature – against Habermas. *Hastings Centre Report*, **36**, 35–42.

Fukuyama, F. (2002) *Our Posthuman Future: Consequences of the Biotechnology Revolution*. Picador, London.

Gottfredson, L.S. (2004) Life, death, and intelligence. *Journal of Cognitive Education and Psychology*, **4**, 23–46.

Gow, A.J., Whiteman, M.C., Pattie, A., Whalley, L., Starr, J. & Deary, I.J. (2005) Lifetime intellectual function and satisfaction with life in old age: Longitudinal cohort study. *British Medical Journal*, **331**, 141–142.

Greenoug, W.T. & Volkmar, F.R. (1973) Pattern of dendritic branching in occipital cortex of rats reared in complex environments. *Experimental Neurology*, **40**, 491–504.

Habermas, J. (2001/2003) *The Future of Human Nature*. Polity Press, Cambridge.

Jennings, B. (2003) The liberalism of life: Bioethics in the face of biopower. *Raritan*, **22**, 132–146.

Juengst, E. (1997) Can enhancement be distinguished from prevention in genetic medicine? *Journal of Medicine and Philosophy*, **22**, 125–142.

Juengst, E. (1998) What does *enhancement* mean? In: *Enhancing Human Traits: Ethical and Social Implications* (ed. E. Parens). Georgetown University Press, Georgetown, Texas.

Juengst, E. (2009). What's taxonomy got to do with it? 'Species integrity', human rights and science policy. In: *Human Enhancement* (eds J. Savulescu & N. Bostrom), pp. 43–58. Oxford University Press, Oxford.

Juengst, E. & Walters, L. (1999). Ethical issues in gene transfer research. In: *The Development of Human Gene Therapy* (ed. T. Friedman), pp. 691–713. Cold Spring Harbour Press, New York.

Just, N. (2011) Enhancement, autonomy and authenticity. In: *Enhancing Human Capacities* (eds J. Savulescu, R. Ter Meulen & G. Kahane), pp. 34–48. Blackwell Publishing, Oxford.

Kaebnick, G. (2000) On the sanctity of nature. *Hastings Centre Report*, **30**, 16–23.

Kaebnick, G. (2007). Putting concerns about nature into context – The case of agricultural biotechnology. *Hastings Centre Report*, **40**, 572–584.

Kaebnick, G. (2008). Reasons of the heart – Emotions, rationality and the 'wisdom of repugnance'. *Hastings Centre Report*, **38**, 36–45.

Kass, L. (2003). *Beyond Therapy: Biotechnology and the Pursuit of Happiness*. The President's Council on Bioethics, Washington, District of Columbia.

Lee, S. (2004) Regulation of muscle mass by myostatin. *Annual Review of Cell Developmental Biology*, **20**, 61–86.

Lee, S. & McPherron, A. (2001) Regulation of myostatin activity and muscle growth. *Proceedings of the National Academy of Sciences USA*, **98**, 9306–9311.

Ljungqvist, A. (2005) The international anti-doping policy and its implementation. In: *Genetic Technology and Sport – Ethical Questions* (eds C. Tamburrini & T. Tännsjö), pp. 13–18. Routledge, London.

Mameli, M. (2004). The role of emotions in ecological and practical rationality. In: *Emotion, Evolution and Rationality* (ed D. Evans & P. Cruse), pp. 159–178. Oxford: Oxford University Press.

Midgley, M. (2000). Biotechnology and morality: Why we should pay attention to the 'yuk factor'. *Hastings Centre Report*, 30, 7–15.

Nielsen, L. (2011) The concept of nature in the enhancement technologies debate. In: *Enhancing Human Capacities* (eds J. Savulescu, R. Ter Meulen & G. Kahane), pp. 19–33. Blackwell Publishing, Chichester.

Nilsson, M., Perfilieva, E., Johansson, U., Orwar, O. & Eriksson, P.S. (1999) Enriched environment increases neurogenesis in the adult rat dentate gyrus and improves spatial memory. *Journal of Neurobiology*, 39, 569–578.

Nussbaum, M.C. (2004) Beyond compassion and humanity: Justice for animals? In: *Animal Rights* (eds C.R. Sunstein & M.C. Nussbaum). Oxford University Press, New York.

Parens, E. (1998) Is better always good? In: *Enhancing Human Traits: Ethical and Social Implications* (ed. E. Parens). Georgetown University Press, Texas.

Parens, E. (2005) Authenticity and ambivalence – Towards understanding the enhancement debate. *Hastings Centre Report*, 35, 35–41.

Parens, E. (2009) Toward a more fruitful debate about enhancement. In: *Human Enhancement* (eds J. Savulescu & N. Bostrom), pp. 181–198. Clarendon Press, Oxford.

Parker, R.A. & Yeates, J. (2011) Assesment of Quality of Life in Equine Patients. *Equine Veterinary Journal*, 44, 244–249.

Pellegrino, E. (2004) *Biotechnology, Human Enhancement and the Ends of Medicine*. Centre for Bioethics and Human Dignity, Illinois.

Powell, R. & Buchanan, A. (2011) Breaking evolution's chains: The promise of enhancement by design. In: *Enhancing Human Capacities* (eds J. Savulescu, R. Ter Meulen & G. Kahane). Blackwell Publishing, Oxford.

Rollin, B.E. (1981) *Animal Rights and Human Morality*. New York, Prometheus Books.

Routtenberg, A., Cantallops, I., Zaffuto, S., Serrano, P. & Namgung, U. (2000) Enhanced learning after genetic overexpression of a brain growth protein. *Proceedings of the National Academy of Sciences USA*, 97, 7657–7662.

Rowlands, M. (1998) *Animal Rights: A Philosophical Defence*. Palgrave MacMillan, Basingstoke.

Sabin, J. & Daniels, N. (1994) Determining medical necessity in mental health practice. *Hastings Centre Report*, 24, 5–13.

Sandel, M. (2004) The case against perfection. *Atlantic Monthly*, 293, 51–62.

Savulescu, J. Sandberg, A. & Kahane, G. (2011) Well-being and enhancement. In: *Enhancing Human Capacities* (eds J. Savulescu, R. Ter Meulen & G. Kahane), pp. 3–18. Blackwell Publishing, Chichester.

Schneider, J.S., Lee, M.H., Anderson, D.W., Zuck, L. & Lidsky, T.I. (2001) Enriched environment during development is protective against lead-induced neurotoxicity. *Brain Research*, 896, 48–55.

Sen, A. (1985) Rights and capabilities. In: *Morality and Objectivity: A tribute to JL Mackie* (ed. T. Honderich). Routledge & Kegan Paul, London.

Singer, P. (1979) *Practical Ethics*. Cambridge University Press, Cambridge.

Tang, Y.P., Shimizu, E, Dube, G.R., Rampon, C., Kerchner, G.A., Zhuo, M., Liu, G., & Tsien, J.Z. (1999). Genetic enhancement of learning and memory in mice. *Nature*, 401, 63–69.

Taylor, C. (1992). *The Ethics of Authenticity*. Harvard University Press, Cambridge, Massachusetts.

VandeVeer, D. (1979) Of beasts, persons and the original position. *Monist*, **62**, 368–377.

Walsh, R.N., Budtz-Olsen, O.E., Penny, J.E. & Cummins, R.A. (1969) The effects of environmental complexity on the histology of the rat hippocampus. *The Journal of Comparative Neurology*, **137**, 361–365.

Wang, H., Ferguson, G., Pineda, V., Cundiff, P. & Storm, D. (2004). Overexpression of type-1 adenlyl cyclase in mouse forebrain enhances recognition memory and LTP. *Nature Neuroscience*, **7**, 635–642.

Wei, F., Wang, G., Kerchner, G., Kim, S., Xu, H.-M., Chen, Z.-F. & Zhuo, M. (2001) Genetic enhancement of inflammatory pain by forebrain NR2B overexpression. *Nature Neuroscience*, **4**, 164–169.

Wolpe, P. (2002). Treatment, enhancement and the ethics of neurotherapeutics. *Brain and Cognition*, **50**, 387–395.

Yeates, J. (2010a) The value of pleasure and pain in welfare ethics. *Animal Welfare*, **19(S)**, 29–38.

Yeates, J. (2010b) The application of veterinary stem cell technologies to dogs and horses. In: *Bioethics and the Global Politics of Stem Cell Science: Medical Applications in a Pluralistic World* (2009) (eds A.V. Campbell and B.C. Capps). Imperial College Press/World Scientific Publishing Co, London.

Yeates, J. & Main, D.C.J. (2008) Positive welfare: A review. *The Veterinary Journal*, **175**, 293–300.

Yeates, J. & Main, D.C.J. (2010) The ethics of influencing clients: Problems and solutions. *Journal of the American Veterinary Medical Association*, **237**, 263–267.

Questions and Answers

Q: What is the RSPCA's position on when enhancement is wrong? [Dr Yeates is now the head of the RSPCA's Companion Animals department.]

A: Our opinion would generally depend on the welfare implications for the individual. The RSPCA does not have an overarching policy on enhancement, partly because it's ill defined. The RSPCA excludes certain types of specific interventions and is opposed to chimeric combinations of animals and humans. Technologies that we don't know that much about or that may have a high amount of risk for limited benefit would also be disapproved of. Similarly, the RSPCA would oppose specific examples like breeding of dogs for aesthetic purposes, that is a cosmetic enhancement, where there is a welfare implication. What I didn't want to do is reduce this simply to an animal welfare discussion of enhancements. There are lots of other moral concepts that are relevant to policy and in terms of how veterinarians and others would want to think about it.

Q: You have laid out the inputs in relation to enhancement but did not touch on people's motivation in enhancing animals. We have enhanced the horse over centuries to create the thoroughbred racehorse for very clear reasons. Why would we want to create intelligent sheep, for example? It seems that we need to understand why we are doing this, what is the end stage for those animals and the duties that we have to them.

A: Regarding the end-stage duties we have to animals, we certainly do have a duty to afford enhanced animals whatever respect they are due based on the moral status that they have because of those enhancements. More intelligent sheep would be due whatever respect is due to animals of that intelligence.

Regarding understanding why we are doing this, the position that motivation is important assumes a precise, valid moral stance. Motivation should not be used to decide whether something is moral. Motivation would be important indirectly to achieve change or important for veterinarians to self-reflect on morality. The legitimacy of the act of enhancing is independent of the motivation of the person doing it, certainly from a policy perspective. In some cases, we might want to talk about 'wanton cruelty', but generally what is important is the acceptability of the act, often in terms of its consequences, especially for animal welfare, rather than the motivation of the person. Motivation is important but not necessarily the centre of our ethical discussion of whether it's right or wrong.

Q: Well let's take extrapolation to the absurd extreme. If we are going to enhance everything to be human, what we've been talking about in terms of conservation and the world actually existing disappears once all the insects have been converted into human beings.
A: I am not sure if wanting to make things human is a common moral goal, except for some forms of perfectionism or specific cases such as scientific work for bio-medical research. But if there is a problem, then there are several different principles that we're bothered about, such as 'naturalness', 'sustainability' and 'we want to make things human'.

Q: There is an important distinction about whether you affect the identity of what you enhance. Some may say *'This poor bulldog should have been bred so that it would have been a healthier animal'*. If it had been bred differently, it would have been a different individual. You criticised utilitarians who can deal with this, but what about other ethical physicians who are focused on individuals? There seems to be an issue that if you're only focused on individuals, there is a problem about the enhancement where the identity of the individual is changed. Accusations such as *'This poor bulldog, you should have bred it otherwise'*, can be answered by replies such as *'No, if you had bred it otherwise, this bulldog would not have existed'*. How in your frame of ethics do you deal with non-identity issues?
A: In the paper, I talk about examples that change either the type of thing an animal is, both in terms of the category and the token. If you're doing something before the animal exists then perhaps you are stopping one animal coming into existence but you are allowing another. From a utilitarian point of view, that's acceptable if the balance is acceptable.

Q: Are you just saying to address this in utilitarian terms?
A: No, that is a bold interpretation. I'm not necessarily suggesting a utilitarian answer to that problem of balancing. Of course, there are other approaches to questions of distributive justice. One might instead choose a John Rawls style

approach of saying there should be a limited minimum standard somewhere, which might be a life worth living perhaps. Utilitarianism doesn't necessarily follow from saying we must address a balance across individuals.

I may not support utilitarian thinking regarding killing animals. That is another case with a problem of balancing. It is harder to say whether we have duties to animals in terms of stopping them being created, because they don't have an identity so it's hard to say who you're harming. There isn't an animal that you are harming, so it's hard to say, '*Well, you've harmed this bulldog that was going to exist and now it's not*'. The reply is '*What bulldog?*' It's very hard to say you are harming one dog and benefiting another. If you can have some philosophically rich idea that this bulldog that would have existed does exist in some sort of modal cross-world or potential way, then you might want to say, '*Here's an individual that I've stopped existing*' but I think that's a struggle for our imagination even if it was ethically the most plausible account.

Q: The frame you set out includes many aspects and a lot of the aspects that are covered in the various talks throughout the two days. So what is actually really valuable about calling it animal enhancement? Aren't you talking more broadly about so many aspects involved with the broad topic of veterinary ethics? Why is talking about animal enhancement so valuable, particularly when you look at the medical field, which is actually quite focused?
A: The medical field isn't necessarily that more focused. The STOA Report, for example, talks about normal conventional treatment being part of enhancement and certainly a lot of the futurists try to draw in other things like diet, education and so forth. So there is a tension between people trying to narrow it down (especially to try and then argue for a moral conclusion) and other people saying, '*Well no, you can't differentiate these in different cases*'.

Perhaps, and this feeds into my final terms of reference, I would agree with your implied suggestion that the term animal enhancement does not really benefit us that much. What we need to do is to talk about specific examples, in which case maybe this over arching term doesn't really necessarily benefit us that much. I'm happy with that conclusion in which case enhancement is just a title in the same way as 'animal welfare' or the title of a book or a talk on 'what I did on my holidays'.

Q: What about migration downwards? Is it animal enhancement, for example, instead to go for the intelligent sheep rather than a dumb chicken?
A: Flaubert said that being 'healthy, selfish and stupid' are the criteria for happiness. So it depends on what we're defining as good and what our definition of enhancement is. We can differentiate between making an animal more able to do something or making an animal better in some sort of outcome-focused way. A dumb chicken is less able to think, but perhaps from an outcome-based view it is happier. Are we just making an animal more something and perhaps that more something will include negative abilities, like the ability not to get disease, not to think, etc., or are we talking about it in terms of the outcomes, animal welfare, *telos*, whatever, naturalness, etc., that we want?

Author's Commentary

The issue of enhancement is clearly complex, and this complexity is not helped by the complexity in how the term is used. I have used a very broad operational definition, but this breadth brings as many dangers as it does benefits, since any definitional choice can influence one's final conclusion. One benefit of a broad definition is that it does not tautologically imply a certain moral conclusion (as would, e.g., a definition of enhancement as 'making an animal better', with a normatively loaded concept of 'better'). But the breadth may still psychologically (or perhaps grammatically) predispose us to a certain conclusion. For example, including education or diet may make us more inclined to approve of enhancement since it is common, contingently necessary (e.g. a condition for developing our own moral agency) and effectively unavoidable (insofar as we have to eat in all bar specific cases).

Perhaps instead of 'enhancement', we should consider particular cases or specific types of case. The many different distinctions in this paper provide a number of ways to cut the enhancement cake into bite-size issues for more focused ethical debate. (I have not examined whether those slices are still too vague for focused ethical debate, so we may face some regress until we reach specific assessments of particular cases.)

Nevertheless, the term enhancement is not useless. People do use it to mean something, at least pragmatically. This highlights the danger of moving from a natural language to an ethical debate. Ethical discussions must usually be couched in language insofar as they are communications. This makes grammar and terminology vital, and analytic philosophy has tried to narrow down terms into (to use scientific concepts) discrete, objectified, reliable units. But we must avoid being overly determined (or hamstrung) by our linguistic choices. There is a middle ground of using words as 'rules-of-thumb' that guide our deliberations without presuming them. To analogise (another danger of analytic philosophy), just as I have to use ink to write this paper, we would not say that this paper should be defined by the ink (it is certainly not all black and white).

This issue is not unique to the topic of enhancement. Perhaps most bioethics tries to categorise moral conflicts and then deal with them as such classes. While some continental (most obviously phenomenologies) and case-based (most obviously casuistries) approaches may look at specific cases, even these tend to imply some generalisation – if only of the basic ideas of phenomenological/casuistic approaches – indeed this implied generality is the obvious reason why people would communicate the results of such approaches. In this, bioethics follows many other stalwarts of modern thinking that use generalisations, not least science.

So let us not get overly despondent about the terminological problems that the animal enhancement debate faces. As with other areas, we can recognise the limitations and follow commonsense guidance to further the debate. I hope the heuristics in the paper provide some guidance.

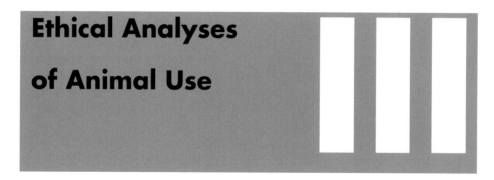

Ethical Analyses of Animal Use

PETER JINMAN

Royal College of Veterinary Surgeons

The final word 'use' in the title is the key to the session. Perhaps the summation of the dilemma and the essence of man is encapsulated in that one word.

In most mainstream religions and societies man is deemed to have dominion over animals, and though there may be species that are revered or respected, man remains, by self-election, the dominant species. Perhaps in a speceist sense, to the victor the spoils!

Setting the boundaries of acceptability for the use of animals by mankind has been, and continues to be, the philosophical and practical legal debate. This debate is informed and led by the advancement of scientific knowledge against a backdrop of an increasingly aware and concerned society acknowledging the sentience of other species and questioning the extent and manner to which man exerts that dominance.

The speakers presenting in this section of the conference reflect on the many ways that man has interpreted the word 'use'; whether as food, companion, for sport or as found in nature, man or his actions have provoked change. The specific breeding of animals to accommodate the needs of man whether it be so as to race faster, pull or carry greater weight or increase the output of man's desired foodstuff, for example milk or meat, has been directed by man. Perhaps in that regard, the ultimate 'use' of an animal remains that carried out by man experimenting with the mental or physical state of a particular sample of a species in the pursuit of knowledge or trialling or testing techniques of intervention or substances that will, if deemed sufficiently successful, prove to be beneficial for man, other animals or the environment.

Veterinary & Animal Ethics: Proceedings of the First International Conference on Veterinary and Animal Ethics, September 2011, First Edition. Edited by Christopher M. Wathes, Sandra A. Corr, Stephen A. May, Steven P. McCulloch and Martin C. Whiting.
© 2013 Universities Federation for Animal Welfare. Published 2013 by Blackwell Publishing Ltd.

In this last context and in the context of this conference about veterinary and animal ethics, the apparent contradiction between the declaration made by all veterinary surgeons when being admitted to the Royal College of Veterinary Surgeons in the United Kingdom and thereby being granted the right to practice becomes all the more perverse:

> *'I promise above all that I will pursue the work of my profession with uprightness of conduct and that my constant endeavour will be to ensure the welfare of the animals committed to my care.'*

Wildlife Medicine, Conservation and Welfare

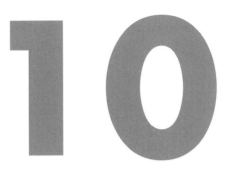

JAMES K. KIRKWOOD

Universities Federation for Animal Welfare

Abstract: The large and growing human population interacts in many ways with, and presents a wide variety of threats to, wild animals at both population (conservation) and individual (welfare) levels. The threats include: various forms of environmental degradation; competition for food, space and other resources; direct killing or disturbance; and introduced predators, competitors and infections. Increasingly, it is taken to be necessary to intervene to manage wild animals in order to tackle or mitigate threats to conservation or welfare. Veterinary science and skills are very relevant to this. However, veterinary medicine developed to meet the economic or emotional needs of animal owners for the treatment of injuries, control of disease and prevention of the premature (as judged by them) death of their domesticated animals. How should veterinary science and medicine be applied to wild animals? And how should judgements be made concerning wildlife management when welfare and conservation objectives may pull in opposite directions?

Keywords: animal, concern, conservation, environment, ethics, killing, medicine, owner, veterinary, wildlife, welfare

10.1 Introduction

Veterinary medicine developed in response to owners' desire and demands for the injuries and diseases that affected their domesticated animals to be treated. Sometimes the motivation to have animals cured will have been partly (or mainly)

Veterinary & Animal Ethics: Proceedings of the First International Conference on Veterinary and Animal Ethics, September 2011, First Edition. Edited by Christopher M. Wathes, Sandra A. Corr, Stephen A. May, Steven P. McCulloch and Martin C. Whiting.
© 2013 Universities Federation for Animal Welfare. Published 2013 by Blackwell Publishing Ltd.

financial – better to pay a small sum to cure a plough horse of its lameness than a large sum to buy a new one. But, no doubt, humans being very fond of animals, the motivation was often primarily, or at least partly, a reflection of emotional bonds with the animal and a desire to alleviate suffering. In the early days of veterinary practice, the main focus of attention was on farm and transport animals, creatures kept for primarily commercial reasons. Now, however, in many countries, more veterinarians are employed in companion animal medicine than in any other branch of veterinary endeavour.

In short, veterinary medicine has its roots in the treatment and control of diseases of individual, owned, domesticated animals. Many of its traditional goals and ethical conventions reflect these particular circumstances. Owners generally, for emotional and/or financial reasons, wish to prevent their animals from dying prematurely (from the owner's point of view). Farmers want the pigs, sheep, cattle and poultry that they raise for meat, to survive until these animals reach slaughter weight; and pet owners generally want their pets to keep them company for as long as possible. Whilst typically in nature, only a small minority of animals survive long enough to approach their maximum possible lifespans, the expectation with pet animals has become that most should. The veterinary care of domesticated, kept animals has been considerably geared towards maximising survival (even if only for the short period until slaughter weight is reached) and, more recently, increasingly towards promoting quality of life.

Modern veterinary medicine readily can be, and increasingly is, applied to wild animals. In addition, for example, to the application of veterinary technology and skills in the detection, diagnosis and monitoring of disease and other threats to wildlife welfare and conservation (e.g. Kennedy 2001; Jepson *et al.* 2005; Miller 2008), and in the use of sedative and anaesthetic drugs to enable handling wild animals for conservation management or research or for other reasons (e.g. Paras 2008), modern veterinary methods are increasingly being used for therapeutic reasons in wild animals. There are safe and effective drugs and surgical techniques that can be applied for treating or alleviating a very wide range of infectious or non-infectious diseases in a wide range of vertebrates (and invertebrates) (e.g. see Mullineaux *et al.* 2003; Fowler & Miller 2007). We have the technology to prevent many deaths through disease and injury and so, should we wish it, to increase average longevities. But, how should veterinary medicine be used in wild animals? For which species? Under what circumstances? And for what, or whose, ends? Who will decide?

The aim of this paper is to review the scale and range of anthropogenic threats to wild animal conservation and welfare and to discuss that, whilst veterinary interventions to tackle or alleviate anthropogenic conservation or welfare problems are likely often to be essential or the case for them to be very compelling, care should be taken to avoid uncritical application of the approaches and tenets of the veterinary care of domesticated animals.

10.2 Anthropogenic Threats to Wild Animal Conservation

The human population is approaching 7 billion and continuing to grow rapidly (US Census Bureau 2011). It seems likely that it will pass 9 billion by the middle of this century, at which point it will have more than trebled in the preceding 100 years. Not only are there very many of us but we utilise resources and produce wastes at biologically unprecedented rates. We maintain huge populations of kept animals: over 23 billion farm animals (FAO 2006) and hundreds of millions of companion animals. Sanderson *et al.* (2002) concluded that 83% of the global terrestrial biosphere was under direct human influence, and Hannah *et al.* (1994) estimated that 36% of the surface was entirely dominated by man. Humans appropriate (utilise or prevent other animals from utilising) about one quarter of the net production (the total plant growth upon which all animals depend) of the earth's lands (Haberl *et al.* 2007).

There is inevitably competition with many other species for space, food and other resources. As is now well understood around the world, because of habitat loss or degradation, pollution, introduced predators or competitors, introduced or facilitated infectious diseases, killing or disturbance and other anthropogenic effects, the viability of many species is under threat (Hilton-Taylor *et al.* 2009). In many species, significant mortality is due to anthropogenic effects (*vide infra*) and Collins and Kays (2011) have pointed out that this may represent a strong selective force for behavioural or morphological changes (i.e. away from the natural genotype).

The percentage of bird species classified as threatened increased from 11.1% in 1998 to 12.2% in 2008 (Vié *et al.* 2009). Of the 5488 mammal species evaluated in the most recent IUCN Red List review, 21% were classified as threatened (IUCN 2008). For reptiles, the corresponding figures were 31% threatened of 1385 species evaluated; for amphibians, 30% threatened of 6260 species evaluated; and for fish, 37% threatened of 3481 species evaluated (Hilton-Taylor *et al.* 2009).

Although there have been some successes, for example, it is thought that 16 species of birds would have become extinct between 1994 and 2004 if not for particular conservation efforts (Butchart *et al.* 2006), overall the outlook for preventing loss of biodiversity is very challenging. Increasingly so, as recent efforts to assess the impact of global warming led to the conclusion that: '*there is growing evidence that climate change will become one of the major drivers of extinction in the twenty-first century*' (Foden *et al.* 2009).

It is clear that without specific efforts to tackle the threats and, in some cases, to actively intervene and to manage species (and their habitats) for their conservation, very many species will be lost. This was perceived only dimly, if at all, 50 years ago. Now it is widely understood. It is to be hoped that widespread loss of species can be averted.

Veterinary contributions towards wild animal conservation have been many and diverse; for example, through research into the causes and impacts of disease and other threats to free-living populations (e.g. Tompkins *et al.* 2002; Kuiken *et al.* 2006; Cunningham *et al.* 2007; Robinson *et al.* 2010) and through development and application of management and disease control methods in free-living and captive populations (e.g. Ensley 1999; Kollias 1999; Sainsbury 2008).

10.3 To Which Wild Animals Do Welfare Concerns Apply?

Concerns about conservation apply to all species: animals, plants, fungi and those in all the many other diverse kingdoms. With perhaps very few exceptions, such as the viruses of smallpox and rinderpest, both of which are thought to be extinct in the wild and which the world was happy to see the back of, there is a general supposition that we should strive to avoid loss of biodiversity.

Concern for welfare, in contrast, applies only to sentient organisms, that is those that have the capacity to be subjectively aware of pleasant and/or unpleasant feelings. For these organisms, there is the possibility that the ways in which we interact with them may make the quality of their lives better or worse from their own points of view. For these animals, the viability of populations is not the only issue, we must consider their feelings also.

The capacity to consciously, subjectively be aware of something is called sentience. We might describe our, human, form of sentience as 'symphonic' because we can be aware of feelings associated with the activity of a wide range external and internal sensors (e.g. sight, sound, warmth, touch, taste, malaise and pain) and also of feelings associated with higher-level, cognitive (thinking) processes (e.g. joy, sorrow, embarrassment and guilt). Some of these kinds of feelings may be unique to humans (e.g. embarrassment perhaps) but many of them may be experienced by other species, some of which may have feelings that humans do not (e.g. those of the echolocation system of bats).

It may be that when sentience first evolved it applied only to one sense (say, taste or vision) and, if so, that there may be some animals for which this remains the case now. Sentience cannot be measured, it can only be inferred, so we do not know where the boundary lies between sentient and insentient organisms. Likewise, we can only infer (not measure) the range of feelings of which organisms are sentient of, beyond drawing facile conclusions, such as that there can be no feelings of colour without some kind of eyes (although, for all we know, bats may have some sound-based imaging with some kind of equivalents to colour, say based on surface texture of objects in their environments).

The great difficulty here, and it is much greater than is generally supposed, is that we do not know where the boundaries of sentient life lie (Kirkwood 2006). The line is, these days, often drawn at or near the border between vertebrates and invertebrates and many modern animal welfare laws reflect this. But, the scientific basis for this is not secure (e.g. see Sherwin 2001). Some authors believe there to be a good case that some invertebrates are sentient, whilst others argue that sentience may be limited to particular (and, according to some, small) parts of the vertebrate tree (Kirkwood & Hubrecht 2001).

10.4 Anthropogenic Threats to Wild Animal Welfare

Until relatively recently, with some notable exceptions, concern for animal welfare has been focused largely on kept animals. Animal welfare science has many of its roots in determining the needs of laboratory and farmed animals and how these needs can be met. The application of the scientific approach to determining how best to keep animals was promoted by, amongst others, Russell and Burch (1959) in their book on *The Principles of Humane Experimental Technique* and by the 'Brambell Committee' (Brambell 1965) *Report of the Technical Committee to Enquire into the Welfare of Animals kept under Intensive Livestock Husbandry Systems*.

There was not, at that time, a corresponding interest in applying the new scientific approaches to assessment of welfare and to the determination of requirements for good welfare, for the benefit of free-living wildlife. In fact, in the enthusiastic pursuit of better health and welfare for farmed animals, the welfare of wild animals was not just overlooked but often routinely and severely harmed. For example, the drainage of ponds and pasture to reduce risks of liver fluke infestation in sheep and cattle may have been good for farm animal welfare but was disastrous for the welfare of wetland amphibians and reptiles.

Another reason for the tendency to overlook the scale of human impacts on wildlife welfare may have been that welfare concerns were sometimes obscured by conservation interests, in so much that it is easy (though often erroneous) to suppose that if a population is viable, there are unlikely to be significant welfare concerns. In fact of course, populations can be sustained in the face of very severe welfare compromises. Myxomatosis, for example, is a very major ongoing welfare problem for European rabbits but does not present a significant threat to the viability of the European population or the species (Sainsbury *et al.* 1995).

Another factor behind the overlooking of wildlife welfare problems may be the tendency for people to rank animal welfare problems not on the basis of their severity and the numbers of animals affected (i.e. as they might be ranked by the animals themselves) but to rank those not caused deliberately as less important than those few that are. The majority of wildlife welfare problems arise as unintended side effects of human actions.

It seems that one of the earliest attempts at a formal study of the nature and scale of anthropogenic effects on wildlife welfare was that undertaken by Sainsbury *et al.* (1995). This looked at a wide variety of anthropogenic welfare problems

Table 10.1   Examples of types of anthropogenic harms to wildlife welfare.

Examples associated with intentional interactions with wildlife
- Injury/failure to kill outright in killing for food (e.g. shooting wildfowl)
- Injury caused in capture or killing for sport (e.g. angling)
- Injury or toxicity caused in population control or management (e.g. warfarin toxicity in brown rat, shooting wounds in red deer)
- Stress and discomfort due to capture for translocation (e.g. black rhino)
- Stress due to capture and marking (e.g. ringing or tagging birds)
- Stress and pain in the course of treatment of wildlife casualties

Examples associated with unintentional interactions with wildlife
- Suffocation of porpoises by-caught in fishing nets
- Poisoning of birds by ingestion of seed-dressings
- Lead poisoning in wildfowl due to ingestion of spent shot
- Stress and pain through effects of introduced infections (e.g. myxomatosis in rabbits, bovine TB in badgers)
- Pain due to injuries caused by road vehicles
- Pain due to injuries caused by collisions with structures
- Electrocution by power lines (birds of prey)
- Malaise due to poisoning by environmental contaminants (DDT, PCBs)
- Starvation and hypothermia due to oiling (sea birds)
- Pain and stress due to injuries caused by domestic cats (garden birds)
- Adverse welfare impacts due to climate change
- Adverse welfare impacts through habitat loss or degradation
- Adverse welfare impacts of introduced predators or competitors

Source: Sainsbury *et al.* (1995). Reproduced with permission from UFAW.

of wild mammals and birds in Europe in terms of the nature of the harm caused to the animals, its intensity and duration and the number of animals affected (Kirkwood *et al.* 1994). Among the conclusions were: '... *it is clear that the welfare of a large number of individuals of a wide range of species is seriously compromised each year as a result of past or present human actions*' and '*those cases which, using our methods of assessment, seem most important in terms of the severity of the harm and the numbers of animals involved are not those that have received the greatest public attention*'.

Almost all anthropogenic wildlife welfare problems arise in one of two ways: (i) as unintended adverse effects associated with deliberate interventions with animals such as culling, harvesting, translocation, marking, etc., and (ii) through adverse consequences of a deliberate or unintended change to the environment such as through loss or degradation of habitat, environmental pollution or introduced infectious disease. Examples are listed in Table 10.1. These are the categories used by Sainsbury *et al.* (1995) in their inquiry into welfare risks to wildlife in Europe. (NB: the intentionality here relates to whether or not the interaction with the animal was intended, not to whether or not harm to welfare was intended – harm to welfare is, with very few exceptions, always an unintended consequence.)

There is no doubt that anthropogenic effects have major adverse impacts on the welfare of very large numbers of wild animals. It is hard to estimate the overall scale of this. Sainsbury *et al.* (1995), in their pilot survey of welfare problems in mammals and birds only, described some particular cases in which the numbers of animals affected in Europe each year were conservatively estimated to be in the 1–10 million and 10–100 million ranges. Worldwide it seems likely that the numbers of wild vertebrates whose welfare is significantly adversely affected by humans is tens and maybe hundreds of billions.

10.5 Responsibility for Wildlife Welfare

It is generally accepted that owners are responsible for the welfare of their kept animals. This stance has a long history and is enshrined by law in many countries. Traditionally, responsibilities for the welfare of wild animals, if any have been recognised at all, have been limited – broadly, to try to avoid causing unnecessary suffering to them.

Hunters often follow quite strong codes and conventions about minimising suffering, for example, regarding the use of appropriate weapons, the need for training and licensing, and adherence to good practice regarding closed seasons, hunting methods, location and despatch of animals not killed outright, and other aspects (e.g. Deer Commission of Scotland 2008; BASC 2011).

There is a general presumption, which in many countries is reflected by legislation, against causing deliberate harm to wild animals and against causing unnecessary suffering in the course of some forms of deliberate, intended, interactions with them. For example, in the EU, there are regulations concerning the conduct of scientific research on wild animals that might cause stress, pain or lasting harm to them (Directive 2010).

Beyond this, the stance regarding the welfare of free-living animals has generally been that it is not our responsibility. This is not just because of the impracticality and impossible scale of attempting to provide for the general welfare of wildlife but because it has been widely considered that we have no obligation to try to prevent or to treat their injuries or diseases – the risks of which are part of animals' natural habitats and ecologies. Animals are as they are, anatomically, physiologically, immunologically and behaviourally, because of natural selection which acts to adapt them to their environments (although anthropogenic effects are likely to be increasingly involved in shaping selection). In the long run, welfare may be best served by not interfering with natural selection, but intervening only where it may be necessary to do so to treat injuries or diseases caused by anthropogenic factors (or to limit suffering by humanely killing moribund animals).

Conventions and regulations regarding interactions with free-living wild animals have generally been such as to give protection from threats arising through our deliberate interactions with them. There are no such clear conventions, let alone regulations, about dealing with situations where anthropogenic welfare problems have arisen as a result of unintended interactions (e.g. see Table 10.1). There is no consistent approach to dealing with these cases.

Because we now greatly influence the fate of very many wild animals, the old distinction between owned and free-living animals, as regards our responsibility for their welfare, is not as clear as it used to be. The quality of the lives of many wild animals is as closely dependent on human activities as that of kept animals. With this, arguably, comes some responsibility for their welfare. If we believe that the welfare of kept animals is important then there is no logic in disregarding our impact on the welfare of wild animals.

The world is feeling its way with this issue at the present time. There is no clear consensus about responsibilities for wildlife welfare and how far these extend. As Sainsbury et al. (1995) pointed out, there has been a movement towards undertaking rigorous environmental impact assessments prior to the implementation of new technologies and developments, to try to foresee and avoid any significant deleterious effects at the population level. Such impact assessments do not usually address welfare impacts per se.

There is no consistent approach to dealing with situations where wildlife welfare is compromised by anthropogenic effects. Sometimes, for example when sea birds are caught in oil spills, there may be efforts to treat them or at least to humanley kill them to minimise suffering. In other cases, for example in the use of anticoagulant rodenticides to control rodents, there has until recently been little public concern, despite evidence that these rodenticides cause marked pain when bleeding occurs into enclosed cavities such as joints, eyes and cranium and, for this reason, have been described as 'markedly inhumane' by the UK's Pesticide Safety Directorate (MAFF 1997).

10.6 Interventions for Wildlife Welfare

Where a wildlife welfare problem is detected, the response may be to (i) do nothing or (ii) treat the animals affected; either option may be followed by (iii) tackle the cause and prevent future cases. For example, the general response to the major welfare problem of myxomatosis in rabbits has been to do nothing. Individuals may humanely kill affected animals they come across in order to limit suffering but there are no efforts to try to tackle the problem at the population level (e.g. by vaccinating wild populations), perhaps because it is perceived to be unfeasible (but there seems to have been little debate about the subject).

Treatment of wild animals that have anthropogenic diseases or injuries is feasible only in a tiny minority of cases and it seems likely that this will remain the case. For example, there is evidence that marine mammals quite frequently become entangled in fishing gear (nets and their associated ropes). Often this results in death by asphyxiation (as the animals are unable to reach the surface to breathe), but in cases where they break free, they may die from very chronic and severe wounds caused by the ropes in which they are entangled (cutting deep into tissues) and from gradual starvation because of their reduced ability to feed (Moore *et al.* 2006). Terrific and heroic efforts have been made to treat some such cases when they have been discovered at sea (Moore *et al.* 2010). There is no doubt, though, that this problem needs to be tackled by prevention and it is to be hoped that ways may be found to prevent such entanglements by modifying net design or deployment (Holy *et al.* 2005). Tackling anthropogenic wildlife welfare problems requires detection of the problems, precise identification of the causes (which is often very difficult) and the development of solutions. Finding resources for this work is not easy.

Interest in the treatment and rehabilitation of wildlife casualties is growing. Some see the role of this work is to address anthropogenic welfare problems, to right the wrongs caused to animals. Others adopt an approach, a paradigm, like that of human and companion animal medicine, and believe it is right, in the interests of preserving the lives of sentient animals, to treat injuries and diseases in wild animals regardless of the cause. In some countries wildlife treatment and rehabilitation is regulated and can only be done, if at all, under licence, in others there are few, if any, controls.

I have previously suggested that respect for life in this context is best served by adopting an approach to wildlife casualties that is guided by concern for species conservation and for the welfare of individuals rather than by aiming simply to save lives (Kirkwood 2005). This is because, generally, food, space and other resources limit population sizes, so saving some animals will tend to be at the expense of others of the same or different species; because the other side of the coin of survival of the fittest is that the less fit do not survive: we should be cautious about interfering with natural selection and compromising selection for evolutionary fitness (e.g. because this may not be good for welfare); and because treatment of wildlife casualties may cause pain and stress. However, even if there was to be some clear consensus that veterinary therapeutic interventions should not generally be applied to wild animals except to tackle anthropogenic problems (to right wrongs caused to them), we should note that, in practice, drawing a clear line between diseases and injuries that have an anthropogenic basis and those that do not can be far from straightforward.

In addition to the growing interest in the treatment of wildlife casualties, there are other large-scale unregulated interventions for wildlife welfare. For example, the provisioning of wild birds. In many countries, some people like to provide garden birds with supplementary food, particularly at times of harsh weather, out of concern for their welfare. Garden bird feeding has become a large industry. In the UK, the total amount of food provided for garden birds is thought to be many tens of thousands of tonnes. The ecological, conservation and welfare effects of provisioning wild birds have, so far, received rather little attention (Dadam 2010).

10.7 Welfare/Conservation Conflicts

Threats to populations and species very often are so because they cause injury, disease and mortality and, so, obviously affect welfare also (Fraser 2010). In these cases, success in alleviating conservation risks is likely to have beneficial welfare effects and *vice versa*. However, concern for the welfare of individual wild animals and concern for viability of populations or species do not always pull in the same direction (see examples below). When they are in conflict, opinions may differ as to whether conservation interests should override welfare concerns or *vice versa* (Kirkwood 2000). Some examples are listed below.

1. Red kites *Milvus milvus* were reintroduced into England and Scotland, after being shot to extinction in these countries over a hundred years ago, by releasing young birds taken from nests in Spain and Sweden (Carter 2007). The best welfare interests of the birds would probably have been to leave them in their native nests but taking and translocating them was good for conservation since it resulted in the re-establishment of large populations within the historic range. Such translocations are increasingly frequently being undertaken for conservation reasons around the world.

2. Brown rats *Rattus norvegicus* and black rats *Rattus rattus* were eradicated from the Island of Lundy (off the Devon coast of the UK) by poisoning them with anticoagulant rodenticides. These rats were predating the nests of sea birds and were killed in order to restore breeding sea bird populations (Lock 2006). This was good for the status of the sea bird populations but at the expense of the welfare of the rats. Control of introduced vertebrate pests in order to conserve island species is a common problem around the world (e.g. Howald *et al.* 2009; Hughes *et al.* 2009).

3. Allowing pet cats freedom to roam may be to the welfare advantage of the cats but, in New Zealand, they can have a deleterious effect on native bird populations. van Heezick (2010) wrote: '*Society needs to ask what it wants in its environment – wildlife or cats – and the job of conservation biologists is to make sure that the informed answer is wildlife. Currently, conservation biologists are pussyfooting around this problem…*'. In the UK, whilst domestic cats have a major impact on welfare of garden birds through scratch and bite wounds (Sainsbury *et al.* 1995), they are not believed to be very important in limiting populations (perhaps because species at risk from domestic cats have long since disappeared from the UK).

4. Captive-bred corncrakes *Crex crex* from Whipsnade Zoo have been successfully reintroduced into the Royal Society for the Protection of Birds Reserve at Nene Washes in Cambridgeshire, UK (RSPB 2008). Bringing wild animals into captivity may have some welfare costs (e.g. in the case of this migratory species, by limiting movements), but can have direct conservation benefits when captive-bred animals are used to reintroduce populations back into their historic range. In some cases, breeding animals in captivity may differ very little from their breeding in the wild and may present little or no threat to welfare. In other cases, captive breeding may involve greater degrees of intervention. For example, using artificial breeding techniques such as electroejaculation, *in vitro* fertilisation and implantation of embryos. In the USA, gaur (*Bos gaurus*) calves have been born to domestic cows (*Bos taurus*) following implantation with embryos from *in vitro* fertilisation of oocytes collected from gaur ovaries *post-mortem* (Johnston *et al.* 1994). In the UK, the Secretary of State's Standards of Modern Zoo Practice (Defra 2004) advocate an ethical review process to consider situations carefully where the use of zoo animals for conservation may not be in the best welfare interests of the individuals involved.

10.8 Dealing with Welfare/Conservation Conflicts

At one end of the spectrum, some may take the view that species conservation is ultimately a greater priority than welfare and that it is justifiable to compromise welfare to achieve a conservation goal. At the other, exactly the opposite view may be held: that welfare should always be prioritised over conservation. However, perhaps the majority position themselves somewhere between the 'pure-bred' environmentalist and individualist positions, believing that decisions should be based on carefully considering and 'weighing' the conservation and welfare aspects.

If this approach is accepted then, in deciding on each case, both welfare and conservation aspects have to be examined thoroughly. The process is not simple or straightforward but judging the conservation value of a proposal, may perhaps be generally more straightforward than judging the welfare aspects.

The conservation case may be relatively simple in some situations where, for example, it can be unequivocally demonstrated that unless action is taken to halt a population decline, there is a very high risk of extinction. Perhaps matters are rarely that simple, but at least, in conservation, the key parameter – population size – can, in principle, be measured objectively.

The welfare side of the balance, however, presents greater conceptual difficulties. We have no direct access to and cannot *measure* how other animals feel (which is what animal welfare is about) but can only make subjective inferences about this. This problem can be minimised by making the bases of our inferences as clear as possible using a two-step process in which subjective welfare inferences are made, based on as much solid objective description of the anatomical, physiological and behavioural effects of the problem as possible. However, the fact is that sometimes people reach very different conclusions. For example, the signs that some interpret as being due to pain or fear in fish are interpreted by others (who do not believe that fish have the brain circuitry necessary to generate conscious perception of feelings) as merely mechanical responses to stimuli.

Because opinions about the way forward with welfare/conservation conflicts not infrequently differ, decisions about whether a procedure for conservation is acceptable in view of its welfare consequences, or *vice versa*, should be made collectively by a group rather than by an individual. Where it decides that an action for conservation should go ahead, the group should also carefully consider steps that should be taken to minimise adverse welfare impacts – using a two Rs approach (after Russell & Burch 1959): *refining* methods and procedures and *reducing* the number of animals affected to the minimum (e.g. translocate no more animals than necessary to achieve the objective).

10.9 Concluding Comments

There has been a great proliferation of situations in which decisions have to be made about wildlife management and the application of wildlife medicine for wildlife welfare and/or conservation, and about how wildlife interests should be balanced with other concerns, for example with the health and welfare of humans or kept animals, where the two are in conflict. As human–wildlife interactions and the pressures on wildlife increase, and as interest in and expectations about animal welfare and conservation continue to develop, we can expect that problems and dilemmas in these fields will intensify.

At present, where these are formally addressed at all, they tend to be dealt with by a variety of bodies, often set up to address particular cases. There might be advantage in establishing national advisory bodies to facilitate the development of expertise and consistent approaches.

References

BASC (2011) British Association for Shooting and Conservation, Codes of Practice: Respect for quarry. Available at: http://www.basc.org.uk/en/codes-of-practice/respect-for-quarry.cfm accessed on 12 June 2012.

Brambell, F.W.R. (1965) *Report of the Technical Committee to Enquire into the Welfare of Animals kept under Intensive Livestock Husbandry Systems.* HMSO. ISBN: 0 10 850286 4.

Butchart, S.H.M., Statterfield, A.J. & Collar, N.J. (2006). How many bird extinctions have we prevented? *Oryx*, **40**, 266–278.

Carter, I. (2007) *The Red Kite*, 2nd Ed. Arlequin Press, Shrewsbury.

Collins, C. & Kays, R. (2011) Causes of mortality in North American populations of large and medium-sized mammals. *Animal Conservation*, **14**. doi: 10.1111/j.1469-1795. 2011.00458.x.

Cunningham, A.A., Hyatt, A.D., Russell, P. & Bennett, P.M. (2007) Emerging epidemic diseases of frogs in Britain are dependent on the source of ranavirus agent and the route of exposure. *Epidemiology and Infection*, **135**, 1200–1212. doi: 10.1017/ S0950268806007679.

Dadam, D. (2010) Wild bird care in the garden: A scientific look at large scale, do-it-yourself, wildlife management. *Animal Welfare*, **19**, 360–362.

Darwin, C. (1859) *On the Origin of Species by Means of Natural Selection, or the Preservation of Favoured Races in the Struggle for Life*. John Murray, London.

Deer Commission of Scotland (2008) Best practice guidance on the management of wild deer in Scotland [Online]. Available at: http://www.bestpracticeguides.org.uk/Default.aspx accessed on 12 June 2012.

Defra (2004) Secretary of State's Standards of Modern Zoo Practice. Department of Environment, Food and Rural Affairs. Available at: www.defra.gov.uk.

Directive (2010) Directive 2010/63/EU of the European Parliament and of the Council of 22 September 2010 on the protection of animals used for scientific purposes. Available at: http://eurlex.europa.eu/LexUriServ/LexUriServ.do?uri=OJ:L:2010:276:0033:0079: EN:PDF accessed on 12 June 2012.

Ensley, P.K. (1999) Medical management of the Californian condor. In: *Zoo and Wild Animal Medicine: Current Therapy 4* (eds M.E. Fowler & R.E. Miller), pp. 277–292. WB Saunders, Philadelphia.

Evans, K. & Adams, V. (2010) Proportion of litters of purebred dogs born by caesarean section. *Journal of Small Animal Practice*, **51**, 113–118.

FAO (2006) FAOSTAT Database Results. Available at: http://faostat.fao.org/faostat/ collections?version=extand hasbulk=0and subset=agriculture (updated on 24 April 06; accessed on 15 July 06).

Foden, W.B., Mace, G.M., Vié, J.-C., Angulo, A., Butchart, S.H.M., DeVantier, L., Dublin, H.T., Gutsche, A., Stuart, S.N. & Turak, E. (2009) Species susceptibility to climate change impacts. In: *Wildlife in a Changing World: An Analysis of the 2008 IUCN Red List of Threatened Species* (eds J.-C. Vié, C. Hilton-Taylor & S.N. Stuart), pp. 77–87. IUCN, Gland, Switzerland. Available at: http://data.iucn.org/dbtw-wpd/edocs/RL-2009-001.pdf accessed on 12 June 2012.

Fowler, M.E. & Miller, R.E. (2007) *Zoo and Wild Animal Medicine: Current Therapy 6*. WB Saunders Co., Philadelphia, Pennsylvania.

Fraser, D. (2010) Towards a synthesis of conservation and animal welfare science. *Animal Welfare*, **19**, 121–124.

Haberl, H., Erb, K.-H., Krausmann, F., Gaube, V., Bondeau, A., Plutzar, C., Gingrich, S., Lucht, W. & Fischer-Kowalski, M. (2007) Quantifying and mapping the human appropriation of net primary production in earth's terrestrial ecosystems. *Proceedings of the National Academy of Sciences of the United States of America*, **104**, 12942–12947.

Hannah, L., Lohse, D., Hutchinson, C., Carr, J.L. & Lankerani, A. (1994) A preliminary inventory of human disturbance of world ecosystems. *AMBIO*, **23**, 246–250.

Hilton-Taylor, C., Pollock, C.M., Chanson, J.S., Butchart, S.H.M., Oldfield, T.E.E. & Katariya, V. (2009) State of the world's species. In: *Wildlife in a Changing World: An*

Analysis of the 2008 IUCN Red List of Threatened Species (eds J.-C. Vié, C. Hilton-Taylor & S.N. Stuart), pp. 15–41. IUCN, Gland, Switzerland. Available at: http://data.iucn.org/dbtw-wpd/edocs/RL-2009-001.pdf

Holy, N., Trippel, E. & King, D. (2005) Altering the chemical properties of nest to prevent bycatch of cetaceans (whales, dolphins and porpoises). Available at: http://www.smartgear.org/smartgear_winners/smartgear_winner_2005/smartgear_winner_2005runner/ accessed on 12 June 2012.

Howald, G., Donlan, C.J., Faulkner, K.R., Ortega, S., Gellerman, H., Croll, D.A. & Tershy, B.R. (2009) Eradication of black rats *Rattus rattus* from Anacapa Island. *Oryx*, **44**, 30–40.

Hughes, B.J., Martin, B.R. & Reynolds, S.J. (2009) Cats and seabirds: Effects of feral domestic cat *Felis silvestris* eradication on the population of sooty terns on Ascension Island, South Atlantic. *Ibis*, **150**(1): 122–131.

IUCN (2008). *2008 Red List of Threatened Species*. Available at: http://www.iucnredlist.org accessed on 12 June 2012.

Jepson, P.D., Bennett, P.M., Deaville, R., Allchin, C.R., Baker, J.R. & Law, R.J. (2005) Relationships between PCBs and health status in UK-stranded harbour porpoises (*Phocaena phocaena*). *Environmental Toxicology and Chemistry*, **24**, 238–248.

Johnston, L.A., Parrish, J.J., Monson, R., Liebfried-Rutledge, L., Susko-Parrish, J.L., Northey, D.L., Rutledge, J.J. & Simmons, L.G. (1994) Oocyte maturation, fertilisation and embryo development in vitro and in vivo in the gaur (*Bos gaurus*). *Journal of Reproduction and Fertility*, **100**, 131–136.

Kennedy, S. (2001) Morbillivirus infections in aquatic mammals. In: *Infectious Diseases of Wild Mammals*, 3rd Ed. (eds E.S. Williams & I.K. Barker), pp. 64–76. Iowa State University Press, Ames, Iowa.

Kirkwood, J.K. (2000) Ethical aspects of interventions for the conservation or welfare of wild-life. In: *Veterinary Ethics – An Introduction* (ed. G. Legood), pp. 121–138. Cassell, London.

Kirkwood, J.K. (2005) Kindness, conservation or keeping alive? The philosophy of veterinary treatment and rehabilitation of wildlife casualties. In: Back to the Wild: Studies in Wildlife Rehabilitation (eds V. Menon, N.V.K. Ashraf, P. Panda & K. Mainkar), pp. 29–33. Wildlife Trust of India (www.wti.org.in).

Kirkwood, J.K. (2006) The distribution of sentience in the animal kingdom. In: *Animals, Ethics and Trade: the Challenge of Animal Sentience* (eds J. Turner & J. D'Silva) (Proceedings of the CIWF Trust Conference, London, March 2005), pp. 12–26. Earthscan, London.

Kirkwood, J.K. & Hubrecht, R. (2001) Consciousness, cognition and animal welfare. *Animal Welfare*, **10**(s), 5–17.

Kirkwood, J.K., Sainsbury, A.W. & Bennett, P.M. (1994) The welfare of free-living wild animals: methods of assessment. *Animal Welfare*, **3**, 257–273.

Kollias, G.V. (1999) Health assessment, medical management, and prerelease conditioning of translocated North American river otters. In: *Zoo and Wild Animal Medicine: Current Therapy 4* (eds M.E. Fowler & R.E. Miller), pp. 443–448. WB Saunders, Philadelphia, Pennsylvania.

Kuiken, T., Kennedy, S., Barrett, T., *et al.* (2006) The 2000 canine distemper epidemic in Caspian seals (*Phoca caspia*): Pathology and analysis of contributory factors. *Veterinary Pathology*, **43**, 321–338.

Lock, J. (2006) Eradication of brown rats *Rattus norvegicus* and black rats *Rattus rattus* to restore breeding seabird populations on Lundy Island, Devon, England. *Conservation Evidence*, **3**, 111–113.

MAFF (1997) Assessment of humaneness of vertebrate control agents. Evaluation of fully approved or provisionally approved products under the control of pesticides regulations 1986. *Pesticide Safety Directorate*, MAFF, London. Available at: http://www.pesticides. gov.uk/psd_evaluation_all.asp

Miller, M.W. (2008) Chronic wasting disease of cervid species. In: *Zoo and Wild Animal Medicine: Current Therapy 6* (eds M.E. Fowler & R.E. Miller), pp. 430–437. WB Saunders, Philadelphia.

Moore, M.J., Bogomolni, A., Bowman, R., *et al.* (2006) Fatally entangled right whales can die extremely slowly. Oceans 2006 MTS/IEEE-Boston, Massachusetts. ISBN: 1-4244-0115-1/06. doi:10.1109/OCEANS.2006.306792

Moore, M.J., Walsh, M., Bailey, J., *et al.* (2010) Sedation at sea of North Atlantic Right Whales (*Eubalaena glacialis*) to enhance disentanglement. *PLoS One*, **5**(3), e9597. doi: 10.1371/journal.pone.0009597

Mullineaux, E., Best, R. & Cooper, J.E. (eds) (2003) *BSAVA Manual of Wildlife Casualties*. British Small Animal Veterinary Association, Quedgeley, Gloucestershire.

Paras, A. (2008) Capture and anaesthesia of otariids in the wild. In: *Zoo and Wild Animal Medicine: Current Therapy 6* (eds M.E. Fowler & R.E. Miller), pp. 312–318. WB Saunders, Philadelphia, Pennsylvania.

Robinson, R.A., Lawson, B., Toms, M.P., *et al.* (2010) Emerging infectious disease leads to rapid population decline of common British birds. *PLoS One*. Available at: http://www. plosone.org/article/info:doi/10.1371/journal.pone.0012215

RSPB (2008) *English Corncrakes Reach 80 Year High*. Available at: http://www.rspb.org.uk/ news/details.aspx?id=tcm:9-192856 accessed on 12 June 2012.

Russell, W.M.S. & Burch, R.L. (1959) *The Principles of Humane Experimental Technique*. Methuen, London.

Sainsbury, A.W. (2008) Medical aspects of red squirrel translocation. In: *Zoo and Wild Animal Medicine: Current Therapy 6* (eds M.E. Fowler & R.E. Miller), pp. 236–242. WB Saunders, Philadelphia, Pennsylvania.

Sainsbury, A.W., Bennett, P.M. & Kirkwood, J.K. (1995) Welfare of free-living wild animals in Europe: Harm caused by human activities. *Animal Welfare*, **4**, 183–206.

Sanderson, E., Jaiteh, M., Levy, M., Redford, K., Wannebo, A. & Woolmer, G. (2002) The human footprint and the last of the wild. *BioScience*, **52**, 891–904.

Sherwin, C.M. (2001) Can invertebrates suffer? Or, how robust is argument-by-anology? *Animal Welfare*, **10**(s), 103–118.

Tompkins, D.M., Sainsbury, A.W., Nettleton, P., Buxton, D. & Gurnell, J. (2002) Parapoxvirus causes a deleterious disease in red squirrels associated with UK population declines. *Proceedings of the Royal Society of London B*, **269**, 529–533.

US Census Bureau (2011) US and world population clocks. Available at: http://www.census. gov/main/www/popclock.html accessed on 5 September 2011.

van Heezick, Y. (2010) Pussyfooting around the issue of cat predation in urban areas. *Oryx*, **44**, 153–154.

Vié, J.-C., Hilton-Taylor, C., Pollock, C.M., *et al.* (2009) The IUCN red list: A key conservation tool. In: *Wildlife in a Changing World: An Analysis of the 2008 IUCN Red List of Threatened Species* (eds J.-C. Vié, C. Hilton-Taylor & S.N. Stuart), pp. 1–14. IUCN, Gland, Switzerland. Available at: http://data.iucn.org/dbtw-wpd/edocs/RL-2009-001.pdf accessed on 12 June 2012.

Questions and Answers

Q: Setting aside pensions for poodles and welfare for wildlife, can I ask your opinion on who we're treating or who we're pandering to when wildlife casualties are treated? Is it the animal or the public?
A: I'm familiar with the difficult dilemma when a member of the public, hoping that successful treatment might be possible, presents a seriously injured casualty wild animal, which, in my view, should be euthanased to prevent further suffering. Each case has to be judged on its merits. When one believes that the kindest course of action is to euthanase, it is important to explain this carefully.

Q: I appreciate what you say about intervening when you can identify an anthropogenic cause of a problem and not doing so when you can't, but how do you make that distinction when we've changed so much in terms of landscape, habitat and so forth? It's becoming blurred where an anthropogenic direct or indirect cause may or may not have occurred; how do you draw the lines these days?
A: I agree with you that deciding whether wildlife welfare problems are natural or anthropogenic is difficult. If there are no facts that make the answer clear and unambiguous, then it has to be a matter of judgement. There is a spectrum. At one end, there are cases that are almost certainly not much to do with anthropogenic effects and, at the other, those which very plainly are. I am suggesting that judgements have to be made, as with many of the matters we're discussing.

Q: We are still struggling with the concept of welfare and what welfare is exactly. Certainly when it comes to wildlife welfare issues, these questions become more important. Just thinking that keeping animals free of any kind of negative state does not really correspond with natural principles. We might see very often that animals choose a negative state in the short term to obtain something more positive in the long term. I was wondering whether you reflected on what a welfare concept for wildlife might be and whether we probably have to reconsider our Five Freedoms approach.
A: It's a good question and I would find it difficult to properly answer it fully, in haste here and now. The concept of the Five Freedoms is valuable in helping us to deal with kept animals but when it comes to dealing with free-living wildlife, you have to think rather differently, particularly with regard to deciding if, and when, interventions for welfare should be made.

Q: I'm a bit concerned about using sentience as the cut-off criterion because, as Aldo Leopold said, *the importance of an individual animal is how it supports the biosphere.* Maybe the biomass of non-sentient beings and their welfare is as, or more, important from a conservation point of view than welfare of sentient animals.
A: My point about sentience is that its presence or absence is what is important in deciding which animals are of welfare concern and which are not (e.g. should we be concerned with the welfare of the sheep or of the parasitic nematodes in its intestine?). All species are arguably equally important from the conservation point

of view. I am not suggesting that we should use sentience in deciding which species to conserve. We generally think that we should be careful to conserve all species, except perhaps the rinderpest virus and the smallpox virus, both of which have been eradicated. But when it comes to deciding to which organisms the concept of welfare applies, then sentience is the critical point. If an animal doesn't have the capacity to feel – to subjectively experience anything – then there is no welfare concern. There may be plenty of good reasons to look after such an animal but concern for welfare is not one of them. It is very difficult to decide where to draw the line and as far as possible organisms should be given the benefit of the doubt.

Q: In moral philosophy, there's a distinction between positive and negative duties. Do we have a negative duty to wildlife in that we have a duty not to cause harm, which fits with anthropogenic habitat destruction, etc., but don't necessarily have positive duties to improve the welfare of all wildlife?
A: We should do all that we can to avoid causing harm to wildlife welfare. In some cases where we have caused a problem, the ideal would be to intervene to ameliorate it and take steps to avoid the problem recurring. However, where welfare is compromised by natural (non-human) agency, perhaps we should generally not intervene.

Q: What is the duty of a veterinarian to wildlife?
A: It depends on the circumstances. A veterinarian presented with an animal must deal with it humanely and, in deciding whether treatment and rehabilitation is possible or whether euthanasia would be kinder, has to take many things into account, for example the animal's condition, the stress of whatever treatment may be necessary, the chances of successful rehabilitation and the possible effects on wild populations.
C: That's the practitioner dilemma. The criterion to which I've always worked is 'can the animal be returned to its normal life, that is can it go back to the wild?'

Q: In New Zealand, there are many whale strandings. Many colleagues think that such whales are committing suicide and should be left alone while others who, sincerely motivated, deeply emotionally involved, will nearly kill themselves to assist these animals. What are your thoughts?
A: Whales strand for a variety of reasons, sometimes because of navigational errors and sometimes because they're ill. If a stranded whale is found to be diseased, then the kind thing might be to euthanase it. If, on the other hand, the signs are that the stranding is due to navigational error then, if the animals can be got back out to sea quickly, that's a kind thing to do.

Author's Commentary

Pet owners often consider their pets to be part of the family and generally want their company for as long as possible. Veterinary medicine is part of the means by which this is achieved and the survival curves of wild and kept animals have come to differ dramatically.

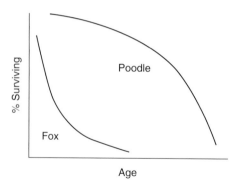

Figure 10.1 Diagram illustrating the difference in the age-related survival curves of wild foxes and of pet poodles. Source: Curves based on data from Armstrong JB (2000) Longevity in the standard poodle. http://www.canine-genetics.com/lifespan.html and Lloyd, HG (1977) In British Mammals. Second Edition. Eds GB Corbett & HN Southern. Blackwell Scientific, Oxford. p319).

Foxes and poodles are very similar animals, with roughly the same adult body size and roughly the same maximum life span (about 15 years). But the survival curves of their populations are very different (Figure 10.1). In the free-living fox, as is typical for many wild animals, mortality is quite high for all age groups, about 50% each year, so only a very few approach old age. As Darwin pointed out, in nature, animals overproduce and because of environmental challenges and competition for resources, often only a few survive to breed. Whereas, buffered from the rigours of life in the wild and from competition with conspecifics, and being the beneficiaries of modern veterinary science and care, many poodles live well on towards the maximum possible lifespan.

Here, then, are two different ways in which a population can be sustained. On the one hand, the 'fit fox' approach of natural selection and on the other, the 'pampered poodle' method that we have engineered. With the former, a larger number of animals can live but each (on average) for a short time. Whereas, in the latter, fewer can live but each for longer. It is not possible, in a world with finite resources, to have both high rates of reproduction and for a large proportion of the population to live for a long time. The pampered poodle strategy is unsustainable without large-scale castration and spaying: we would be chest-deep in poodles the world over in a few years if they all lived to old age and bred freely.

Which is better way of filling the available niches? The net amount of pleasure and pain associated with the 'fit fox' and 'pampered poodle' strategies may be about the same. The fact that the poodle survival curve is the shape it is, suggests that our default assumption is to think that that is how it should be, that ideally all poodles should live to old age. Otherwise why would we have engineered it to be that way? Does that mean we think natural selection's approach is wrong?

Darwin (1859), being very aware that natural selection was an uncomfortable idea in a society that had tended to see life as part of a divine and benevolent purpose, strove to soften the blow for his readers. He wrote: *'we may console ourselves with the full belief that the war of nature is not incessant, that no fear is felt, that death is generally prompt, and that the vigorous, the healthy and the happy survive and multiply'*.

Death is not always quick and painless but it may tend often to be fairly quick for wild animals. This is the case for small birds suddenly snatched by hawks and for voles suddenly snatched by kestrels or owls. Is sustaining a population the 'fit fox' way worse than sustaining one the 'pampered poodle' way? The latter is certainly not without its hazards, all poodles have to die eventually and there is no guarantee that the process will be painless. Also, once we humans start to take over from natural selection in deciding which individuals should live and breed, the long-term welfare consequences can be serious (the UFAW web site on genetic welfare problems in companion animals provides many examples: http://www. ufaw.org.uk/geneticwelfareproblems.php).

I have suggested elsewhere that it is important to be clear, when dealing with wildlife casualties, whether it is being done for welfare or conservation reasons as this is likely to influence both the judgements about what is ethically acceptable and the practical approaches (Kirkwood 2005). The question is, in the application of veterinary science for wildlife welfare (as opposed to conservation), should we favour the 'fit fox' model, that is tending to intervene only to prevent suffering by euthanasing injured or diseased animals that would otherwise die more slowly? Or, should we favour the 'pampered poodle' approach and try to treat diseases and injuries and to prevent deaths (until later)?

The last of the questions put to me after my presentation (see above) goes right to the heart of the difficulty. Natural selection's approach to whales that become stranded means that only those that do not become stranded survive to breed. This process (over millennia) has already resulted in whales being very well (but not yet perfectly) adapted and equipped to avoid stranding. We can presume that as long as very strong selection pressure for not stranding continues, such cases may tend (over very long timescales) to become ever less likely. Our first instinct faced with stranded whales might be that if the stranding appears to be due to a navigational error and the animals can be returned quickly to the sea, then that is the obvious and kind thing to do.

That remains my view. However, making any interventions to save wildlife casualties that can be ascribed to natural causes is straightaway to take a step in the pampered poodle direction which, if rolled out on a large scale, would be likely to result in future populations being less well adapted. For example, the current bizarre situation that 90% of Boston terriers cannot be born naturally but have to be delivered by Caesarean section (Evans & Adams 2010) has come about because of interventions to save dogs in what were, initially, rare cases of birth difficulties. The present strange situation is because the very strong selection pressure against pups being too big to be born has been relaxed through the almost routine use of Caesareans. Arguably, such situations can be managed to some extent in domesticated animals but we could not manage them in wild animals. There is therefore a strong case for being careful in managing wildlife into the (hopefully) very far future, not to uncritically apply medical interventions. I suggest that, with wildlife, we have to a greater extent to be careful, when acting for the benefit of one individual (say to treat a wildlife casualty), to take account of the effects, over the long term, on the welfare of all the rest of the population.

Where an animal population sustains itself at the carrying capacity of the environment, if we intervene to save some individuals then others are likely to be disadvantaged. Alternatively, if we decide to euthanase a casualty rather than treating it and returning it to the wild, then its niche is likely to become occupied by another that otherwise would not have had the chance to survive. We can save particular individuals if we choose to do so but, generally, this is likely to be at the expense of others so that, at the population level, there may be no net effect on welfare or population viability.

However, although there may be a valid argument on welfare grounds for adopting the 'fit fox' approach with self-sustaining populations and for intervening only to euthanase to prevent unnecessary suffering rather than trying to treat wildlife casualties, the fact is that often that approach does not feel right (at least not to everyone). Depending on the species, there are often powerful emotional drives that argue that it is better to attempt treatment rather than to euthanase. There may be no rational basis for the differences in attitudes to rats and seals that are apparent when it comes to dealing with casualties (there is no reason to suppose that their capacities for suffering differ), but these different attitudes and their consequences are nevertheless real. In dealing with wildlife, we often find ourselves involved with a complex mix of interests, some rational and some not: some of the head, and some which, although of the heart, may be just as, if not more, forceful. Here again, as suggested in the conclusion to the main paper above, there is a case for national bodies that can seek informed consensus and provide advice.

Veterinary Ethics and the Use of Animals in Research: Are They Compatible?

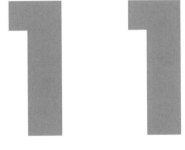

COLIN GILBERT[1] AND SARAH WOLFENSOHN[2]

[1]The Babraham Institute
[2]Seventeen Eighty Nine

Abstract: Veterinarians have an ethical responsibility to use their professional skills to improve welfare and alleviate suffering of animals, irrespective of the context of their lives. Laboratory animals are bred and reared for clearly defined purposes, some of which may result in harm. Balanced against these harms are potential benefits that may accrue to medicine (including veterinary medicine), fundamental scientific knowledge or other purposes deemed to be justifiable. While this situation exists, the active involvement of the veterinary profession is essential to provide clinical care for intercurrent diseases of laboratory animals, to assist in the management of any harms resulting from experiments and to advise on matters such as animal husbandry and staff training. In addition, veterinarians should apply their expertise in contributing to the detailed ethical debates that determine whether or not, and how, experiments may be conducted.

Keywords: conduct, debate, environment, ethics, harm, husbandry, laboratory animals, medicine, veterinarian, veterinary ethics, welfare, 3Rs

Veterinary & Animal Ethics: Proceedings of the First International Conference on Veterinary and Animal Ethics, September 2011, First Edition. Edited by Christopher M. Wathes, Sandra A. Corr, Stephen A. May, Steven P. McCulloch and Martin C. Whiting.
© 2013 Universities Federation for Animal Welfare. Published 2013 by Blackwell Publishing Ltd.

11.1 Historical Perspectives

Animal use in science dates back to Erasistratus and Herophilus in the third century BC and Galen in the second century AD (Schiller 1967). Ground-breaking experiments that demonstrated the circulation of the blood (Harvey 1628) would not be countenanced today owing to their method of animal use, yet underpin modern cardiovascular physiology. Religious thinkers such as Saint Cuthbert, Saint Francis of Assisi and followers of Jainism had already emphasised the importance of kindness to animals, but when the philosopher Jeremy Bentham asked in 1789: 'The question is not can they talk, nor can they reason, but can they suffer?' then the modern concept of animal welfare was born (Bentham 1789). The subsequent rise of the anti-vivisection movement encouraged the development of self-regulation. In 1831, Marshall Hall developed 'five principles for experimental research' and in 1871 the British Association for the Advancement of Science developed a moral code of practice. Neither was readily universally adopted. For example, an article in *The Lancet* (Anon 1902) put forward reasons why it was '*impossible for the medical man to argue with anti-vivisectionists of the more rabid order*' who were '*trying to wreck the labours of the truly charitable*'. With opinions polarising, increasing levels of violent protests, especially from the 1960s, reinforced a bunker mentality as laboratories using animals closed their doors to visitors. Some breeding centres were forced to close, with the unintended consequence of increased transport times for animals (Wolfensohn & Maguire 2010). The principles of Reduction, Refinement and Replacement in animal experiments, proposed by Russell and Burch (1959), took time to gain their now almost universal acceptance and for necessary improvements to follow, many of which were formalised in the UK by the Animals (Scientific Procedures) Act of 1986. Today, the welfare of laboratory animals continues to be strongly debated. Most observers agree that constructive dialogue has increased the quality of both animal welfare and research output, whereas simple hostility has been counterproductive. Attitudes to laboratory animals will undoubtedly alter in the future as our moral and cultural perspectives change.

11.2 Scale of Usage

A summary of laboratory animal usage within the 27 states of the EU can be found at http://ec.europa.eu/environment/chemicals/lab_animals/reports_en.htm, from which Figure 11.1 is taken. The total number of animals used for experimental and other scientific purposes in 2008 (with one Member State reporting for 2007) was 'just above 12 million'.

Since 2005, the percentage of animals used for research and development for human medicine, dentistry and veterinary medicine has dropped from 31% to

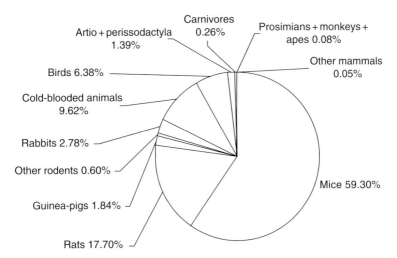

Figure 11.1 Percentages of animals used by classes in the Member States (Gilbert, 2010). Used with permission.

23%, whereas that of animals used for fundamental biological research has increased from 33% to 38%. Animals used for toxicological and other safety evaluation for different products or environmental test schemes amounted to 9% of the total. Primates represented 0.1% of the total, equating to 9600. For comparison, in the USA (according to the USDA) 69 990 primates were used in 2007. Clinical research demand for primates in the USA is set to continue (Hayden 2008).

11.3 Public Perceptions

The polling company Ipsos MORI has been asking the public in the UK about their views on animal research since 1999 (Ipsos MORI 2010). Amongst their findings, as reported by the organisation Understanding Animal Research (http://www. understandinganimalresearch.org.uk/your_views), was that throughout this time, more than 80% of respondents accepted the need for animal research provided that certain conditions were met:

- there is no unnecessary suffering;
- the research is for serious medical or life-saving purposes; and
- there is no alternative.

Much of the existing regulatory process is built around a desire to satisfy these caveats. The MORI poll showed that, since 2005, a majority of the surveyed population *expect that the rules in Britain on animal experimentation are well enforced*. A significant, and often vocal, minority of the population are opposed to any use of animals in research. Campaigning organisations such as the BUAV argue that *'Harming animals in the name of science is morally indefensible'* (http://www.buav.org/humane-science).

Many interactions between man and animals involve animals being used in ways which they would be unlikely to choose for themselves. Some animal suffering can arise from human behaviour that is negligent or is at best ignorant of animals' needs. Some interactions are overtly selfish, such as the over-exploitation, by humans, of companion and sporting animals in competitions. Some may be driven by a misplaced aesthetic sense that motivates cosmetic mutilations. Activities such as organised dog fighting are plainly cruel. In contrast to the many examples in which animals suffer pointlessly at the hands of humanity, usage of laboratory animals in experimental procedures is purposeful and is ethically scrutinised in advance. However, this process leads to the harms that might occur being pre-meditated. This may lie behind some accusations directed towards scientists using animals as being at best unemotional, ranging to inhumane and abusive. While animal research has historically received public criticism similar to activities such as hunting, fishing and factory farming, the moral case for carefully controlled research using animals is much more defensible. And yet, an individual animal's perception of pain and suffering is the same whatever the context or 'reason' for its life. A laboratory animal will not have the benefit of knowing that its harm is in 'a good cause' nor can it give permission, so the value of any knowledge resulting from an experiment cannot be the only determinant of whether it can be justified. A system to compare life experiences of laboratory animals with farm, companion or wild animals has been proposed (Figure 11.2).

11.4 Ethical Standpoints

The philosophical case for unimpeded use of animals for research is usually based around a concept of the superiority of humans over other species. Where the research is for medical purposes, the moral obligation of humans to prevent the suffering of other humans is also cited. Others argue that all living creatures have inherent value and hence moral rights. It would seem contradictory that a species could be similar enough to humans for experimental data to be useful, yet different enough for any suffering to be morally acceptable. Further, the moral status of a 'subject of a life' would include the right never to be treated merely as a means to the ends of others (Regan 2004).

There is general agreement in the scientific community that progress through animal experimentation is expensive, bureaucratic and subject to animal-induced variability and that, aside from any ethical issues, it is rarely the method of choice. Extrapolation between species is a common cause of reducing confidence in experimental conclusions. However, these constraints alone are not enough to ensure that animals are only used when essential. Any justifiable use of animals must

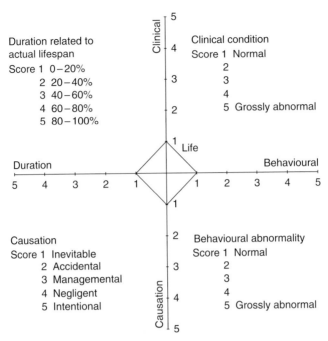

Figure 11.2 Welfare illustrator grid for assessing animal welfare across sectors through the comparison of four-sided figures derived from plotting the scores of component parameters of separate events which challenge an animal's welfare. Source: Wolfensohn & Honess (2007). Reproduced with permission from UFAW.

include an acceptance that animals are not merely tools. For many biomedical advances, animal research has indisputably been part of the pathway to progress – but that is not the same as saying that animal research was *necessary* for that progress. Indeed some would say that advances have been made despite animal research. The crucial question is – how great are the benefits that *only* animal research can deliver?

Scientists who use animals would argue that an ability to balance or set aside the short-term price of agreeing to cause harm to animals for a long-term gain that is judged to be greater demonstrates moral responsibility, as they are acting as moral agents (Nuffield Council on Bioethics 2005). However, in order to perform statistically sound experiments animals usually need to be 'grouped' and this has an unintended effect of 'depersonalising' the group's members. In addition, when animals might suffer, there is a natural tendency towards emotional detachment on the part of handlers and experimenters alike, for the protection of their own emotions. Both of these tendencies should be resisted in good laboratories by remembering the principle that 'good welfare results in good science' and must be based on understanding the individual as well as the group. Naturally, anti-vivisectionists find these arguments hard to accept.

Porter (1992) suggested that research scientists should follow Schweitzer's principle of 'respect for all life' and become anti-vivisectionists at heart. This apparent contradiction would act as an internal regulator of experimental design under the guidance of ethical tool kits, one of which he proposed. The 3Rs of reduction, refinement and replacement, first proposed by Russell and Burch (1959), have grown to become a popular shorthand against which to judge ethical tool kits and are discussed in more detail below.

One consequence of the need for experimental planning is the creation of a convenient framework for assessment of likely harms and potential benefits. This has been seized upon by all sides of the debate, apart from abolitionists, as a means to judge the merits of any given proposal. The resulting mechanisms for practical ethical appraisal are more advanced than in most other spheres of veterinary work. For example, the ethical framework around using prosthetic limb replacements for companion animals is in an early stage of construction (McCulloch 2011).

As we have already seen, majority opinion today is a reluctant acceptance of the need to use animals in certain circumstances (although these differ markedly between individuals) and a wish for independent regulation such that scientific users of animals are answerable to society at large. The argument turns on whether society is prepared to set aside current and future benefits that may arise from animal research on the basis of a moral obligation to the species used.

The philosophy that best describes the balance of public sentiment is utilitarianism. Crucially, utilitarianism does not rule out any harms as a matter of principle. However, parts of the regulatory framework of both the UK and EU override utilitarianism in an attempt to mirror majority public opinion of ethical 'lines in the sand'. These elements arise from the philosophy of deontology which argues that some actions should be seen as moral duties to be adhered to whatever the consequences. A problem with mixing these two approaches is knowing when to apply each principle and in particular how to manage cases on the margins. This may be illustrated by the following examples.

1. At what point in the phylogenetic tree should animals fall under ethical considerations and legal protection? At present the UK law protects all living vertebrates plus *Octopus vulgaris*, whereas EU directive 2010/63/EU includes all cephalopods. This suggests that these species matter, whereas the remaining do not. Other species considered for inclusion during drafting of the latter legislation included decapod crustaceans, some spiders and insects such as honey bees. Complexity (number of synapses) of the brain is not always a helpful measure of sentience or suffering (Hubrecht, in preparation) and the evolutionary tree has many examples of convergent as well as divergent evolution. Natural selection produces species that are best fitted to their environment, not those that are the most sentient. The idea that there is a link between degree of evolutionary development and capacity to suffer is a gross oversimplification, but is used as

a basis for regulation. A purely ethical approach to regulation might be to confer the benefit of the doubt for any species where sentience is disputed.

The UK effectively banned the use of great apes in regulated procedures in 1997, and in 2010, EU directive 2010/63/EU (Article 8) agreed unless (Article 55) 'exceptional and scientifically justifiable reasons' become apparent. It could be argued that by taking a deontological standpoint, the UK encouraged others to follow suit, but there is a lack of international endorsement as the USA continues to allow the use of apes. In addition, the regulatory caveat of Article 55 produces an uncomfortable ethical position that might provocatively be described as 'conditional deontology'.

2. During the drafting of EU directive 2010/63/EU, calls were made for a ban on experiments involving severe or prolonged suffering, irrespective of the perceived need or justification. In effect, the harm–benefit balance would have deontological limits applied. Problems with this approach include how to define 'severe and prolonged suffering' and how to act in the unlikely event of overriding need, such as a lethal human pandemic. In Directive Article 15, it states that '*a procedure is not performed if it involves severe pain, suffering or distress that is likely to be long-lasting and cannot be ameliorated*' but again this is subject to the force majeure arguments of Article 55 which allows the 'line in the sand' to be circumvented.

3. Selling cosmetics that have been tested on animals was banned throughout the EU in 2009. The reduction in the use of animals for this purpose has been widely welcomed. However, a difficulty arises on the margins of defining a cosmetic. Substances such as botulinum toxin have a license for only medical use but are also used for primarily cosmetic purposes; batches are tested for potency using animals. Should sun blocks which reduce the risk of skin melanomas be classed as cosmetics or medicines?

4. Special protections are offered under UK law for research dogs, cats, equids and non-human primates. The reason is more to do with the special emotional attachment that humans have for these species than any scientific grounds. No special protections are offered for species with probably overlapping degrees of sentience such as pigs, sheep, dolphins, foxes or even crows. Should not all sentient species be protected equally?

11.4.1 Utilitarianism

Once deontological exclusions have been applied, the remaining uses of laboratory animals are usually judged according to principles of utilitarianism, a development of consequentialist reasoning. Consequentialism argues that the value of an action is determined by its outcome. To go forward, the harms and benefits of any action need to be known and compared and the balance of benefit over harm should be greater than any other feasible option. Utilitarianism, espoused by philosophers such as Bentham and Mill, further argues that there is a moral duty to maximise the balance of benefits to harms (Nuffield Council on Bioethics 2005). Within the arena of laboratory animal research, this has become the cornerstone of ethical judgements in the use of laboratory animals. The system has the perceived advantage of each proposal receiving case by case attention with no preconceptions.

An objective harm–benefit analysis must multiply the value of a hoped-for benefit by the likelihood of achieving it, before weighing that estimate against the predictable harms. However, a major problem for any utilitarian analysis is that the (anticipated) benefits and harms are measured in different units, the old problem of comparing apples and oranges. This, as is well known to philosophers, is part of the problem of seeking to make ethics a matter of quantification. Jeremy Bentham had the understandable intention of making ethics 'scientific' (in terms of the science of his day), but J.S. Mill was amongst those who recognised that different kinds of pleasure and pain simply cannot be counted together in any precise way. In the light of this difficulty, it is a good thing that the ethical review process in the UK requires the presence of a number of experts plus lay members to provide balance and increase public confidence (RSPCA & LASA 2010). This variety of experts can help a committee to appreciate the variety of harms and benefits involved, and offset any crude attempt at precise quantification.

Potential benefits are easy to overestimate. It is difficult for proponents of a particular project to remain objective, particularly when career progression is involved. Harms may be easier to predict but are difficult to measure. Limiting harms effectively is directly dependent on local standards of animal care put in place by management and the competence of staff to adhere to those standards.

11.5 Measuring Harms and Benefits

11.5.1 Measuring benefits

Predicting beneficial outcomes of experiments before they have been conducted is fraught with difficulty. If outcomes were known in advance, then experiments would be redundant. The nature of scientific enquiry depends more upon testing the reliability (or 'falsifiability') of a hypothesis than proving unequivocal truths (Popper 1963). However, scientific history is full of instances where progress in fundamental knowledge, using animals, has been shown after the event to have been crucial for advances in medicine and human quality of life. Treatments for life-threatening diseases such as polio, diabetes and smallpox are often cited. Some of this progress might have been achievable by other means, but we cannot know this.

The funding for research using laboratory animals arises from three main sources: Government grants (national or international), charities and the biomedical and chemical industries. The first two categories usually require peer-reviewed grant applications, a process which examines claims of potential benefits. However, industry-driven research ultimately requires a return on investment, which to some extent skews the selection of research area as well as placing demands on efficiency.

Controversial purposes for animal use in recent years have included the following:

- A UK defence research laboratory used anaesthetised pigs to study blast lung injuries caused by explosions. Justification included improved care for victims of bomb blasts. However, an RSPCA spokesman said: *'For many, such a use of animals represents a distressing example of the price animals can end up paying as a result of humans'* inhumanity towards other humans' (http://news.bbc.co.uk/1/hi/england/wiltshire/8507616.stm). In this instance, the ethical arguments for the use of animals overlapped with those on the morality of warfare and politics of terrorism.
- Therapies for avoidable lifestyle diseases caused by smoking, alcohol or overeating. One in four people in the developed world are obese. Should this be addressed through using animals in basic research into addiction leading to drug development or by social efforts to improve human behaviour?
- Toxicity testing of materials such as food additives, pesticides, industrial and household chemicals. A large range of tests are required by laws (which vary between nations), measuring different elements of hazard, including acute versus chronic exposure, effects on different organ systems (eyes, skin, blood, internal organs, etc.), and different stages of life (adults, infants, pregnancy), pharmacokinetics, metabolism into other potentially toxic by-products and carcinogenicity. The details of these tests are beyond the scope of this paper but are well described on http://alttox.org/ttrc/tox-test-overview/. Attempts to improve the process and reduce both animal use and suffering are receiving much attention currently but the numbers of animals used in these tests are still large (www.epaa.eu.com).

11.5.2 Measuring harms

The modern concept of welfare which is now promoted by the Farm Animal Welfare Council (FAWC 2009) is that of *a life worth living, from the animal's point of view*, or, even better, *a good life*. Good standards should also apply to animals used in the laboratory, and in order to ensure that animals can be valid subjects for research, it is necessary to protect their health and welfare. A judgement of the quality of life of experimental animals against the benefits to other animals, or humans, is the basis of the harm–benefit analysis. It is much more than simply the prevention of cruelty: quality of life should be used for decision making and to do this a quality of life balance sheet can be prepared (Wathes 2010).

Proper welfare assessment allows feedback on changes affecting the animal's welfare, but if this is simply an academic exercise, it does nothing for the animal. Decisions must be taken. The outcome could be to do nothing, but if so, there must be reasons why. All those who interact with laboratory animals must accept responsibility in delivering animal welfare; monitoring is simply the tool that demonstrates whether it is working or not.

Suffering can be divided into direct suffering, which occurs as a result of the specific procedure carried out, and contingent suffering, which the animal undergoes as a result of being held in a laboratory environment (Russell & Burch 1959). For example, the way in which a test substance is administered, how much blood is taken, how the animal is restrained or trained, what anaesthesia is used, levels of post-operative care, side effects such as nausea, all constitute direct suffering. Contingent suffering results from such things as housing, husbandry, transport or social hierarchy and may include fear, boredom or discomfort.

Measurement of harms can use behavioural and endocrine data, together with analysis of production records. Schemes for objective assessment of adverse events have been published (Morton & Griffiths 1985; Carstens & Moberg 2000). A pain-scoring system for rodents using facial expressions has recently been reported (Langford *et al.* 2010). Behavioural approaches to pain measurements have the advantage that they include a component of cognition and integrated 'feelings' which methods based purely on neurochemical measurements find more difficult. In its simplest form, persistent attempts to flee and/or showing defensive aggression are clear signs of welfare costs. However, individual variation in temperament includes 'stoical' characteristics that may conceal responses.

Individual measures of welfare are most valuable when considered in conjunction with other welfare-related parameters. The welfare assessment matrix (Wolfensohn & Honess 2007; Honess & Wolfensohn 2010, Figure 2) combines the clinical condition of the animal, behavioural deviations, the duration of the incident and the quality of the environment and shows how a grid can illustrate the temporal component of suffering. Since it is cumulative suffering that matters to the animal's quality of life, as much as single incidents, the points of suffering can be added up over a period of time to determine when a limit has been reached. The matrix must include contingent as well as direct suffering to truly reflect cumulative harms and allows an evaluation of the animal's quality of life. It can demonstrate the true welfare implications of research and the effect of refinements, both at the planning stage and when reviewing finished work to ensure that harm–benefit scoring remains valid.

Rearing animals for humane killing to provide tissues for *in vitro* studies represents the majority of laboratory animal usage. It can be argued that if death is not preceded by any premonition of the event, or any perception of pain, it does not affect welfare. On this basis, the reporting of statistics of animals used in experiments does not include animals reared, housed and killed by an approved method, providing no procedures were performed during life. This logic holds providing that (a) the quality of husbandry can be shown to be such that the animals have (enjoyed) a life worth living; (b) the animals' genetic background and phenotype are not intrinsically harmful and are compatible with their surroundings; (c) it is accepted that animals are not conscious of death or the potential for future life experiences; and (d) death was indeed painless and free from fear. Euthanasia, if carried out competently, may be easier for the animal than those parts of a procedure that may have caused pain, suffering or distress. On the other hand, performing euthanasia can be the most difficult part for the researcher and coping with death of research animals can take its toll on the emotions of those involved (Pekow 1994; Halpern-Lewis 1996). Killing an animal is never a pleasant task; but it does not have to be unpleasant for the animal, provided it is carried out competently and humanely.

Decisions and actions on euthanasia must be made promptly if suffering is to be prevented. Collection of reliable data is essential since, without that, any suffering caused would be pointless and unethical, as the animal would have been used without purpose. Well-designed experiments should detect early signs of distress, allowing the definition of a point at which adequate data have been obtained, but any animal suffering is minimised (Morton 2000). The precise time at which to kill the animal must be based on accurate clinical judgement, assessing the degree of suffering against the potential loss of data. To go beyond what is required for a scientific outcome may cause unnecessary suffering and is therefore inhumane.

11.5.3 Sentience and the dilemma of species choice

Sentience has been defined in many ways, but a critical part of the argument seems to be that for an animal to be sentient an experience must 'matter' to them in a manner which exceeds a reflex response (e.g. a pin prick). Measuring sentience will always be difficult because it is a private matter. Although we may instinctively believe that less complex animals have lower levels of sentience (and by inference may be less able to suffer), the actual evidence for this is far from complete. UK legislation requires that suffering is minimised by using *animals that have the lowest degree of neurophysiological sensitivity'* (HMSO 1990). However, research results derived from animals that are distant from humans in evolutionary terms often bear a greater burden of proof that they are relevant to humans, leading to greater animal numbers or more complex procedures being used. The most relevant species to study conditions that occur in human beings must be humans themselves, but ethics rightly limits the use of humans in research.

11.6 The Rise of the 3Rs

First proposed by Russell and Burch (1959), the successful application of the 3Rs has improved the use of laboratory animals and in some areas enabled progress without animal use at all. In 2004, a UK government initiative established the National Centre for the Replacement, Refinement and Reduction of Animals in Research (www.nc3rs.org.uk/). EU directive 2010/63 makes explicit reference to the 3Rs and requires that *'member States should contribute through research and by other means to the development and validation of alternative approaches'*. Brief examples are given below.

11.6.1 Replacement

Alternatives are often argued not to be 'the real thing', but nor are live animal models. In the field of toxicity testing, USA's National Academy of Sciences (2007) put forward a vision of replacement using high throughput *in vitro* screening assays, tests in 'lower' organisms, systems biology, functional genomics and transcriptomics as well as predictive *in silico* approaches. Practical moves towards replacement amongst regulatory authorities include the Organisation for Economic Co-operation and Development (OECD) guidelines accepting the use of artificial human skin as a replacement for living skin in the testing of chemical irritancy (OECD 2010). Groups such as the European Centre for the Validation of Alternative Methods (ECVAM), the European Partnership for Alternative Approaches (EPAA), the Centre for Alternatives to Animal Testing – Europe and the In Vitro Testing Industrial Platform have risen to prominence in recent years as impetus (and funding) has increased the rate of discovery and application of alternatives to chemical and drug safety testing.

11.6.2 Reduction

When animals cannot be replaced, proper planning of experiments is required in order to produce reliable data with the fewest and most suitable animals. The application of statistical methods such as power analysis and blocking and the use of inbred strains of animal to reduce variation have been espoused for many years (Festing *et al.* 2002) with some success, but it remains frustrating that surveys of published data continue to show improper designs or a lack of uptake of these ideas (Kilkenny *et al.* 2009).

11.6.3 Refinement

Refinement can improve welfare by acting on both direct and contingent suffering. The search for refinement must be continual to take advantage of technological advances. Current examples of refinement in action include (1) the almost universal application and continuous updating of anaesthesia and analgesia methods, (2) a refined non-surgical technique involving trans-cervical instillation of genetically altered embryos into the uterus of surrogate recipients, potentially rendering laparotomies redundant for many thousands of mice (Green *et al.* 2009) and (3) a recent paper (Hurst *et al.* 2010) showing that the usual method of capturing and picking up mice (by the tail) results in anxiety compared with cupping and may impinge on welfare.

A key requirement for the 3Rs is sharing accurate data. There remains a reluctance from scientists and publishers to use print space to report negative results or experimental 'failures', which, if overcome, would avoid needless repetition (Magalhaes-Sant'Ana *et al.* 2009). Sufficient detail on animal care for experiments to be reliably repeated without errors is often lacking (Kilkenny & Altman 2010). The ARRIVE (Animals in Research: Reporting In Vivo Experiments) guidelines are a welcome initiative designed to correct this deficiency (Kilkenny *et al.* 2010).

11.7 Ethics and the Drug Discovery Process

Research programmes targeting diseases of the developed world tend to dominate drug company portfolios. Costs of achieving marketing authority skew research and development choices away from niche treatments for rare conditions, diseases of poverty and the less significant animal diseases, although regulatory initiatives on so called 'orphan drugs' have attempted to address this. Modern society is also highly risk averse and expects new drugs to be safe. Historically, paracetamol did not undergo the stringent toxicity testing before its introduction that now occurs: it is currently the most common drug seen in self-poisoning in the UK (Sheen *et al.* 2002). Other drugs such as Vioxx (Merck) were developed in the modern competitive pharmaceutical industry and then withdrawn following litigation by groups of side-affected individuals (Chu 2005). Biomedical companies are increasingly sensitive to reputational damage and financial loss arising from treatments that have harmful side effects for even a small subset of patients. In consequence, testing potential new medicines has become an attritional process. The fact that unsafe drugs get through the process while some efficacious drugs are probably lost because of safety concerns can be used as an argument to suggest either that the system is inherently flawed or that more extensive testing is required.

How safe should a substance be relative to its efficacy? Since the level of confidence is to some extent related to the quantity and quality of animal tests, this is an ethical question. A reduction in safety guarantees would require a cultural change, perhaps including patients being asked to sign waivers for treatments on a 'buyer beware' basis. This is unpalatable yet, despite the increasing rate of validated *in vitro* replacements, large numbers of animals are used to support the current imperfect system. Greater openness would help to address this problem.

11.8 Openness

Modern society demands accountability in laboratory animal use. If this use is truly defensible and ethically robust, it should be more transparent. Labelling drugs and household substances to show if animals were used during development could be part of this. This would build trust, assist those who do not wish to use products derived from experiments involving animals and increase uptake of the 3Rs. However, some patients may refuse important treatment.

Campaigners in the UK have historically played a vital role in bringing about legislation to control animal research. Martin's Act of 1822 against cattle cruelty, the Cruelty to Animals Act 1876 and the Animals (Scientific Procedures) Act 1986 all owed an enormous amount to campaigners bringing the issues into the public arena. Activism has directly influenced the research of some groups (Cressey 2011) and different parts of the scientific community have either adopted greater public openness or been driven to regrettable but understandable secrecy. Animal cruelty has no doubt occurred in the history of research and anti-vivisectionists have rightly called attention to it. Establishment in 1999 of the Local Ethical Review Process owes much to the importance placed on animal welfare and the ethics of animal research. There is now a degree of peer pressure in many establishments to ensure that the welfare of animals is paramount, both for its own sake and for the management of wider reputational risks. The modern research community generally puts the ethics of animal experimentation at the heart of all its work, and the aim for the future must be not only to maintain this high standard but also to continue openly to seek improvement.

11.9 Conclusion: The Role of the Veterinary Profession

Within the veterinary profession, the use of laboratory animals appears to have a lower profile than some other ethical issues. In a 2010 welfare prioritisation survey from the British Veterinary Association (BVA), only 1 of 12 issues listed (rodent husbandry) referred to laboratory animals. However, all veterinary clinicians need medicines for their patients and must rationalise the use of laboratory animals to acquire knowledge leading to better treatments for other animals. In effect, along with human clinicians and all those who accept recommended treatments, they are end-users of the system.

The veterinary profession as a whole has a responsibility to provide clinical care and preventive medicine for laboratory animals and should therefore also engage in the ethical debate. Some veterinarians may use their skills to conduct procedures on behalf of other scientists. In addition, veterinarians may shift between more traditional forms of veterinary work and practice in a research environment and need to accommodate both in their ethical outlook. The Royal College of Veterinary Surgeons code of professional conduct states that '*my constant endeavour will be to ensure the welfare of the animals committed to my care*' (RCVS 2010, Part 1A (2)). This creates a potential dilemma when dealing with experimental animals as their welfare may be unavoidably compromised in a premeditated way. Although responsibility for limiting animal suffering remains with researchers themselves, vets can and should be assisting in promoting a culture of care. Veterinarians with careers as research scientists with responsibility for their own programmes of research should engage independent veterinary advice for any animals they use. There are occasions when the role of a laboratory animal vet is challenging, if refinements are not being implemented vigorously (Lloyd *et al.* 2008). The skill-sets of veterinarians should make them of particular value in refining techniques.

End-users of animals and any derived reagents provide the demand that leads to their supply. Local ethical responsibility needs to be matched by delegated responsibility for such animals before they are delivered. Auditing of suppliers is one means to ensure ethical standards as well as other measures of quality, and veterinarians are well placed to assist in this process.

BVA policy states that '*The veterinary profession has a legal and ethical duty to care for animals used in research*'. Acceptance or refusal of programmes of work rests with regulatory authorities, but good science and good animal welfare are closely interrelated (Nuffield Council on Bioethics 2005). The laboratory animal veterinarian has an important contribution within laboratories to remind all sides of this truth. The functioning of the Ethical Review Process in the UK has been recently reviewed (RSPCA & LASA 2010) and includes mandatory involvement of a vet with 'expertise in laboratory animals'. Veterinary participation can provide assurance that the quality of science has been adequately balanced against welfare.

Veterinarians should endeavour to ensure that each animal under their care has a life that is worth living, whether in producing food, offering companionship, enhancing the diversity of our ecosystems or advancing science. The veterinarian can add value by ensuring that animals are used with the best possible welfare, that humane endpoints are applied, that risks are appropriately managed and that public perception is accurate.

Acknowledgements

The authors are grateful to Dr Geoffrey Butcher of the Babraham Institute and Professor Michael Langford of the University of Cambridge for their helpful scrutiny of the text.

References

Anon. (1902) The anti-vivisection question. *The Lancet*, **159**(4101), 978–979.

Bentham, J. (1789) *An introduction to the Principles of Morals and Legislation*, Latest edition. Adamant Media Corporation Boston, Massachusetts, 2005 ISBN 1402185642, ISBN 978-1402185649.

Carstens, E. & Moberg, G.P. (2000) Recognizing pain and distress in laboratory animals. *ILAR Journal*, **41**, 62–71.

Chu, W.L. (2005) Vioxx scandal points to deeper industry issues. Available at: http://www.outsourcing-pharma.com/Preclinical-Research/Vioxx-scandal-points-to-deeper-industry-issues

Cressey, D. (2011) Battle scars. *Nature*, **470**, 452–453.

FAWC (2009) *Farm Animal Welfare in Great Britain: Past, Present and Future*, 70pp. Farm Animal Welfare Council, London. Available at: http://www.fawc.org.uk/pdf/ppf-report091012.pdf

Festing, M.F.W., Overend, P., Das, R.G., Borja, M.C. & Berdoy, M. (2002) *The Design of Animal Experiments. Laboratory Animal Handbook No. 14*. Royal Society of Medicine Press, London.

Gilbert, C. (2010) *Report from the Commission to the Council and the European Parliament: Sixth Report on the Statistics on the Number of Animals used for Experimental and other Scientific Purposes in the Member States of the European Union*. SEC (2010) 1107, Brussels, Belgium.

Green, M.A., Bass, S. & Spear, B.T. (2009) A device for the simple and rapid transcervical transfer of mouse embryos eliminates the need for surgery and potential post-operative complications. *BioTechnicques*, **47**(5), 919–924.

Halpern-Lewis, J.G. (1996) Understanding the emotional experiences of animal research personnel. *Contemporary Topics*, **35**, 58–60.

Harvey, W. (1628) *Exercitatio Anatomica de Motu Cordis et Sanguinis in Animalibus* [Translated]. Available at: http://www.fordham.edu/halsall/mod/1628harvey-blood.html

Hayden, E.C. (2008) US plans more primate research. *Nature*, **453**(7194), 439.

HMSO (1990) *Guidance on the Operation of the Animals (Scientific Procedures) Act 1986*. ISBN: 0102182906.

Honess, P. & Wolfensohn, S. (2010) A matrix for the assessment of welfare and cumulative suffering in experimental animals. *Alternatives to Laboratory Animals*, **38**(3), 205–212.

Hubrecht, R. (in preparation) Species choice and animal welfare. In: *The Welfare of Animals Used in Research*.

Hurst, J.L. & West, R.S. (2010) Taming anxiety in laboratory mice. *Nature Methods*, **7**(10), 825–828.

Ipsos MORI (2010) Available at: http://www.ipsosmori.com/DownloadPublication/1343_ sri-views-on-animal-experimentation-2010.pdf

Kilkenny, C., Parsons, N., Kadyszewski, E., Festing, M.F.W., Cuthill, I.C., Fry, D., Hutton, J. & Altman, D.G. (2009) Survey of the quality of experimental design, statistical analysis and reporting of research using animals. *PLoS ONE*, **4**(11), e7824. doi:10.1371/journal.pone.0007824.

Kilkenny, C. & Altman, D.G. (2010) Improving bioscience research reporting: ARRIV-ing at a solution. *Laboratory Animals*, **44**, 377–378.

Kilkenny, C., Browne, W.J., Cuthill, I.C., Emerson, M. & Altman, D.G. (2010) Improving bioscience research: The ARRIVE guidelines for reporting animal research. *PLoS Biology*, **8**(6), e1000412. doi: 10.1371/journal.pbio.1000412.

Langford, D.J., Bailey, A.L., Chanda, M.L., *et al.* (2010) Coding of facial expressions of pain in the laboratory mouse. *Nature Methods*, **7**, 447–449.

Lloyd, M.H., Foden, B.W. & Wolfensohn, S.E. (2008) Refinement: Promoting the 3Rs in practice. *Laboratory Animals*, **42**, 284–293.

Magalhaes-Sant'Ana, M., Sandoe, P. & Olsson, I.A.S. (2009) Painful dilemmas: The ethics of animal-based pain research. *Animal Welfare*, **18**, 49–63.

McCulloch, S. (2011) The Bionic Vet: We don't know where to draw the line. *Veterinary Times*, **41**(4), 14.

Morton, D.B. (2000) A systematic approach for establishing humane endpoints. *Institute for Laboratory Animal Research Journal Online*, **41**(2).

Morton, D.B. & Griffiths, P.H.M. (1985) Guidelines on the recognition of pain, distress and discomfort in experimental animals and an hypothesis for assessment. *Veterinary Record*, **116**, 431–436.

National Academy of Sciences (2007) *Toxicity Testing in the 21ˢᵗ Century: A Vision and a Strategy*. The National Academies Press, Washington, District of Columbia.

Nuffield Council on Bioethics (2005) *The Ethics of Research Involving Animals*. ISBN: 1 904384 10 2.

OECD (2010) *In Vitro Skin Irritation: Reconstructed Human Epidermis Test Method. OECD Guideline for the Testing of Chemicals No. 439*. OECD, Paris. Available at: http://iccvam.niehs.nih.gov/SuppDocs/FedDocs/OECD/OECD-TG439.pdf

Pekow, C.A. (1994) Suggestions from research workers for coping with research animal death. *Laboratory Animals*, **23**, 28–29.

Popper, K. (1963) *Conjectures and Refutations*. Routledge and Kegan, London.

Porter, D.G. (1992) Ethical scores for animal experiments. *Nature*, **356**, 101–102.

RCVS (2010) *Guide to Professional Conduct*, London.

Regan, T. (2004) *The Case for Animal Rights*. University of California Press, Berkeley, California.

RSPCA & LASA (2010) *Guiding Principles on Good Practice for Ethical Review Processes*. A Report by the RSPCA Research Animals Department and LASA Education, Training and Ethics Section (ed. M. Jennings). Available at: http://www.rspa.org.uk/sciencegroup/researchanimals/reportsandresources/ethicalreview

Russell, W.M.S. & Burch, R.L. (1959) *The Principles of Humane Experimental Technique*. Methuen, London.

Schiller, J. (1967) Claude Bernard and vivisection. *Journal of the History of Medicine*, **22**, 246.

Sheen, C.L., Dillon, J.F., Bateman, D.N., Simpson, K.J. & MacDonald, T.M. (2002) Paracetamol toxicity: Epidemiology, prevention and costs to the health-care system. *Quarterly Journal of Medicine*, **95**, 609–619.

Wathes, C. (2010) Lives worth living? *Veterinary Record*, **166**, 468–469.

Wolfensohn, S. & Honess, P. (2007) Laboratory animal, pet animal, farm animal, wild animal: Which gets the best deal? *Animal Welfare*, **16(S)**, 117–123.

Wolfensohn, S. & Maguire, M. (2010) What has the animal rights movement done for animal welfare? *Biologist*, **57**, 22–27.

Questions and Answers

Q: Obviously, it's not possible to re-home laboratory animals after their experimental life has come to an end and so they're euthanised humanely. Could they be given a short period where they can live a good life before euthanasia? Not only would this be beneficial to the animals involved but it would also benefit those who are against laboratory research.

A: We work with research dogs and cats. It's standard policy to re-home all our animals. Part of my role is to socialise and habituate our animals to a home environment so that they integrate well when they're re-homed.

It is not entirely true to say that animals from laboratories cannot be re-homed: some can be and are. One of the duties of veterinarians in UK laboratories is to determine if welfare would be compromised if an animal was to be re-homed. This is a difficult decision because if animals have become accustomed to a routine, they may well be institutionalised to some extent; their ability to adapt to a new environment may be limited. The idea of a routine post-experimental cooling off period is appealing. Sentimentally I agree, providing that the animals derived a clear benefit. Some financiers of experiments would be less likely to agree but if there was a groundswell of opinion from the general public, then I think the idea should be looked at.

Q: You talked about the veterinarian's role in measuring harm and in assessing animals as candidates for re-homing. How does this work fit into the tripartite licensing system?

A: The responsibilities of laboratory animals veterinarians in the UK include advice on the ethical review process, the 3Rs, suitability of animal models, surgical techniques, post-operative care, recognition of pain, suffering and distress, humane endpoints and euthanasia. These are in addition to the routine diagnosis and treatment of disease. These responsibilities are now being harmonised throughout the European Union through a recent legislative directive. Veterinarians can be particularly helpful as an 'honest broker', while always considering the animals first. The logo of the Laboratory Animal Veterinary Association is a set of scales tilted towards a mouse and away from a human, which sums this up quite nicely. The tripartite system of regulation in the UK involves separate authorisations of projects, people and places. Veterinarians have responsibility to advise on all three strands.

Q: The UK seems to have fairly strict regulations about the use of laboratory animals. There is a well-developed ethical review process and bans on the use of the animals, either in place or coming into place, for various purposes. Yet according to published data, the number of animals being used is rising. Do you think this indicates a failure of the system?

A: The number of animals used in scientific procedures in the UK has risen to above 3.5 million from a low point around the turn of the millennium of just above 2.5 million procedures. The majority of this increase is due to the increased use of genetically modified organisms, particularly fish and mice. Their inclusion in the statistics is a matter of debate, as many are reared solely to be killed humanely for tissue collection. I believe that these genetically modified animals should not be removed or re-categorised unless it can be confidently established that they are not suffering as a consequence of their genetic modification. The increase in animal use means that the issue is not going away: we need to redouble our efforts to reduce, replace and refine the use of experimental animals.

Q: Keeping animals in poor conditions means that our long-term baseline data are poor. In the USA, there is a refusal to change conditions because they're still working with those long-term baselines. Work by Hanno Würbel shows that attempts to standardise conditions are counterproductive; providing varied conditions and diversity of housing and diversity of conditions for animals is better at standardising results.

Institutional Animal Care and Use Committees in the USA provide a good model for case-by-case analysis. However, they do not usually provide an overview of whether a particular type of research ought to be going on at all. I would suggest that they ought to consider at least annually the broad questions rather than just case-by-case questions.

A: I'm very impatient of an inertia that argues that *'we've always done it this way therefore we can't improve animal care because it will mess up our data'*.

Q: Ethical decisions should satisfy the majority of society and should be made independently of animal users. However, animal-using scientists can play an important role in ethics committees because they can talk about the quality of their studies. Do you agree?

A: The current construction of ethical review committees in the UK includes scientific users of animals, scientific non-users of animals, veterinarians, administrators, animal care staff and lay members. Scientific users of animals should be part of the decision-making process but should not make the final decisions.

Production Animals: Ethical and Welfare Issues Raised by Production-focused Management of Newborn Livestock

12

DAVID J. MELLOR

Massey University

Abstract: Urban consumers raise concerns about the animal welfare costs of farming practices that were originally devised, at least in part, to maximise the availability and minimise the financial cost of animal-derived products. Familiar examples are the high-density management of pigs and poultry, nutritional inadequacy in high-yielding dairy cows and the transport and slaughter of livestock. However, a potentially sensitive issue that is receiving growing attention is the impact of production-orientated breeding strategies, induction of birth and neonatal management on the mortality and welfare of newborn farm animals. The potent image of debilitated, dying or dead newborns raises questions such as: How much neonatal death may be justified by the natural hazards of birth? Is financially or production-driven breeding for greater litter size, which is accompanied by an inevitable increase in mortality rate, acceptable?

Veterinary & Animal Ethics: Proceedings of the First International Conference on Veterinary and Animal Ethics, September 2011, First Edition. Edited by Christopher M. Wathes, Sandra A. Corr, Stephen A. May, Steven P. McCulloch and Martin C. Whiting.

Should healthy newborns be euthanised in anticipation of almost certain poor welfare later? In what ways might the genetically pre-programmed, culturally reinforced human emotional commitment to care for and protect vulnerable young influence ethical thinking about the management of newborn farm animals? These questions are considered by referring to examples of production-orientated approaches used in the dairy, sheep and pig industries.

Keywords: animal welfare, calves, concern, consumer, cost, cow, environment, ethics, euthanasia, husbandry, lambs, livestock, neonatal mortality, pig, piglets, production, sheep, slaughter

12.1 Introduction

During the early decades of the last century, sound scientific knowledge of the biology, husbandry and clinical management of animals was quite limited. Yet, at the time, science offered the prospect of providing an objective basis for improving the efficiency, consistency and level of productivity of farm livestock and their veterinary care (Fraser 1999; Mellor *et al.* 2009). Accordingly, there followed seven to eight decades during which primary industries and governments committed substantial financial resources to such scientific endeavours, exemplified by the establishment and subsequent support of numerous agricultural and veterinary research institutes and university faculties or schools worldwide. The outcome was an exceptional increase in the understanding of animal functionality and how that could be manipulated for practical, economic, health and other purposes. This information, now regarded as established knowledge, is available in a large number of scientific texts on animal behaviour, husbandry, nutrition, physiology, breeding, microbiology, immunology, pathology, clinical practice and other such disciplines (Mellor *et al.* 2009).

Among the numerous enthusiastic participants in this enterprise were many fundamental scientists who derived immense satisfaction from discovering or clarifying previously unknown details of and interactions between body mechanisms. At the same time, many applied scientists derived equally great satisfaction from successfully deploying that fundamental knowledge to solve practical, husbandry and/or clinical problems. Yet, on another level, they considered their activities to be dispassionate and value-free exercises in logic because, in accord with the dominant view at the time, they were involved in the objective acquisition of new knowledge and the equally objective application of that knowledge to serve whatever purposes were then considered to be legitimate (Mellor & Reid 1994; Mellor 1998). Predominant criteria of legitimacy related to the utility of the animals and their products (Fraser 2008; Mellor *et al.* 2009), as there was then little or no consideration given to today's ideas about sentience and the capacity of animals to experience negative or positive subjective, emotional or affective states (Green & Mellor 2011; Mellor 2012). Typically, a problem was defined in utilitarian terms, the relevant functional mechanisms were identified if known or researched if not, and then ways of manipulating those mechanisms were devised to solve the problem. This was an immensely successful approach as virtually every practical science-based, animal-related development considered at the time to be worthwhile was of this type. Thus, animal-based scientists were confident about their aims and proud of their achievements, which were applauded by farmers who often benefited from adopting their recommendations. Today, however, some of the consequences of this approach are considered to have been adverse (Fisher & Mellor 2008; Fraser 2008; Mellor et al. 2009). For instance, successfully pursuing the productionist paradigm of 'more is better' is now understood to have had some undesirable effects on animal behaviour, physiology, health and welfare, genetic diversity and the environment (Fisher & Mellor 2008).

Although such adverse outcomes were often unforeseen consequences of well-intentioned scientific activity (Mellor et al. 2009), 25–35 years ago their existence increasingly led to questioning of the scientists' view that such work could be regarded as value free, and this questioning was intensified as greater notice began to be taken of credible ethical challenges to the conduct of animal-based science itself (e.g. Singer 1990, first edition 1975). As animal-based science to that point had been largely two-dimensional, with its primary focus on the acquisition and application of knowledge, it was recognised that a third ethical dimension needed to be introduced because these ethical challenges demanded ethical responses (Mellor & Reid 1994). At the time, this was intellectual territory to which most scientists had little exposure (Rollin & Kesel 1990; Tannenbaum 1991). However, engagement with the values context of animal-based science was considered to be essential if its practitioners were to retain the confidence of the lay public when addressing increasing societal concern about what constituted acceptable use of animals for human purposes, including their use in science (Mellor & Reid 1994; Mellor 1998). During the same period, animal welfare science was emerging as a discipline in its own right (Mellor & Bayvel 2008), and it became apparent that application of its findings to the formulation of minimum standards in farm animal welfare codes required scientists, veterinarians, regulators, farmers, animal advocates and others to make value judgements based on ethical thinking (Tannenbaum 1991; Sandøe & Simonsen 1992; Fraser 1999, 2008; Sandøe et al. 2003; Mellor et al. 2009).

Familiar areas of concern arising from contemporary farming methods that were developed largely as outlined above include the welfare consequences of the high-density management of pigs and poultry, the often compromised health and inadequate nutrition of very high-yielding dairy cows, the use of painful husbandry procedures (mutilations) and the transport and slaughter of livestock (Webster 2005; Grandin 2010). Although scientists and others are currently exploring ways of avoiding, correcting or effectively managing such problems, the spectrum of perspectives canvassed in discussions of such livestock production activities now increasingly includes ethics (e.g. Turner & D'silva 2006; Armstrong & Botzler 2008; Tulloch 2011). Thus, in general terms, there is interest in exploring how ethical considerations may inform decisions about what are and are not acceptable farming practices. A major purpose of the present paper is to contribute to these discussions by using specific examples drawn from an area that has not been subjected to much analysis of this type to date, namely, the impacts of breeding strategies, the induction of birth and/or the extent of neonatal intervention on the mortality and welfare of newborn livestock, in particular dairy calves, lambs and piglets. Farmers will need to show that they are aware of the implications of such multidimensional thinking on these matters if they wish to retain public support for their methods. Images of debilitated, dying or dead newborns presented with increasing regularity by the media are particularly potent. They heighten public concern about neonatal suffering on farms and generate opprobrium directed at those farmers whose statements focus on the economic losses they sustain, thereby wrongly suggesting indifference to the suffering such newborns may experience (Mellor 2010a).

12.2 Production-Orientated Neonatal Management Issues

In this section, a science-based productionist perspective on several management approaches that have impact on the survival potential or require the purposeful euthanasia or slaughter of calves, lambs and piglets will be outlined as a prelude to the next section in which consideration will be given to some ethical and animal welfare issues that these approaches raise.

12.2.1 Induced calves

Non-therapeutic induction of birth in a small proportion of animals has been used to improve management efficiency by synchronising calving and lactation across individual herds (Taverne & Noakes 2009). It has also been used in pasture-based dairy systems, such as those prevalent in New Zealand, to maximise milk production by manipulating calving dates so that the changing nutritional demands of the cows coincide more closely with suitable pasture growth patterns (Taverne & Noakes 2009). The method, based on a detailed knowledge of the hormonal control of birth in ruminants (Thorburn & Challis 1979), was probably first used to terminate pregnancy in diseased or injured cows (therapeutic inductions) before it began to be used to enhance husbandry efficiency and economic returns from milk (production-driven inductions). It involves the injection of hormones into the mother, principally corticosteroids (Taverne & Noakes 2009), which act on the uterus directly and, after entering the fetal circulation, also act on fetal and placental tissues (Challis & Thorburn 1975). The aim is to simulate the normally occurring pre-birth surge in fetal cortisol release which triggers a cascade of changes in other hormones that are required both for the pre-birth maturations of fetal tissues (Mellor 1988; Liggins 1994) and for the onset, progression and completion of labour (Thorburn & Challis 1979; Liggins 1994). The desired outcome of premature birth is usually achieved, but there are several complications, some of which affect the calves (Taverne & Noakes 2009). These complications usually occur because pre-birth maturation of fetal tissues, including the lungs, is insufficient. The closer the proximity of induction to the time of natural birth, the fewer the maturational impediments to calf survival and *vice versa* (Taverne & Noakes 2009). Most induced newborn calves with immature lungs initially struggle or lift their heads and repeatedly gasp for breath until they die, behaviour which is suggestive of asphyxial suffering. The fact that such calves cannot suffer if they never successfully breathe air and therefore remain unconscious (Mellor 2010b), gives little reassurance to those observers who are strongly affected by seeing these calves as they are dying. Indeed, a strongly adverse public perception of the state of induced calves led to the New Zealand dairy industry's commitment to implement a phased marked reduction in non-therapeutic inductions and contributed to the National Animal Welfare Advisory Committee strongly discouraging the practice (Anonymous 2010). Finally, even when calves of this type and other more mature calves that do breathe successfully are humanely and expeditiously killed, that act itself can have negative emotional impact on those directly involved and any observers (Mellor 2010b; Mellor *et al.* 2010).

12.2.2 Bobby calves

Dairy cows are maintained in order to provide milk and milk-derived products for human consumption. The birth of calves is essential to initiate lactation, but when viewed strictly in terms of the production imperatives of maximising milk yield and efficient management of dairy farms, calves are an inconvenience. Nevertheless, there are some financial incentives to committing time and resources to promote calf survival, health and growth. For example: the first milk (colostrum), which must be excluded from the bulk milk collected by dairy companies, is used to enhance the survival potential of all calves; some female calves are retained in the herd to replace culled mature cows; other calves may be reared elsewhere for dairy beef; and the remainder, so-called bobby calves, are usually slaughtered within 5–10 days of birth to provide veal-like meats and other products (Stafford *et al.* 2001; Anonymous 2010). In dispassionate managerial terms, therefore, bobby calves may be seen to be surplus dairy animals which are born, live a few days, and are then disposed of by slaughter at the earliest time that regulations permit. Yet, such calf disposal is rarely dispassionate, especially with calves killed on farm, but some farmers may be spared from the full emotional impact of that when it is done by others at slaughter plants located elsewhere.

12.2.3 Lamb mortality

Much sheep farming activity revolves around the annual birth of lambs that, eventually, will be slaughtered for meat, kept for wool or retained as replacements. The dominant objective is to rear as many healthy lambs per ewe as genetics, land area, farm topography, climate, feed availability and quality, facilities, husbandry constraints and affordable veterinary care will permit. Neonatal lamb mortality has a significant impact on this objective because each year an average of 10–25% of lambs reportedly die within the first 3–7 days after birth, most of them within the first 1–2 days (Mellor & Stafford 2004). However, between different farms in a particular region, the range can be as wide as 5–70% (Alexander 1984). Among the numerous interacting factors that are known to increase the mortality rate (Alexander 1984; Mellor 1988; Mellor & Stafford 2004; Dwyer & Lawrence 2005; Dwyer 2008) are a birth weight below the breed norm and elevated litter size, such that twins and especially triplets are at greater risk than are singletons. Superimposed upon this are the deleterious effects of cold exposure, especially when the weather is wet and windy as well. A number of strategies have been used successfully to minimise lamb losses (Fisher & Mellor 2002). At one end of the spectrum, breeds of sheep are chosen that have undergone rigorous selection for ease of lambing and minimal shepherding in extensive environments. These breeds have a smaller average litter size as well as demonstrable physical, physiological and behavioural traits underlying a predisposition for enhanced lamb survival (Fisher & Mellor 2002; Dwyer & Lawrence 2005). Such breeds are more commonly used in hill country or other inaccessible or potentially inhospitable areas where shepherding is hindered. At the other end of the spectrum, the breeds used have been selected genetically in contexts of intensive shepherding and provision of shelter, interventions that have been deployed to help minimise the potentially higher lamb losses in these breeds (Mellor 1988; Eales et al. 2004). In general, these ewes have higher average litter sizes, give birth more slowly and mother their lambs less intensely, while their newborn lambs often weigh less, are slower to stand and then suck from the udder, exhibit less active bonding behaviour and are less cold resistant (Fisher & Mellor 2002; Dwyer & Lawrence 2005). Other chosen combinations of breed, intensity of shepherding and provision of shelter occupy intermediate positions on this spectrum of management approaches (Fisher & Mellor 2002). Despite considerable success in reducing overall lamb losses across this spectrum (Fisher & Mellor 2002; Mellor & Stafford 2004), significant mortality rates appear to be unavoidable. A constructive analysis of the wider implications of this should show farmers how strictly productionist perspectives can and should be modulated in ways that would help to assuage public concern about these annual lamb death events (Mellor 2010a).

12.2.4 Piglet mortality

Pre-weaning piglet mortality rates have markedly decreased over time, reportedly averaging about 35% in 1924 and 13–15% in 2000 (Lay et al. 2002). Factors contributing to this decline include improved knowledge of sow nutrition, environmental impacts (including cold), disease prevention and treatment, hygiene and the major specific causes of piglet mortality, knowledge which was successfully applied to the development of better husbandry approaches, farrowing facilities and veterinary care. Nevertheless, mortality rates remained significant. During more recent decades, one 'productionist' objective of pig breeding programmes has been to increase litter size at birth in order to maximise the number of piglets weaned per sow per year (Grandinson *et al.* 2002). However, as greater litter size gives rise to more stillborn piglets as well as to higher mortality rates among live born piglets between birth and weaning (Grandinson *et al.* 2002; Lay *et al.* 2002; Borges *et al.* 2005), this objective, if successful, may be achieved at the cost of greater piglet mortality. Mean litter size now appears to be around 10–12, ranging in individual sows between 6 and 18 (Grandinson *et al.* 2002; Borges *et al.* 2005), a mean of 3–12% of piglets are stillborn (Borges *et al.* 2005) and a mean of 12–35% die between birth and weaning (Varley 1995; Lay *et al.* 2002). Functional predisposing factors include prolonged farrowing/dystocia, low birth weight, starvation, disease and maternal undernutrition, and sow behavioural factors include overlying or crushing, savaging and, in outdoor units, abandonment of piglets (Varley 1995; Fraser & Broom 1998; Grandinson *et al.* 2002; Lay *et al.* 2002; Borges *et al.* 2005; Andersen *et al.* 2007). As with lamb mortality, it seems that significant levels of piglet mortality are unavoidable.

12.3 Ethical and Animal Welfare Issues

The primary purpose of this section is to stimulate discussion about ethical and related animal welfare issues raised by the 'productionist' perspectives outlined above, not to draw definitive ethical conclusions.

Birth 'in the wild' is hazardous. It is normal for a proportion of newborn and very young animals to die. It is unsurprising, therefore, that significant rates of mortality are also found in domesticated animals (Mellor & Stafford 2004). Although it is not immediately obvious what rates of on-farm mortality may be justified ethically by the natural hazards of birth, it is clear that some level of neonatal death is unavoidable even when the very best care is provided. However, usual mortality rates will be higher than this minimum because the management system (extensive/intensive), facilities (outdoor/indoor), available time and cost constrain the provision of care, so the best that would be possible in ideal circumstances is not practically achievable on farms. Yet, knowledgeable application of science-based strategies for managing the dam and offspring before, during and after birth has been correctly credited with keeping mortality rates lower than they would be otherwise (Eales *et al.* 2004; Mellor & Stafford 2004). From an ethics-of-care perspective (Sandøe *et al.* 2003), therefore, it may be argued that an acceptable minimum would be the neonatal mortality rate remaining after the conscientious application of validated current methods designed to maximise survival. If so, one implication of the declared 'productionist' breeding objective of increasing the litter size of various strains of sheep and pigs (Grandinson *et al.* 2002; Stafford & Gregory 2008), which will predictably increase neonatal mortality rates unless additional specialised post-natal care methods are adopted, would be a heightened ethical obligation to assiduously apply these remedial measures. However, any such additional neonatal deaths may be regarded as less acceptable than others because they can be avoided simply by not adopting this breeding strategy.

A major reason for concern about neonatal mortality is the expectation that before death the young will suffer (Mellor & Stafford 2004; Dwyer 2008). However, that will not be the case in young that remain unconscious before death, because consciousness is a prerequisite of suffering. There is now compelling evidence that farm animal fetuses remain in unconscious states throughout late pregnancy and birth, and that newborns only become conscious once they successfully breathe air (Mellor & Diesch 2006; Mellor 2010b). Thus, unconsciousness would be expected to prevent welfare compromise in immature calves that cannot expand their lungs following induced birth and in piglets that die before or during birth or die immediately after birth before they start to breathe. That is reassuring from a welfare perspective. In contrast, most calves, lambs and piglets that die after a natural birth breathe successfully, become conscious and thereafter may experience welfare compromise in forms that include breathlessness, chilling distress, hunger, sickness, pain and/or separation anxiety (if they have bonded with their mothers) (Mellor & Stafford 2004; Dwyer 2008). These states will be experienced while consciousness is maintained, but hypothermia, which commonly precedes death of newborn and young animals, dulls consciousness and may thereby provide some relief (Mellor & Stafford 2004). Nevertheless, quite unpleasant experiences may dominate the short lives of these young animals. Although it has been suggested in terms of utilitarian ethics that experiencing a 'decent' or 'good' life might reasonably compensate mature animals for being slaughtered in order to provide the products for which they are reared (Sandøe *et al.* 2003; Lund & Olsson 2006; Yeates 2011), no such compensation appears to be applicable to those young that die spontaneously after short unpleasant lives, even when their carcases may provide commercial returns as occurs in New Zealand.

These observations raise the question of what role euthanasia might have in reducing or preventing suffering in newborns. Of course, euthanasia would rarely be possible with hands-off, extensively managed flocks of sheep kept in fairly inaccessible areas, but, as already noted, the breeds used in these circumstances often achieve higher rates of lamb survival in the absence of shepherding (Fisher & Mellor 2002; Dwyer & Lawrence 2005). Moreover, intervention with such breeds may disturb ewe–lamb bonding and increase lamb losses (Fisher & Mellor 2002). On the other hand, the accessibility of intensively and semi-intensively managed livestock increases the opportunity, and possibly the obligation, to employ euthanasia. For instance, it may be argued that induced calves that are struggling to breathe and clearly will not survive should not be left to die of their own accord, especially if there is any likelihood that they may become conscious. Nor should any conscious calf, lamb or piglet, born naturally, whose survival is unlikely because of serious functional impairment or debility and the absence of effective remedies. In practice this would require clear decision criteria for the implementation of euthanasia and may be justified ethically in terms of minimising harm. However, a form of what might be called anticipatory euthanasia may be more questionable. This is where the most vulnerable newborns in a litter would be euthanised, despite being in a reasonable state at the time, in order to prevent them from suffering later through failure to compete for milk with stronger litter mates. For example, the smallest or weakest of triplet lambs or of piglets in litters of more than about 12–14 could be euthanised. This would tend to improve both the welfare and the production potential of the remaining members of the litter. Such anticipatory euthanasia might be more acceptable in sheep and pigs managed semi-intensively where it would be difficult to intervene again after giving immediate care at birth. However, it may be deemed to be less acceptable among more easily accessed intensively managed animals where cross fostering of selected newborns onto other dams may be carried out successfully (Eales *et al.* 2004; Andersen *et al.* 2007). Hand rearing is also an option with intensively managed lambs (Eales *et al.* 2004) and is usual with most dairy calves (Anonymous 2010).

In fact, the usual on-farm approach with accessible newborns is to provide whatever care is possible practically and economically in light of the available facilities, knowledge, skills and time. Moreover, caring for newborns using well-validated methods under favourable circumstances can be very successful (e.g. Eales *et al.* 2004; Andersen *et al.* 2007). A strong motivation to engage in such activity rests on our inherited ancestral drive or desire to care for and protect newborn human infants as well as the vulnerable young of other species (Mellor *et al.* 2010). This emotional drive, which is culturally reinforced and is undoubtedly felt by farmers and lay members of the public alike (Mellor 2010a), is concordant with ethics-of-care thinking (Sandøe *et al.* 2003). Interestingly, an associated strong reluctance to avoid harming newborns helps to explain why many farmers evidently prefer to let weak or debilitated young die 'naturally' rather than take the active step of euthanising them, despite the fact that, judged in terms of minimising suffering, euthanasia would often be the preferable option.

In concluding this brief analysis, it might be argued that ethically it is not reasonable to expect farmers to do better than nature and avoid neonatal death or debility altogether. However, the decision to domesticate farm animals for human purposes reasonably brings with it an ethical obligation to apply our current knowledge to minimise suffering. Thus, matters should not be made worse, for example by adopting questionable breeding objectives, and positive neonatal outcomes should be promoted by conscientiously deploying the most effective and practicable care methods available in each circumstance. Moreover, the culturally reinforced, genetically pre-programmed human drive or desire to care for and protect vulnerable young should be acknowledged as a strong motivating emotion. In light of this, it is recommended that consideration be given to whether or not this emotionally compelling drive or desire should impose on farmers (and others) a greater ethical obligation to more assiduously care for and protect newborn and young animals than older ones.

Acknowledgements

I thank James Battye, Tamara Diesch and Kevin Stafford (Massey University), Mark Fisher (Ministry of Agriculture and Forestry [MAF], New Zealand) and numerous other colleagues with whom I discussed some of the ideas outlined here. I am also grateful to David Bayvel of the Animal Welfare Standards Directorate, MAF (New Zealand) for approving partial financial support for the completion of this review, and to Corrin Hulls (Massey University) for practical assistance with its preparation.

References

Alexander, G. (1984) Constraints to lamb survival. In: *Reproduction in Sheep* (eds D.R. Lindsay & D.T. Pearse), pp. 199–209. Australian Academy of Science and Australian Wool Corporation, Canberra, Australia.

Andersen, I.L., Tajet, G.M., Haukvik, I.A., Kongsrid, S. & Bøe, K.E. (2007) Relationship between postnatal piglet mortality, environmental factors and management around farrowing in herds with loose-housed, lactating sows. *Acta Agriculturae Scandinavica, Section A*, 57, 38–45.

Anonymous. (2010) *Animal Welfare (Dairy Cattle) Code of Welfare 2010.* National Animal Welfare Advisory Committee, Ministry of Agriculture and Forestry, Wellington, New Zealand.

Armstrong, S.J. & Botzler, R.G. (eds) (2008) Animals for food. In: *The Animal Ethics Reader*, 2nd, Ed. pp. 215–296. Routledge, Oxford.

Borges, V.F., Bernardi, M.L., Bortolozzo, F.P. & Wentz, I. (2005) Risk factors for stillbirth and fetal mummification in four Brazilian swine herds. *Preventive Veterinary Medicine*, 70, 165–176.

Challis, J.R.G. & Thorburn, G.D. (1975) Prenatal endocrine function and the initiation of parturition. *British Medical Bulletin*, 31, 57–62.

Dwyer, C.M. (2008) The welfare of the neonatal lamb. *Small Ruminant Research*, 76, 31–41.

Dwyer, C.M. & Lawrence, A.B. (2005) A review of the behavioural and physiological adaptations of hill and lowland breeds of sheep that favour lamb survival. *Applied Animal Behaviour Science*, 92, 235–260.

Eales, F.A., Small, J. & Macaldowie, C. (2004) *Practical Lambing and Lamb Care: A Veterinary Guide*, 3rd Ed. Blackwell Publishing Ltd, Oxford.

Fisher, M.W. & Mellor, D.J. (2002) The welfare implications of shepherding during lambing in extensive New Zealand farming systems. *Animal Welfare*, 11, 157–170.

Fisher, M.W. & Mellor, D.J. (2008) Developing a systematic strategy incorporating ethical, animal welfare and practical principles to guide the genetic improvement of dairy cattle. *New Zealand Veterinary Journal*, 65, 100–106.

Fraser, D. (1999) Animal ethics and animal welfare science: Bridging two cultures. *Applied Animal Behaviour Science*, 6, 171–189.

Fraser, D. (2008) *Understanding Animal Welfare: The Science in its Cultural Context.* Wiley-Blackwell, Oxford.

Fraser, A.F. & Broom, D.M. (eds) (1998) Early behaviour and parental behaviour. In: *Farm Animal Behaviour and Welfare*, pp. 198–255. CAB International, Wallingford.

Grandin, T. (ed.) (2010) *Improving Animal Welfare: A Practical Approach*. CAB International, Wallingford.

Grandinson, K., Lund, M.S., Rydhmer, L. & Strandberg, E. (2002) Genetic parameters for the piglet mortality traits crushing, stillbirth and total mortality, and their relation to birth weight. *Journal of Animal Science*, 52, 167–173.

Green, T.C. & Mellor, D.J. (2011) Extending ideas about animal welfare assessment to include 'quality of life' and related concepts. *New Zealand Veterinary Journal*, 59, 263–271.

Lay, D.C., Matteri Jr. R.L., Carroll, J.A., Fangman, T.J. & Safranski, T.J. (2002) Preweaning survival in swine. *Journal of Animal Science*, 80, E74–E86.

Liggins, G.C. (1994) The role of cortisol in preparing the fetus for birth. *Reproduction Fertility and Development*, 6, 141–150.

Lund, V. & Olsson, A.S. (2006) Animal agriculture: Symbiosis, culture or ethical conflict? *Journal of Agricultural and Environmental Ethics*, 19, 47–56.

Mellor, D.J. (1988) Integration of perinatal events, pathophysiological changes and consequences for the newborn lamb. *British Veterinary Journal*, 144, 552–569.

Mellor, D.J. (1998) How can animal-based scientists demonstrate ethical integrity? In: Ethical Approaches to Animal-Based Science (eds D.J. Mellor, M. Fisher & G. Sutherland), pp. 19–31. Australian and New Zealand Council for the Care of Animals in Research and Teaching, The Royal Society of New Zealand, Wellington, New Zealand.

Mellor, D.J. (2010a) Farmer and public perspectives on neonatal lamb mortality. *Welfare Pulse*, 6, 12–13.

Mellor, D.J. (2010b) Galloping colts, fetal feelings and reassuring regulations: Putting animal welfare science into practice. *Journal of Veterinary Medical Education*, 37, 94–102.

Mellor, D.J. (2012) Animal emotions, behaviour and the promotion of positive welfare states. *New Zealand Veterinary Journal*. doi: 10.1080/00480169.2011.619047.

Mellor, D.J. & Bayvel, A.C.D. (2008) New Zealand's inclusive science-based system for setting animal welfare standards. *Applied Animal Behaviour Science*, 113, 313–329.

Mellor, D.J. & Diesch, T.J. (2006) Onset of sentience: The potential for suffering in fetal and newborn farm animals. *Applied Animal Behaviour Science*, 100, 48–57.

Mellor, D.J. & Reid, C.S.W. (1994) Concepts of animal well-being and predicting the impact of procedures on experimental animals. In: *Improving the Well-being of Animals in the Research Environment* (eds R.M. Baker, G. Jenkin & D.J. Mellor), pp. 3–18. Australian and New Zealand Council for the Care of Animals in Research and Teaching, Glen Osmond, South Australia.

Mellor, D.J. & Stafford, K.J. (2004) Animal welfare implications of neonatal mortality and morbidity in farm animals. *The Veterinary Journal*, 168, 118–133.

Mellor, D.J., Diesch, T.J. & Johnson, C.B. (2010) Should mammalian fetuses be excluded from regulations protecting animals during experiments? *Alternatives to Animal Experimentation*, 27(Special Issue), 199–202.

Mellor, D.J., Patterson-Kane, E. & Stafford, K.J. (2009) *The Sciences of Animal Welfare*. Wiley-Blackwell, Oxford.

Rollin, B.E. & Kesel, M.L. (eds) (1990) *The Experimental Animal in Biomedical Research. Volume 1. A Survey of Scientific and Ethical Issues for Investigators*. CRC Press, Boca Raton, Florida.

Sandøe, P. & Simonsen, H.B. (1992) Assessing animal welfare: Where does science end and philosophy begin? *Animal Welfare*, **1**, 257–267.

Sandøe, P., Christensen, L.G. & Appleby, M.C. (2003) Farm animal welfare: The interaction of ethical questions and animal welfare science. *Animal Welfare*, **12**, 469–478.

Singer, P. (1990) *Animal Liberation*, 2nd edn. Thorsons/Harper Collins Publishers, Hammersmith, London.

Stafford, K.J. & Gregory, N.G. (2008) Implications of intensification of pastoral animal production on animal welfare. *New Zealand Veterinary Journal*, **56**, 274–280.

Stafford, K.J., Mellor, D.J., Todd, S.E., Gregory, N.G., Bruce, R.A. & Ward, R.N. (2001) The physical state and biochemical profile of calves on arrival at a slaughter plant. *New Zealand Veterinary Journal*, **49**, 142–149.

Tannenbaum, J. (1991) Ethics and animal welfare: The inextricable connection. *Journal of the American Veterinary Medical Association*, **198**, 1360–1376.

Taverne, M. & Noakes, D. (2009) Parturition and the care of parturient animals including the newborn. In: *Veterinary Reproduction and Obstetrics*, 9th edn. (eds D.E. Noakes, T.J. Parkinson & G.C.W. England), pp. 154–193. Saunders/Elsevier: London.

Thorburn, G.D. & Challis, J.R.G. (1979) Endocrine control of parturition. *Physiological Reviews*, **59**, 877–888.

Tulloch, G. (2011) Animal ethics: The capabilities approach. *Animal Welfare*, **20**, 3–10.

Turner, J. & D'silva, J. (eds) (2006) *Animals, Ethics and Trade: The Challenge of Animal Sentience*. Earthscan Publications Ltd, London.

Varley, M.A. (1995) Introduction. In: *The Neonatal Pig: Development and Survival* (ed. M.A. Varley), pp. 1–13. CAB International, Wallingford.

Webster, J. (2005) *Animal Welfare: Limping Towards Eden*. Blackwell Publishing Ltd, Oxford.

Yeates, J.W. (2011) Is 'a life worth living' a concept worth having? *Animal Welfare*, **20**, 397–406.

Questions and Answers

Q: In your exploration of the ethical issues related to neonatal mortality from a New Zealand perspective, you appear to have dodged the biggest ethical issue of all, namely, the induction of birth of dairy cows in order to coincide lactation with the onset of spring grass growth.

A: Non-therapeutic inductions are being phased out. I understand that the rate is now approaching 5%. Dairy calves present a difficulty. They fall into the category of unwanted newborns because managing them intrudes into the efficient running of a farm. If inductions are to be done at all, they must be done very carefully. However, the New Zealand dairy industry has made much progress in phasing out the practice because members of the public regard it as unacceptable; the industry is responding in a commercial way to that pressure.

Q: In Denmark, we have a big political problem with pig breeding. For a while, Danish pig breeders were so efficient that relative piglet survival to day 5 increased, which met the productionist objective, but this occurred at the cost of an increased stillbirth rate. Now, your principle appears to discount stillborns: they don't matter because they don't feel anything. You only count those that are born alive. This approach will come out positive on your measure because there is an increased relative survival rate to day 5. So you think that's fine, even though the public hates it because they see piles of dead piglets, but according to your principle it should be fine as long as the relative mortality of those that are born alive actually decreases. **A:** You may have misunderstood me. In the paper, I quoted the percentage of stillborns from Danish work. My point here is one of emphasis. I'm focusing on the welfare issue, not the ethical or moral issues related to the numbers born that never get a reasonable life. In welfare terms, stillborn piglets are not a problem because they've died before they've had any chance to breathe and therefore experience anything.

Q: Then they're no problem?
A: In welfare terms, they're not a problem, but in terms of the impact of the total breeding process, of course there is an issue.

Q: What kind of issue?
A: Inevitably, there would appear to be in any domesticated species, a proportion that are going to die for others to live. Maybe the breeding structure of pigs needs to be re-managed to decrease litter sizes so that there is not a significant proportion of runts that are going to die *in utero*, before or during the birth process, and, linked to that, so that most fetal and newborn piglets are larger and have a greater survival capacity right through to birth and beyond.

Q: In South Africa, we are trying to drive non-lethal predator growth, but we get serious opposition, mainly from the farming communities. You mentioned briefly this issue of predation. In some countries, it's regarded as a massive issue. Now we've got a conundrum because the farmer wants to make profits, the conservationist wants to keep the animals in due numbers, and there is the welfare of both predated animals and predators.
A: This is an extremely difficult question. I don't know the answer. There are three competing interests. If anyone else has constructive ideas on how to manage three competing interests that appear to be very compelling, I'd welcome their thoughts.

Q: I was interested in your remark that you found it reassuring that animals that hadn't breathed wouldn't suffer. Bull calves in the dairy industry are an issue because they're effectively a by-product and we're often concerned about what happens to them. Would it be logically right, from what you were saying about the importance of the onset of breathing, to suggest that we should identify those calves *in utero* and deliberately induce parturition at a stage at which we could be confident they wouldn't be capable of breathing and therefore couldn't suffer?
A: The answer is 'No' because the solution is to look after bull calves properly once they've arrived and breathed. There is no need for a long ethical analysis here. Just look after the calves properly.

Q: But they're unwanted. We kill about 30% of our bull calves in the UK in the first week alone.

A: Do it humanely and before they suffer. This may seem rather dispassionate, but the reality in the New Zealand dairy industry, as in the UK, is we don't want the calves. We want to drink the milk. We don't want the calves drinking it. What we do in New Zealand is to manage the calves for the first five to ten days, depending on how long it takes, until they are strong enough to be transported to the abattoir where they're slaughtered, or we direct them into bull beef production.

C: That's possibly better than some of the systems here where they're immediately put down once they're born.

Q: You've made an inherent assumption that the newborn needs to be breathing to be conscious. There are conscious fetal feelings, so the point at which stillborns die is important. They may well have gone through a traumatic birthing process to die just before it is complete. The other thing you've not addressed is the impact on the welfare of the dam.

A: I suspected that the question of prenatal unconsciousness would come up. Unfortunately we don't have time for a full account of this here. The environment of the brain *in utero* is utterly different from its environment *ex utero*. There are at least eight neuroinhibitory factors operating uniquely *in utero* which maintain the fetus in continuous, unconscious sleep-like states until after it is born.

Q: We have to have reasonable codes of practice based on science and common sense; they exist both in New Zealand and the UK. You said that it is not reasonable to expect farmers to do better than nature. That can't be right because farming sheep, for example, is completely different to what happens in nature because of breeding. Suffolk and Scottish Blackface sheep are completely different beasts. We expect farmers of Suffolks to do a great deal better than nature does and that's an obligation that we place on them. And this idea that we have these wonderful green, free-range systems and because it's natural, everything is beautiful is not something which you should promote.

A: What I was actually referring to was the perspective of the urban person who has had little or no contact with the reality of farming life, who thinks that any lamb that dies is a travesty and a reason for not managing sheep on farms. I was approaching this issue from a completely different direction. I agree with you, of course, and have made the same point in my paper. As you may know, I have actively researched this area for about 20 years until the late 1980s in Scotland. Over the last 50 years, scientists have worked hard to improve the way we manage newborns in order to help farmers who can now successfully keep lamb mortality rates down from 50% to about 10–15%, 15–20% and 20–25% in the UK, New Zealand and Australia, respectively. In this way, farmers are already doing better than nature.

Companion Animals

13

SANDRA A. CORR

University of Nottingham

Abstract: Many animals are kept as companions: it is the nature of the relationship, and not the species, which identifies an animal as a 'companion animal' (Kristensen 2008). This paper considers aspects of keeping cats and dogs as human companions, reflecting on the equality of the human-companion animal bond, and the issues arising as a result of a shared lifestyle. The perception of the cat or dog as a member of the family is considered in the context of owners' expectations of veterinary treatment, with particular reference to the potential for 'overtreatment'. As a result, it is apparent that the way we keep and treat companion animals gives rise to a number of conflicts of interests and ethical dilemmas, which deserve to be discussed and dealt with, in the same way that we have for decades discussed and dealt with dilemmas and conflicts of interests relating to other forms of animal use.

Keywords: cats, companion animals, dogs, ethics, human-companion bond, owners, veterinarians

13.1 Introduction

The role of cats and dogs as human companions (or 'pets') has evolved over thousands of years, from initially hunting and protecting food stores to their current place as family members. The entitlement of a person to keep a cat or dog is rarely challenged and minimally regulated, in contrast, for example, to keeping farm animals. While anti-cruelty legislation has been in place for some time, there is

Veterinary & Animal Ethics: Proceedings of the First International Conference on Veterinary and Animal Ethics, September 2011, First Edition. Edited by Christopher M. Wathes, Sandra A. Corr, Stephen A. May, Steven P. McCulloch and Martin C. Whiting.
© 2013 Universities Federation for Animal Welfare. Published 2013 by Blackwell Publishing Ltd.

currently little legislation to protect companion animals against 'normal' use that may adversely affect their welfare. The recent Animal Welfare Act 2006 moves the focus beyond simply preventing harm, to making it a requirement that certain positive provisions be made. Nonetheless, a pet remains a piece of property in the eyes of the law, and ultimately can be dealt with or disposed of as the owner wishes, as long as 'unnecessary' cruelty is not involved.

The lack of specific legislation may reflect a belief that companion animals are kept for pleasure and therefore the majority will be well looked after. A recent report by one of the UK's leading welfare charities (People's Dispensary for Small Animals, PDSA) challenges this. In the report, they estimate that there are approximately 12 million cats, 8.3 million dogs and 1.7 million rabbits in the UK, and surprisingly for a nation of pet lovers, the report suggests that the majority were: *Stressed. Lonely. Overweight. Bored. Aggressive. Misunderstood ... but loved*' (PDSA Animal Wellbeing (PAW) Report 2011). If this is truly representative of the life of the majority of our pets, then we must consider the ethical dilemmas raised by keeping animals as companions and ask whether keeping pets is simply another form of animal use.

13.2 Domestication of Cats and Dogs

There is significant scholarly controversy over how and why different species of animals became domesticated, but it is generally believed that dogs were the earliest species to be domesticated, as long as 12 000 years ago. From the original wolf-like hunting companion, there are now estimated to be as many as 400 pure breeds of dogs in the world (Gamborg 2008). Original selection may have taken place based on simple criteria such as friendliness or obedience; however in later decades, selection has been based on 'breed standards', for example traits that are considered physically appealing or based on tradition. Unfortunately many of the traits adversely affect the dog's health and welfare, for example the obstructive airway problems seen in brachycephalic dogs such as Bulldogs. Such breed-related problems have recently received much media attention and will not be considered further here.

Cats are estimated to have been domesticated from 3000 BC and arguably retain more of their *telos*, as Rollin (1993) calls the original nature of the animal (the 'cat-ness' of the cat, or 'dog-ness' of the dog). By nature cats are solitary hunters, and as a result may be better able to fend for themselves as feral or stray animals than dogs. Although feral and stray animals are of a concern, humans seem generally more accepting of cats than dogs in this role (at least in some parts of the world), which may suggest that we apply different ethical principles to cats and dogs in some situations.

The question of whether domestication can be viewed as a special kind of human–animal social contract is also the subject of much debate. Contractarianism is defined as the theory that moral norms come into existence and are subsequently justified through a mutual agreement (McQueen & McQueen 2010). Much of the debate therefore revolves around whether animals were collaborators in the process of domestication, whether domestication can truly be considered a contract in the social sense (as both parties are clearly not free and equal individuals who understand and consent to it) and whether it really is a win-win situation for both parties (Palmer 1997). On the last point at least, domestication may be considered acceptable unless taken to the extreme, for example breeding dogs with genetic defects that cause suffering to either the dog (physical), the owner (emotional or financial) or to both. With the same proviso, domestication may be acceptable from a utilitarian perspective (the greatest good for the greatest number); Gamborg (2008) proposes that it may even be our duty to improve companion animals through selective breeding. Domestication of cats may be more acceptable than dogs from a 'respect for nature' perspective, which holds that we have a duty to protect not just individual animals, but the species to which they belong, as cats retain their original nature to a greater extent. Conversely, it has been argued that if we have significantly altered an animal's *telos* through domestication, such that they are better suited to their new lives, that may make it more acceptable (Rollin 1993), as long as their *telos* is not simply suppressed through lack of opportunity. From an animal rights perspective, it is less clear how domestication would be viewed, although in principle this ethical perspective opposes most forms of animal use.

13.3 The Role of Cats and Dogs in the Family: The Human-Companion Animal Bond (CAB)

People's relationships with their pets differ. Many owners consider them to be family members, others use them to portray a certain image (e.g. by keeping a large aggressive dog), and for others they are possessions, to be disposed of when the novelty has worn off or they become too expensive to keep.

The human-companion animal bond traditionally refers to the relationship where pets are treated, to variable extents, as member of the family. The cats and dogs live indoors and share people's lives in a specific way, unlike other domesticated animals such as sheep and cows. Described by some as 'furry children', they have a 'boundary' status (neither child nor animal) and share our lives (homes, food, hobbies, settee, bed) in way that even our closest relatives, the non-human primates, do not. We know them well as individuals (their likes and dislikes, temperaments, natures) and have an interest in their happiness, rather than just their health. This relationship provides many emotional benefits for the humans, including companionship, unconditional 'love', constancy and lack of judgment, as well as physical benefits such as safety, relaxation and promoting activity. Studies have shown that the elderly who have a pet have a lower risk of stroke and heart attack, reduced blood pressure and cholesterol levels, better social interactions (in people with dementia) and make less visits to their GP (SCAS 2011). In some cases, the owner may become very dependent on their pet, for example lonely, socially isolated people, and the longevity of a pet permits the development of a strong relationship and a common history (Kristensen 2008). Many people put their pets' interests before their own, be it walking the dog in the rain or foregoing the family summer holiday to pay for an expensive operation. Conversely, a vulnerable client may form a strong emotional attachment to a sick animal (Morgan 2008), and insist on treatments being pursued at all costs, irrespective of the animal's best interests. There may even be a degree of reciprocity in the relationship on an emotional level: our pets interact with us, and two-way communication is possible through an understanding, on both sides, of certain types of vocalisations and body language (e.g. tail wagging and purring or barking).

It is also interesting to consider the CAB in the context of dangerous or fighting dogs. Arguably, keeping dangerous dogs or fighting dogs reflects an animal being treated as a possession, rather than a family member. However, a form of the CAB still exists, in that such dogs have been suggested to give status to individuals who perhaps perceive themselves to otherwise have little status in society (Grant 2010). The pattern of people who abuse animals progressing to abusing other humans is well recognised.

Although humans benefit in many ways from keeping companion animals, as Singer (2010, p. 81) says, there is no logical reason why a being's right to protection from physical harm should be conditional on what that being can give back, quoting as an example, babies or the mentally handicapped. Equally, while there is no doubt that the CAB benefits both parties, it remains potentially skewed in favour of the human and, as discussed by Kristensen (2008), it remains largely at the discretion of the human to maintain or break that bond, for example by re-homing the animal or having the animal euthanised. Interestingly, while dogs rarely break the bond with their owner, it is not unusual for cats to do so by re-homing themselves with neighbours; however clearly the nature of the 'bond' as perceived by the cat is different from that perceived by the owner.

13.4 Ethical Issues Arising from a Shared Lifestyle

As discussed previously and highlighted in the PDSA report, the companion animal bond does not necessarily guarantee good welfare for the animal. Companion animals share our routines: in common with ourselves, we may under-exercise them and overfeed them. As Sandøe and Christiansen (2008a) comment, having a close relationship with humans is no guarantee that an animal's welfare is assured: the owner may unintentionally jeopardise the animal's health or welfare through ignorance, for example treating it as a human rather than an animal of the species in question with its particular needs, or failing to understand natural behaviours for which the animal is inappropriately punished. Equally, they make the point that keeping the animal on its own terms rather than primarily on the owner's may be incompatible with the relationship the owner wants to have with the animal. In this context, it is worth considering two common examples of how we affect pets' lives either unconsciously (obesity resulting from overfeeding and under-exercising) or consciously (neutering) to make pet ownership more convenient for us.

Canine obesity is currently considered to be one of the most significant issues affecting canine welfare in the UK, and as such, is a top welfare priority for the RSPCA (2011). Although inappropriate diet or overfeeding is often the result of misplaced good intentions, the end result, an adverse effect on welfare, is the same. Preference theory suggests that to have a good life, it is necessary to achieve what one wants or strives for, and there is no denying that most dogs love to eat. However, the urge to eat results from impulse-driven preference rather than informed preference being satisfied, and so obesity cannot be defended based on preference theory (Sandøe & Christiansen 2008b). Obesity can exacerbate many other conditions such as osteoarthritis and heart disease, and so the benefits of loosing weigh are clear, however very few owners will persist with a diet plan for long enough for their dog to lose weight. A prolonged period of unsuccessful dieting has an adverse effect on the quality of life of both the animal (hunger) and the owner (guilt, frustration). This is reflected in a survey of 153 veterinary practices by Bland *et al.* (2010) on owners' opinions on the cause and management of obesity: 97% of the cases were attributed to human-related factors (dietary/exercise management), and the most common reasons owners of obese dogs gave for resistance to weight loss management were anthropomorphic, such as the '*animal might suffer*'. As Kristensen (2008) comments, this is an example of situation where it may be difficult for an owner to change without changing their lifestyle or establishing two separate lifestyles.

In contrast, neutering a pet is a conscious decision. Neutering is promoted by vets and major pet charities as an essential part of responsible animal ownership. The proposed benefits relate directly to the animal (avoiding repeated pregnancy and potential dystocia, reduced rate of certain types of tumours, fighting, wandering, etc.) and through the 'greater good' argument (avoidance of strays and euthanasia of unwanted animals). With good analgesia and surgical skill, the suffering associated with the procedure should be minimal, and therefore neutering may be considered acceptable from an avoidance of greater suffering perspective. However, others argue that avoidance of suffering is only one aspect of a good life, and there must be something of positive value in life to make it worth living, which Bentham (1789) describes as pleasure. This is encompassed in the theory of hedonism; that a good life is one in which there are more positive and few negative experiences. This should be balanced with the perspective that it is also important that the animal lead a natural and full life, that is nurturing and fulfilling the animal's nature, or *telos*. The theory of 'perfectionism' expands this concept to incorporate the importance of being able to fulfil species-significant potential. However it could be argued that neutering is a way of changing, rather than frustrating, the *telos* of an animal (Sandøe, personal communication). As Sandøe and Christiansen (2008b) ask, is a good life for a family cat one in which it just eats, sleeps and hangs around the family house or one in which it lives a full and risky cat life? Each of my two cats (neutered, siblings) demonstrates a different preference. Whether, on balance, neutering can be considered to be acceptable remains to be determined.

13.5 Ethical Issues Arising from Pets as 'Furry Children': The Importance of the Individual

When pets are considered as members of the family, most owners have expectations of their level of healthcare, and uniquely, will spend far more on their pet than its monetary value. In this context, it is arguably easier for vets to follow the major principles of medical ethics: doing no harm (non-malfeasance), the desire to do good (beneficence) and be fair (justice) and to respect the individual (autonomy), than it is, for instance, when dealing with farm animals.

The concept of 'patient advocacy' promotes the treatment that is most likely to provide the greatest benefit with the least risk, irrespective of the owner's wishes and financial constraints. In reality, it is the client who ultimately determines what happens to their animal, and only in cases of cruelty can the vet disregard the owner's wishes, and have legal protection. As Morgan (2008) comments, professionals are not hired by animals, they are hired by people who require their services as a direct result of owning and/or using animals. However, the client's decisions will be heavily influenced by the advice given to them by the vet, and respect for the autonomy of clients varies. Fettman and Rollin (2002) state that the '*challenge for veterinarians is to provide enough information and recommendations to facilitate adequate informed consent from the owner without compromising the health of the patient, nor imposing personal preferences that may impose acceptance of a level of risk against the client's own inclinations*'.

13.5.1 Ethically, whose interests should take priority?

Considering the question from various ethical perspectives will, not unusually, produce a different answer. A relational view would regard the CAB to be the most significant factor, that protecting/preserving the specific relationship between that owner and their animal is the most important concern. This will not necessarily predetermine the outcome, however, as Kristensen (2008) discusses: the animal becoming sick may strengthen this bond (the owner caring for and nurturing it) or weaken it (if the animal can no longer fulfil the role the owner requires of it). Arguably, therefore, the bond still works in favour of the human. The latter situation may actually reflect more of a contractarian view, which would hold that the interests of the animal are of indirect concern, only in as much as they affect the owner, for example who can no longer share long walks with their dog. In contrast, the animal rights view, that the animal itself is all that matters, potentially disadvantages the owner. A utilitarian view would of course advocate a more equal consideration of equal interests, to include those of the animal, owner, other family members and vet.

13.5.2 What would the animal choose?

A similar situation is faced by doctors treating patients who cannot make informed decisions for themselves: the very young, the old and senile, the mentally impaired or comatose. In such cases, 'best interests' are used: the decision is based on '*the action that is likely to produce the greatest balance of benefit over harm for the individual*' (Berger 2011). Berger describes broadly shared interests as being free of distressing physical symptoms, being free of excessive psychological, emotional and existential suffering, to have dignity preserved and to live in a state that is generally regarded as not worse than death. While it may be possible to identify 'best interests' for a fellow human being, how does one know whether an animal would choose a life in which it was no longer physically intact, for example, whether a hemiplegic dog would choose a life in a cart over euthanasia?

13.5.3 Is palliative care ethical?

Palliative care is described as treatment that relieves the symptoms of a disease or condition without dealing with the underlying cause (OED Online). Palliative care is common in human medicine, and the most difficult decisions deal with whether complications in palliative care should be treated (Löfmark *et al.* 2007). They describe the importance to patients of gaining a little time, for example if there are children involved or if the patient is trying to survive for a special occasion before dying. Palliative care of terminally ill companion animals is often undertaken to give the owners extra time to come to terms with losing their pet, although it is not always in the best interests of the animal.

13.5.4 Does the end justify the means?

The greater or more prolonged the suffering, the better the eventual outcome must be to counterbalance it. However, if as Singer (2010, p. 73) states, many animals have no conception of themselves and live from instant to instant without seeing themselves as distinct entities with a past and a future, then it is difficult to believe that they would choose any suffering, if they could not imagine a future where the suffering had ended. It has been argued that if an animal has no concept of death and no explicit desire to stay alive, then the quality of life is more important than the quantity, and this perspective is supported by animal welfare legislation (McKeegan 2011). In contrast, should an animal be deprived of future happiness, just because it cannot anticipate it – the same could be said of young children?

13.5.5 Overtreatment and 'heroics'

Calman (2004) suggests that social ethics acts in the opposite direction to evolution (survival of the fittest) and that doctors can be seen as the main agents for interfering with nature. The same could be said of vets, as advances in veterinary medicine close the gap between human and animal healthcare. In human medicine, a study on ethically problematic treatment decisions reported that overtreatment (having done too many investigations or given unnecessary treatments) was more common in most specialties than undertreatment (having done too few investigations or withdrawn necessary treatments), psychiatry being the exception (Saarni *et al.* 2008).

But when does treatment become overtreatment? 'Overtreatment' may be defined in a number of different ways, including: a treatment that results in a poorer quality of life than no treatment or euthanasia, one that is chosen in favour of a cheaper but equally effective treatment, or a treatment or test that makes no difference to the animal's condition or quality of life. Advances in veterinary medical care, fuelled in part by pet insurance, mean that animals that were previously euthanased can often be saved, and geriatric medicine (and the associated tendency for pre-emptive or routine screening diagnostics) is a rapidly growing specialty. Intensive care can save animals that would previously have died, but may leave them with significant incapacity – a situation reflected in human neonatology units. As Yeates (2010) stated, animals cannot represent their own interests and must rely on their caregivers, some of whom may have personal interests in overtreatment. Likewise vets, in pursuing academic satisfaction or profitable business, may be biased when advising owners, who may then feel guilty, overwhelmed with choices or simply unaware that they can refuse the treatment. Various studies of human patients have shown that between 19.1% and 56.1% of patients do not know that they have the right to refuse the treatment recommended by the physician (Deveci *et al.* 2005; Erer *et al.* 2008).

Equally, Norton *et al.* (1995) reject the justification of a particular action '*helping to benefit humans and other animals*', arguing that humans have implicitly taken on an obligation to cater for the needs of domestic animals, and cannot therefore sacrifice the individual for the greater good. This ethos is reflected in the veterinary declaration, although the practice is inconsistent: procedures such as blood transfusions are becoming increasingly routine, but cannot be justified as being in the interests of the donor animal. A more extreme example is that of feline renal transplants, which involve the removal of a kidney from a healthy donor cat.

In the case of novel or 'heroic' procedures, it is not possible to determine whether the procedure is in the best interests of the animal until it can be compared to the best currently available alternatives, which is not possible until the procedure has been performed (perhaps many times) and the outcomes, complications and eventual success rates are known. A 'catch 22' situation. As a result, it is difficult for an owner to give truly informed consent, and the owner may be influenced by the interests of the individual veterinarian.

It is possible that many of the changes in veterinary care are driven by the fact that for many years veterinary schools have attracted academically high achievers with high expectations. Combined with more recent changes in the veterinary curricula highlighting the need for business skills, IT and entrepreneurship, there may also be a change in veterinary-focused motivations towards profit, career development, 'heroism', public relations or avoiding litigation, as suggested by Yeates (2010). These developments present modern vets with interesting ethical challenges.

13.6 Euthanasia

Euthanasia is defined as being a gentle and easy death or the action of inducing a gentle and easy death (OED Online). Arguably, the practice of euthanasia is the most significant difference between human and veterinary medicine: as Singer (2010, p. 83) asks, when we say life is sacred, does this only apply to human life? Some doctors have expressed a belief, in this context, that animals are treated more humanely than humans. Although passive euthanasia is quietly condoned in human medicine, active euthanasia is generally not (except in Holland and Switzerland, or countries with the death penalty). The 'acts and omissions' doctrine proposes an important moral distinction between performing an act that has certain conse-quences, for example resulting in the death of a severely disabled child, and omitting to do something that has the same consequences (Singer 2010, p. 206). Conversely, active euthanasia is commonplace in veterinary practice, and perhaps as a result, passive euthanasia (of a suffering animal) is unusual.

In both human and animal medicine, concern is increasingly raised over whether preservation of life at all costs is in the best interests of the patient. In a survey of nurses and physicians on transference from curative to palliative care (Löfmark *et al.* 2007), none of the respondents felt that the decisions were made too early, but some thought that they often were made too late. Berger (2011) states that many human patients expressed a preference for death over continued life in a dependent and non-capacitated state, and even more strongly than for living with physical suffering. Although these preferences may be based on certain reflective capacities that animals do not have, it is possible that some ill or disabled animals could feel frustration about no longer being able to act in certain ways.

Different ethical issues may be raised by the euthanasia of healthy animals. If an animal is incapable of conceiving of itself as existing over time, Singer (2010, p. 91) suggests that we need not take into account the possibility of it worrying about the prospect of its future existence being cut short. However there is evidence that some animals have a concept of self and time, for example some apes recognise them-selves in a mirror, and have used sign language to refer to past and future events (Singer 2010, p. 112). Equally, as previously discussed, the fact that an animal cannot know it has happiness ahead of it (in the same way as a small child would not) does not necessarily justify depriving it of the chance to experience it. From a utilitarian pers-pective however, it could be argued that no wrong is done if the animal that is killed humanely is replaced by one living an equally pleasant life. The alternative to eutha-nasing a healthy animal may be to re-home it, but this does not guarantee that its life will be long and satisfying, rather than short and miserable. Further ethical issues are raised by the policy of 'no-kill' shelters – that no healthy animal will ever be euthanised, no matter how unlikely it is to be successfully re-homed.

13.7 Conclusion

The ethical issues around keeping cats and dogs as companions have not been widely considered, perhaps because we have assumed that pets generally have lives worth living, most of the time. As our understanding of animal behaviour evolves, it becomes apparent that the way we keep and treat companion animals gives rise to a number of conflicts of interests and ethical dilemmas. These deserve to be discussed and dealt with, in the same way that we have for decades discussed and dealt with dilemmas and conflicts of interests relating to other forms of animal use.

Acknowledgements

The author is very grateful to Clare Palmer and Peter Sandøe for providing helpful comments on this manuscript.

References

Bentham, J. (1789) A utilitarian view. In: Animal Rights and Human Obligations (eds T. Regan & P. Singer), 1989, pp. 25–26. Prentice-Hall, Englewood Cliffs, New Jersey.

Berger, J.T. (2011) Is best interests a relevant decision making standard for enrolling non-capacitated subjects into clinical research? *Journal of Medical Ethics*, 37, 45–49.

Bland, I.M., Guthrie-Jones, A., Taylor, R.D. & Hill, J. (2010) Dog obesity: veterinary practices' and owners' opinions on cause and management. *Preventative Veterinary Medicine*, 94, 310–315.

Calman, K.C. (2004) Evolutionary ethics: Can values change. *Journal of Medical Ethics*, 30, 366–370.

Deveci, S.E., Ogeturk, A., Ozan, T., Tokdemir, M. & Açik, Y. (2005) Awareness about patient's rights amongst patients admitting to a primary level health care facility. *Journal of Medical Ethics*, 13, 174–178.

Erer, S., Atici, E. & Erdemir, A.D. (2008) The views of cancer patients on patient rights in the context of information and autonomy. *Journal of Medical Ethics*, 34, 384–388.

Fettman, M.J. & Rollin, B.E. (2002) Modern elements of informed consent for general veterinary practitioners. *Journal of the American Veterinary Medical Association*, 221, 1386–1393.

Gamborg, C. (2008) Animal breeding and biotechnology In: *Ethics of Animal Use* (eds P. Sandøe & S.B. Christiansen), Chapter 9, pp. 137–152. Blackwell Publishing, Oxford.

Grant, D. (2010) Quoted in: Inner City Life – Inner city pressure: Status dog culture in spotlight. Fearon, R. Veterinary Times, Oct 25.

Kristensen, A.T. (2008) Companion animals. In: *Ethics of Animal Use* (eds P. Sandøe & S.B. Christiansen), Chapter 8, pp. 119–136. Blackwell Publishing, Oxford.

Löfmark, R., Nilstun, T. & Ågren Bolmsjö, I. (2007) From cure to palliation: Concept, decision and acceptance. *Journal of Medical Ethics*, **33**, 685–688.

McKeegan, D. (2011) Quoted in: BVA Congress Report – Where do you draw the line on treatment? *Veterinary Record*, **167**: 636–637.

McQueen, P. & McQueen, H. (2010) *Key Concepts in Philosophy*, p. 36. Palgrave Macmillan, Hampshire.

Morgan, C. (2008) Role of veterinarians and other animal science professionals. In: *Ethics of animal use* (eds P. Sandøe & S.B. Christiansen), Chapter 4, pp. 49–65. Blackwell Publishing, Oxford.

Norton, B., Hutchins, M., Stevens, E.F. & Maple, T.L. (1995) *Ethics on the Ark: Zoos, Animal Welfare and Wildlife Conservation*. Smithsonian Institution Press, Washington, DC.

OED Online. Available at: http://www.oed.com/ (accessed on 20 May 2011).

Palmer, C. (1997) The idea of the domesticated animal contract. *Environmental Values*, **6**, 411–425.

PDSA (2011) PDSA Animal Wellbeing (PAW) Report 2011 – The State of Our Pet Nation. The People's Dispensary for Small Animals.

Rollin, B.E. (1993) Animal production and the new social ethic for animals. In: *Food Animal Well-Being* (ed. Purdue Research Foundation), pp. 3–13. Conference Proceedings and Deliberations. US Department of Agriculture and Purdue Office of Agricultural Research Programs, West Lafayette, Illinois.

RSPCA (2011) Available at: http://www.rspca.org.uk/allaboutanimals/pets/general/obesity (accessed on 28 June 2011).

Saarni, S.I., Halila, R., Palmu, P. & Vänskä, J. (2008) Ethically problematic treatment decisions in different medical specialties *Journal of Medical Ethics*, **34**, 262–267.

Sandøe, P. & Christiansen, S.B. (2008a) The changing face of animal ethics. In: *Ethics of Animal Use* (eds P. Sandøe & S.B. Christiansen), Chapter 1, pp. 1–14. Blackwell Publishing, Oxford.

Sandøe, P. & Christiansen, S.B. (2008b) What is a good animal life? In: *Ethics of Animal Use* (eds P. Sandøe & S.B. Christiansen), Chapter 3, pp. 33–49. Blackwell Publishing, Oxford.

SCAS (2011) Society for Companion Animal Studies. Available at: http://www.scas.org.uk/1851/benefits-of-the-bond.html (accessed on 10 June 2011).

Singer, P. (2010) *Practical Ethics*, 2nd edn. Cambridge University Press, Cambridge.

Yeates, J.W. (2010) When to euthanase. *Veterinary Record*, **166**, 370–371.

Questions and Answers

Q: You said that veterinarians can influence clients, and they can. The PDSA report concluded that the veterinary profession hasn't done a very good job of influencing its clients. What could be done? For example, should we be teaching our veterinary students not just communication skills but actually 'influencing skills' and the ethics of influencing?

A: Yes, but we must differentiate between individual veterinarians who may have an agenda and the veterinary population as a whole.

In surgery rounds with veterinary students, I say, '*Don't think so much about the health but look at this animal and see how you could make it feel better*', because often veterinary students are so fixated on, for instance, giving the animal morphine at the exact time that it requires it, that they don't notice that it's got unnecessary bits of elastoplast and mucky eyes and all the things that are more about absence of positives as much as anything else. For example, we default to putting collars on to stop animals pulling drips out when in fact they might really need to give themselves a good groom.

We should better educate our students. We can put as much about ethics as we want into an undergraduate curriculum but unless the 'role models' demonstrate to the students that it's okay to talk about ethical aspects of treatment, I don't think that message is going to get through because students are very good at kind of compartmentalising things. I could stand at surgery rounds and could have an intense argument in front of the students about the best way to treat a cruciate rupture. I could say, '*Why did you do that procedure?*' and it wouldn't become at all scary for anyone, but if I said to a colleague, '*Ethically defend what you did to that animal*' that would be inappropriate. So I don't know that we're actually demonstrating very well from the top down but we're certainly pushing it into the curriculum from the bottom up.

Q: Your comments about neutering are very interesting. Veterinarians promote the benefits of a procedure rather than the negative side, but sadly we also have to take account of the human factor. We are selective about the dogs that we neuter. Humans are very good at taking the line of least resistance, and perhaps won't keep their dogs on a lead or keep them in, with consequences for the number of stray dogs. For example, we had over 120 000 stray dogs in the UK last year, of which 7000 were killed while in the care of the local authorities.

Perhaps we ought to make it more difficult for people to access companion animals so that they know how to look after them. My concern is more stray animals, more animals killed and perhaps go back to this dreadful practice that used to happen 50 years ago of litters of puppies and kittens literally being killed at birth.
A: Client education or owner education is fundamental but I'm going to pre-empt those in the audience who think that it's outrageous that we have to exert that control by 'invading' the animal and performing a fairly major surgical procedure. I'm not sure about the population of strays in countries like Sweden, but it doesn't seem to be a problem there and they don't default to neutering. I accept your perspective and I know it's controversial but wonder if there isn't a better solution.

Q: I was thinking about your equation [owner + animal = veterinarian]. The owner has interests and the animal has interests. In your equation, the veterinarian has no interests, implying that what they decide to do was a product of the animal's and owner's interests. This is probably not always the case.
A: I agree.

Q: It's been quite interesting working at Edinburgh because the clinicians themselves have asked for a clinical ethical review committee to be set up. As yet we haven't really used it, although we've done some retrospective looking at cases that have caused concern. What was interesting was one of the comments that was made that at a veterinary school: you are expected to be cutting edge and many of the advances are obviously because people did over-treat. I was interested in the idea of a cost-benefit analysis, not necessarily for the owner but for future animals.

A: Some veterinary schools are very good at doing just that. For instance, in the United States there's work on joint replacements in animals, for example, elbow joints. These were audited by the universities which had performed them, that is to look at the cases, work out what was working well or not so well, refine the procedure and publicise the improved technique. When the body of specialists and appropriate people determined that the procedure was working satisfactorily, they ran training courses: only when you'd been trained in the techniques and certified as competent, could you then perform them. What concerns me a little, and I don't want to fixate on one particular example, but for the bilateral amputee cat with prosthetic limbs, I don't know how many cats had that procedure that failed, how many procedures that particular cat had, whether that cat is on constant analgesia; clearly, it doesn't walk normally. I'd like to think of myself as an evidence-based practitioner: I'd like to know that before I'd even contemplate recommending that to my owners. I'm not comfortable with the way that sort of thing is becoming sensationalised in the press. Chris Lawrence at the Dogs Trust made a telling comment as well – that if we're selling these procedures as the 'gold standard' without a real body of evidence, you're also making ordinary owners who can't really afford that kind of level of novel therapy feel bad, that somehow they're not taking good enough care of their animals.

Q: A lot of parents and others believe that there are benefits of pet ownership to children and young people in terms of things like responsibility and empathy. Do you think those benefits are real, or do they just allow apparently bad habits and practices to be transmitted from generation to generation? And if they were realised, do you think those human interests trump perhaps the solitary rabbit in order to achieve them?

A: I'm afraid that I don't know.

Ethical Analysis of the Use of Animals for Sport

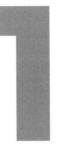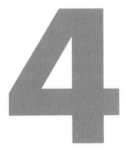

MADELEINE CAMPBELL

Hobgoblins Equine Reproduction Centre

Abstract: In recent years, there has been increasing public and media interest in the welfare of sporting animals before, during and after their competition careers. Regulatory bodies have responded by introducing rules that have undoubtedly improved the lifetime welfare of sporting animals. However, improvements in welfare do not suffice to address the fundamental underlying ethical issue of whether we are at all justified in using animals for sporting purposes, given that there is no absolute need for man to do so and that there are invariably associated risks of stress, morbidity and mortality for the animals. If we do accept that the use of such animals can be ethically justified, should that acceptance be unconstrained, or should we set limits on sporting use? Associated questions of professional ethics for veterinarians treating competition animals relate to the core issue of whether a veterinarian's responsibility is primarily to the animal or to the owner/trainer/team presenting that animal. This paper suggests a hybrid ethical view, which argues in favour of both the continued use of animals for sport and limitations for that use based on respect for *telos* and physiological norms. It concludes that the pre-eminent current ethical question about sporting animals is: '*Just because the animal is prepared to do as we ask, should we ask it?*'

Keywords: competition, dog, ethics, greyhound, horse, injury, owner, sport, *telos*, veterinarian, welfare

Veterinary & Animal Ethics: Proceedings of the First International Conference on Veterinary and Animal Ethics, September 2011, First Edition. Edited by Christopher M. Wathes, Sandra A. Corr, Stephen A. May, Steven P. McCulloch and Martin C. Whiting.
© 2013 Universities Federation for Animal Welfare. Published 2013 by Blackwell Publishing Ltd.

14.1 Introduction

For the purposes of this paper, a narrow definition of 'sport', which includes activities in which man pits animal against animal in regulated direct competition but excludes activities such as hunting, bullfighting and dogfighting has been adopted. The range of sporting events for which animals are used by man is diverse, and to consider the ethics and related welfare issues of each sport individually would be an enormous undertaking. This paper aims instead to use examples from some animal sports to illustrate ethical problems which relate to all of them.

14.2 Welfare Issues of Animals in Sport

Public interest in the welfare of sporting animals has increased in recent years has been reflected in, and to some extent driven by, media coverage. The intense debate surrounding the deaths of two horses and the ban of the winning jockey for overuse of the whip in the Grand National race in England in April 2011 typified this interest (Hancock 2011; Lysaght 2011). Welfare issues affecting sporting animals may be divided into those affecting them before, during and after their competition careers. Some considerations, for example housing and feeding, span all three periods. Generally, the expectation is that high-value competition animals will be well looked after at least until their competitive career is over, since good care maximises the chance of competitive success. This expectation is broadly in line with Rollin's argument that when animals have an economic worth and are treated as individuals, it follows that welfare standards are good (Rollin 2006a). However, there is an obvious argument to be made that the way in which competition animals are housed (e.g. racing greyhounds which may spend up to 23 hours a day in kennels; Saddlebred horses which are shod in a way that precludes turning them out or racing pigeons which are housed in overcrowded conditions) denies them the freedom to express normal behaviour (FAWC 1979). One could make the theoretical argument that, since racing and competing animals have been bred for purpose, this is a non-identity problem (Parfit 1984): for the individual animal existing as a free-ranging, extensively managed member of its species was never an alternative option, and that being so its existing life, albeit deficient in terms of ability to express normal behaviour, is nonetheless, taken in the whole, worth living (FAWC 2009). In practice, however, awareness that extended periods of confinement not only represent a welfare concern but may also contribute to poor performance is increasing, thanks in part to the stance taken by some leading professionals such as the dressage rider Susanne Meisner and veterinarian Gerhard Heuschmann, who have built their businesses around the argument that horses need time to stretch and to express normal behaviour if they are to become successful athletes (Heuschmann 2009).

The two most prominent welfare issues relating to the early part of sporting animals' lives are the rate of attrition before an animal reaches competition age and the effect on injury rates of training and racing whilst the musculoskeletal system is still immature. Donoughue's independent review of the greyhound industry in Great Britain (2007) recognised that: '... *there is a welfare issue surrounding animals which do not ever make the grade: a large number of puppies are unaccounted for each year between earmarking and registration*'. Similar concerns have been expressed about the incidence of wastage amongst racehorses (Jeffcott *et al.* 1982; Wilsher *et al.* 2006). Indiscriminate breeding of 'second-rate' race horses and dogs contributes to the problem of animals for which homes and purpose must then be found. Within both the thoroughbred racehorse and greyhound industries, policies have been enacted to attempt to re-home animals which are unsuitable for racing, as well as those at the end of their careers. Some organisations, such as the many local greyhound re-homing charities and equine charities such as the Re-homing Ex-racehorses Organisation Scheme (HEROS) are run on a voluntary basis, whilst some such as the National Greyhound Racing Club's (NGRC) Retired Greyhound Trust are associated with a regulatory body. The Greyhound Board of Great Britain's (GBGB 2010) Rule 18 sets out the responsibilities of greyhound owners and includes the requirement to make (specified) acceptable arrangements for a retired greyhound. However, it only covers animals racing at licensed tracks, and even then: '*Taken together, the BGRB [British Greyhound Racing Board] initiatives and the welfare charities re-home [only; emphasis added] about a half of the dogs which retire from racing. Some others are personally re-homed by their owners and trainers. We do not know what happens to the rest*' (Donoughue 2007). Media reports of greyhounds being sold to research laboratories, offered to a university as teaching subjects and sent to 'euthanisation specialists' suggest that, though the efforts of the authorities are to be applauded, the end-of-career welfare issues for some sporting animals at least remain unresolved (Foggo 2006, 2008; Jeory 2010; Qureshi 2010).

During the period of its life in which a sporting animal is in training, there are a number of potential welfare issues. The big-money events in both horse and greyhound racing, such as the Derby, are run for young animals. Sporting industries are structured so that the victorious animal usually retires to stud shortly thereafter, thus maximising breeding revenue. Considerable interest has been devoted to the question of whether training and competing animals at an age when their musculoskeletal system is immature predisposes them to (sometimes catastrophic) injury, which could be avoided if the industry was restructured so that maximal prize money was offered for older animals. Donoughue (2007) reported: '*It has been suggested to us that a racing career starting at 15 months may be too early for the health of the dogs. We have seen no evidence to support this view but it seems likely that this is because no formal, targeted research into the issue has been undertaken*'. For Thoroughbred racehorses, such peer-reviewed research exists. The results, however, are not straightforward to interpret since different studies show a varying effect of age dependent upon the type of injury investigated (Bailey *et al.*

1997; Reed *et al.* 2011) and the type of race (Ely *et al.* 2009), and are frequently confounded by differences in racing surface, trainer and training regime. The balance of evidence suggests, however, that for both bone and tendon injuries, exercise during musculoskeletal immaturity is protective (Smith *et al.* 1999; Verheyen *et al.* 2005; van Weeren *et al.* 2008), and therefore that increasing the age at which animals commence training and compete would not necessarily improve welfare.

Another area into which research has been conducted in relation to both horse and greyhound racing in an attempt to improve welfare is the effect of racing surface on injury rate and type (Zebarth & Sheard 1985; Bloomberg & Dugger 1991; Gillette 1992; Cook 1998); this work has recently been extended to horses competing in other disciplines such as dressage (Murray *et al.* 2010). The findings may not always be easy to translate into practice: for example, since many greyhound injuries are incurred at corners (Bloomberg 1989), running greyhounds on a straight rather than an oval track might improve welfare, but oval tracks provide better spectator viewing. Nonetheless, there seems to be a general and increasing recognition, both on the part of the responsible authorities and of the public, that there are welfare issues associated with mainstream animal sporting events, and an increasing willingness to address such issues. Removing or ameliorating specific *welfare* issues, however, does not address the fundamental *ethical* question which underlies all uses of animals for sport, which is whether we are in any way justified in using animals for sporting purposes given that there is no absolute need to do so and that there are associated risks of stress, morbidity and mortality for the animals.

14.3 The Ethics of Using Animals for Sport

14.3.1 Is there any ethical justification for using animals in sport?

It is a fact of life that humans use animals, whether as a source of food, in medical experiments, as companions or for sport, and implicit in this use is a recognition that animals matter less than humans (Sandøe & Christiansen 2008). Society's views on what constitutes a defensible use of animals, however, change over time. Thus, for example, previously accepted use of animals to test cosmetics is now rejected by a large part of the population and (correspondingly) by many of the main manufacturers of such products. Use of animals for 'sport', too, has changed over time: 'competitions' such as dogfighting which at one time were the norm are nowadays regarded as ethically unacceptable. How, then, are we to determine what sporting use of animals is, and is not, ethically acceptable, or indeed whether such use is acceptable at all? On a utilitarian view, many of our uses of animals are justified on the grounds that the benefit to humans outweighs the loss to animals. Thus, one can argue that there is a benefit to humans in eating meat, and to developing new drugs, and that the use of production and laboratory animals can be justified on these grounds. One can claim that, providing that the animals are well looked after and have *a life worth living* (FAWC 2009), this is ethically acceptable. Superficially, such an argument is hard to make in the case of using animals for sport since the benefit to humans is not related to nutrition or to health but merely to vicarious pleasure or to economic gain. High-level sport, whether the athlete be human or animal, invariably and inevitably involves physiological stress, injury, illness and occasionally even death. The benefit to humans of using animals for sport is not *necessary* and yet the loss to animals is inevitable and unavoidable. Maybe in a utilitarian argument, then, there can be no justification for ever using animals for sport: the downside to the animals could not be outweighed by the upside to humans. One would surely also conclude that the use of animals for sport was ethically unjustifiable if one took an animal rights view (Regan & Singer 1989), since the use of animals in sport essentially treats individuals (particularly those which are discarded as too slow or too old) as lacking in independent value and as a means to an end (which might be winning the prize money or selling the semen).

The practical situation, however, is less clear than either of these theoretical arguments and, in my opinion, necessitates the adoption of a hybrid view which allows for the use of animals in sport whilst attempting to preserve their dignity and *telos* (Rollin 1981). It is an oversimplification to argue that the benefit to humans of using animals in sport is unnecessary. Whilst that argument might hold true on an individual level, it does not do so in terms of society as a whole. The small sum of money which my husband won by betting on a horse in the Grand National could not possibly be considered significant to his welfare. However, modern day animal sport as an industry represents a source of employment, both direct and indirect, for many thousands of people. In the UK alone in 2009, horse racing provided ~20 000 direct full-time jobs and ~70 000 indirect full-time jobs. The employment provided by the equine industry as a whole equalled that provided by agriculture (British Horse Industry Confederation, BHIC 2009). Modern day animal sport is considered by some to be as economically relevant as farming. In that context, the same utilitarian justifications may be made for using animals for sport as may be made for using them for farming: we know that there are welfare issues associated with both of these types of use, yet we believe that the associated benefit to human welfare in terms of increased living standards outweighs the loss of welfare to animals. If one is prepared to accept this as a starting premise (and those with animal rights views are unlikely to do so), then the logical view to adopt when considering the use of animals in sport is surely a hybrid one, which has a utilitarian basis but recognises the rights of animals to a certain level of protection of their Five Freedoms (FAWC 1979); to have *a life worth living* (FAWC 2009); and to maintain their dignity throughout their life (Regan & Singer 1989) (this last point being particularly relevant to the question of what happens once an animal's competitive career is over). Within this framework, the question becomes not whether we should use animals in sport at all, but rather whether we are prepared to accept that the ethical justifications for doing so are unconstrained.

14.3.2 Should we put limits on the use of animals for sport (and, if so, how do we decide what those limits are)?

Many of the sporting events in which humans engage animals mimic what the animal would do in its natural environment. Horses in a field often canter around and give the impression (in so far as we can tell) of enjoying doing so. My pet greyhound, every time I flatten our sand riding arena, runs flat out around the perimeter apparently for fun and in a good imitation of a dog racing on a track (though, perhaps in a subconscious attempt to avoid injury, she does change direction). It is often said by horsemen that a horse can perform all of the advanced dressage movements without the help (hindrance) of a rider, and one has only to watch a horse turned loose in deep snow to see that that is true. However, the same horse is unlikely to voluntarily put its neck in a position of hyperflexion (FEI 2010) and hold it there for some minutes. Perhaps, then, one test of what it is fair to ask an animal to do for sport is to consider whether it would do that activity naturally? However, the mere fact that an animal can do an activity naturally may not be sufficient justification for us asking that animal to do it. Horses and rabbits can both jump considerable heights if forced to do so by a predator. They are unlikely, however, to do so unprovoked. Is it therefore reasonable for humans to ask horses to show-jump? Is it reasonable for humans to ask rabbits to show-jump (Brooke 2009)? Does making these demands of animals violate their *telos* even if they are able and apparently willing to do what we ask of them? The ability to jump is an inherent talent shared by horses and rabbits, and therefore part of their *telos*, yet, in my opinion, watching show-jumping rabbits on www.YouTube.com inspires in some a feeling of ethical unease which watching 'Horse of the Year Show' rarely does. That may be, however, because we are accustomed to watching horses – and not rabbits – show-jumping rather than because there is any true ethical difference in what they are being asked to do.

There has been significant recent media coverage about the use of whips in horse racing, as a result of which the manager of Towcester racecourse has announced that all future races will be run under 'hands and heels' rules (Armytage 2011). What is it about the use of a whip that members of the public, many of whom are happy to condone horse racing in general terms, find unacceptable? One rider and former racehorse owner explained her dislike of the whip as being due to the feeling that the horse was winning not as a result of its natural talent but out of fear. This sentiment is another way of arguing that the limit which ought to set on what it is acceptable to ask animals to do relates to their natural abilities or part of their *telos*: when what we are asking exceeds that limit (in this case, can only be elicited by the imposition of fear), it becomes ethically unacceptable.

Extending this argument, competitions which clearly involve an animal being tested beyond the limits of its physiological capabilities also become unacceptable. A day spent at a short-distance endurance competition normally results in an impression of horses which are competing within their 'physiological comfort zone', and is generally accepted as not representing a welfare issue. In contrast, the deaths of two endurance horses during the World Equestrian Games in Jerez in 2002 from metabolic failure associated with fatigue was criticised (Mesoly 2002) and resulted in a recommendation following on from the Sixth International Conference on Equine Exercise Physiology (Marlin 2004) that standards of veterinary monitoring during competitions be improved to ensure that detection of the early signs of stress and fatigue is prompt and results in elimination and treatment for the horses. There is a clear ethical distinction being drawn here between undertaking endurance competitions at all (ethically acceptable) and 'allowing' horses in endurance competitions to be pushed beyond their physiological limits.

14.3.3 The role of lay people in setting ethical standards in animal sport

In most forms of animal sport, the potential welfare issues which result from an animal being pushed past its physiological capabilities and make the competition ethically unacceptable can be ameliorated by correct training. Conversely, the expectations of trainers, owners and members of the public can frame a sport in a way which many find ethically unacceptable because the animals involved are being produced in a manner which seems to go beyond the realm of what is natural (to defy their *telos*). Competition Saddlebreds and Tennessee walking horses provide good examples. Both breeds are (naturally) high-stepping and extravagant, and these characteristics are rewarded in ridden competition. Training techniques, such as the use of stacked, weighted shoes, can cause sheared heels, quarter cracks and laminitis, and fetlock chains, which have the potential to cause lesions. Similarly, reward of a highly carried tail in competition has perpetuated the practice (which has been banned by some breed societies) of surgical 'nicking' of the retractor muscles on the underside of the dock followed by setting the tail set so that when the muscles and ligaments heal, it is carried higher. The healed tail cannot be tightly clamped by the horse. Such procedures can surely not be considered acceptable under any ethical view other than a strictly contractarian one in which animal suffering is not an ethical issue *per se* (Sandøe 2008, p. 19).

Breeders, too, have a role to play. Like trainers, breeders operate in an industry driven by profit and understandably breed horses with characteristics which mimic those of the horses which are already winning. In the case of American Quarter Horses, belief amongst breeders that there was an association between desirable muscle characteristics and the hyperkalemic periodic paralysis gene resulted in breeding horses which were prone to periodic paralysis and an unwillingness to undertake genetic screening. The welfare and ethical issues surrounding such practices have been recognised by the American Quarter Horse Association, which has now established a 'premium level' for those breeders who agree to test for genetic diseases. One breeding-related practice, which evidently violates the principle that each animal has individual worth, is the practice of breeding nurse mares to provide foster mothers for expensive foals whose mothers have died or rejected them. Surrogate nurse mares are sent to racing stables to nourish valuable foals, whilst their own foals may be left to struggle with malnutrition or are sometimes euthanised.

The general public also has a role to play in helping to determine the limits of what is ethically acceptable in animal sport. Much of the comment surrounding the deaths of two horses in the 2011 Grand National resulted from the fact that, due to a veterinary decision that the interests of fallen horses were best served by initial treatment on the course rather than by removing the horses, television viewers were able for the first time to see the stricken horses on the ground. Some argued that the television crews should not have filmed such aerial views. However, since animal sport is to a large extent driven by what the public wants to see, it is surely morally correct that the public should be fully informed about the reality of the events which they are supporting. This is analogous to the argument that those who eat meat should do so in full understanding of the processes which have brought meat to their plate (Coetzee 1999).

14.3.4 Ethical issues for the veterinarian dealing with sporting animals

The ethical issues that tend to preoccupy members of the public and of the media who are interested in sporting animals are generally acute issues such as death or injury during a competition and long-term issues such as the fate of the animals. The veterinarian working with sporting animals has to deal with these and additional issues that relate to the ongoing treatment of competition animals. However good the precautions and consideration for welfare, injury is unavoidable in athletes of any species. Veterinarians dealing with acute situations may sometimes be called upon by the owner to euthanase an animal which they believe could be treated and conversely to salvage an animal which they think will (ultimately) have an unacceptable quality of life. In superficially similar situations, veterinarians may find themselves agreeing to owners' wishes and then being faced with very different public reactions in terms of ethical acceptability. Thus, the veterinarians who 'salvaged' Grand National winner Aldaniti after a career-threatening injury were applauded at the time for their (successful) efforts, whereas those who tried to salvage Barbaro for breeding after his catastrophic injury were criticised for having acceded to the owner's allegedly financially driven wishes and treated the horse beyond what some considered ethically acceptable in terms of suffering (Richardson 2007).[1]

Rollin (1978) describes the fundamental question of veterinary ethics as: does the veterinarian have primary allegiance to the animal or the owner? Rollin (2006b) argues that it is unethical for a veterinarian to treat a horse with a painkiller in order that the horse may compete although its lifespan may be shortened. Yet, many veterinarians 'patch up' animals in order that they may continue to compete.

---

[1] Dr Richardson stated in his lecture that he at no time believed that Barbaro's owners allowed financial considerations to outweigh their concern for the horse's welfare.

In a utopian world, one would have an enforceable rule whereby any animal which was injured in training or competition had to be retired to live out its natural lifespan. Many believe this to be unrealistic: the alternative is most likely euthanasia because the owner cannot afford to keep more than one horse and wants one which he/she can ride. In that scenario, the fact that the horse's lifespan has been shortened is undeniable, whereas if it is treated it may still enjoy some useful pain-free years during which it will be well cared for.

Treatment of competition animals is a fact of sporting life, just as is treatment of human athletes (though with the obvious difference that human athletes consent to their treatment). That being so, we need to somehow establish principles to determine which treatments are ethically acceptable and which are not. Using the hybrid utilitarian-*telos* view outlined above, we could argue that a treatment is acceptable if it is likely to have a beneficial effect for the humans associated with the animal and, based on evidence-based medicine, has the potential to improve the animal's condition rather than just to mask pain and disease. Thus stem cell treatment of tendon injuries, which promote tendon repair (Taylor *et al.* 2007) would be ethically acceptable, whereas 'firing' tendons (McCullagh & Silver 1981; Hayward & Adams 2001) would not. The situation is less clear-cut when the short-term and long-term effects of treatment may differ, resulting in both beneficial and detrimental effects, as is the case with equine intra-articular steroid injections (McIlwraith 2010).

Individual veterinarians and veterinary bodies are also faced with ethical issues relating to an animal's fitness to compete and drug testing. At licensed greyhound tracks, just as for FEI equestrian sports, animals are checked by a veterinarian before and sometimes during an event to ensure that they are sound and fit to compete. There are also clear policies on permitted medications and on dope testing. This serves the dual purpose of safeguarding both animal welfare and the betting public's right to assume that competitions are being run on merit. In other sports such as polo, the level of veterinary involvement is much lower and medication and dope-testing rules are more relaxed: comparative research on the incidence of injury in animal sports with and without a high degree of veterinary supervision and drug testing might inform good practice in animal sport.

Veterinary involvement and drug monitoring will never completely overcome the ethical issues associated with trainers and owners who try to cheat by using drugs designed for other purposes or painful training aids to influence their animal's performance. Examples include the use of human drugs such as Ritalin to modify equine behaviour and the application of topical substances to horses' legs in training so that hitting a pole is made more painful ('hypersensitisation'). However proactive are the responsible authorities in trying to prevent such practices (FEI 2011), and however vigilant are event veterinarians in trying to detect them, there will be always be some who strive to gain unfair advantage in sport by cheating; this undermines the ethical basis of competition and training.

14.4 Conclusion

The use of animals for sport can only be ethically justified if, on balance and over the whole of its lifetime, the animal has *a life worth living* (FAWC 2009). This should include not only the periods before, during and after its competition career but also the animal's death. Many would agree with Regan and Singer that animals have individual worth, and yet still believe that providing a humane death is morally right for those cases where there is no good alternative once their competitive life is over. If society wishes to keep sporting animals, then society in general and veterinarians in particular must undertake to identify and address welfare issues wherever we can (no matter how financially unpopular); to constantly update and review what is good practice in sport in the light of the evidence base; to be honest about what happens to the animals before, during and after their competition careers; and not to shy away from advocating responsible euthanasia.

In considering our use of animals for sport in the twenty-first century, we should always bear this in mind and should constantly question: *'Just because the animal is prepared to do as we ask, should we ask it?'*

References

Armytage, M. (2011) Towcester racecourse to ban jockeys from using the whip in races at the track. *The Telegraph*, 21 April.

Bailey, C.J., Reid, S.W.J., Hodgson, D.R., Suann, C.J. & Rose, R.J. (1997) Risk factors associated with musculoskeletal injuries in Australian Thoroughbred racehorses. *Preventive Veterinary Medicine*, 32, 47–55.

BHIC (2009) *BHIC Briefing – Size and Scope of the Equine Sector*. BHIC, High Holborn, London.

Bloomberg, M.S. (1989) Racing greyhound track injuries. In: *Proceedings of the International Racing Greyhound Symposium*, Florida, pp. 3–12.

Bloomberg, M.S. & Dugger, W.W. (1991) Incidence and characteristics of orthopaedic injuries of the racing greyhound between 1984–1990 at six racetracks in Florida. In: *Proceedings of the 7th International Canine Sports Medicine Symposium*, Florida, pp. 8–17.

Brooke, C. (2009) Pictured: The show-jumping rabbits who are 'hop' favourites to win pet talent contest. Mail On-line, 1 May. Available at: http://www.dailymail.co.uk/news/article-1175432/Pictured-The-showjumping-rabbits-hop-favourites-win-pet-talent-contest.html

Coetzee, J.M. (1999) *The Lives of Animals*. Princeton University Press, Princeton, New Jersey.

Cook, A. (1998) Literature survey of racing greyhound injuries, performance and track conditions. *Journal of Turfgrass Science*, 74, 108–113.

Donoughue, B. (2007) *Independent review of the greyhound industry in Great Britain. A report by Lord Donoughue of Ashton for the British Greyhound Racing Board and the National Greyhound Racing Club*. HBLB, London. Available at: http://www.greyhounds-donoughue-report.co.uk

Ely, E.R., Avella, C.S., Price, J.S., *et al*. (2009) Descriptive epidemiology of fracture, tendon and suspensory ligament injuries in National Hunt racehorses in training. *Equine Veterinary Journal*, **41**, 372–378.

FAWC (1979) Press Statement 5th December. Available at: http://www.fawc.org.uk/pdf/fivefreedoms1979.pdf (accessed on 20 April 2012).

FAWC (2009) Farm animal welfare in Great Britain: Past, present and future. Available at: www.fawc.org.uk/pdf/ppfreport091012 (accessed on 9 February 2010).

FEI (2010) Press Release. *Round Table Conference Resolves Rollkur Controversy*. Available at: http://www.fei.org/disciplines/dressage/press-releases/fei-round-table-conference-resolves-rollkur-controversy (accessed on 20 April 2012).

FEI (2011) http://www.fei.org/veterinary/hypersensitivity-in-equestrian-competition (accessed on 28 May, 2012).

Foggo, D. (2006) Killing field of the dog racing industry. *The Sunday Times*, July 16.

Foggo, D. (2008) Greyhound breeder offers slow dogs to be killed for research. *The Sunday Times*, May 11.

GBGB (2010) Rules of Racing [online]. Available at: http://www.gbgb.org.uk/files/GBGB%20Rules%20of%20Racing%20December%202010.pdf

Gillette, R.L. (1992) Track surface influences on the racing greyhound. *Greyhound Review*, April.

Hancock, M. (2011) Use of the whip in horseracing. Early Day Motion 1938, Available at: http://www.parliament.uk/edm/2010-11/1938 (accessed on 20 April 2012).

Hayward, M. & Adams, D. (2001) The firing of horses. A review for the Animal Welfare Advisory Committee of the Australian Veterinary Association. Available at: http://www.gungahlinvet.com.au/papers/Firing_of_Horses_01 (accessed on 20 April 2012).

Heuschmann, G. (2009) *Dressage moderne: un jeu de massacre?* Belin, Paris, France.

Jeffcott, L.B., Rossdale, P.D., Freestone, J., Frank, C.J. & Towers-Clark, P.F. (1982) An assessment of wastage in Thoroughbred racing from conception to maturity. *Equine Veterinary Journal*, **14**, 85–198.

Jeory, T. (2010) Agony of caged greyhounds. *The Sunday Express*, May 30.

Lysaght, C. (2011) *British Horseracing Authority must take the lead in whip ban debate*. *The Guardian*, Sport Section, p. 9.

Marlin, D. (2004) Endurance research to improve welfare. *Horse and Hound*, 6 July issue. Available at: http://www.horseandhound.co.uk/news/397/56280.html (accessed on 20 April 2012).

McCullagh, K.G. & Silver, I.A. (1981) The actual cautery – Myth and reality in the art of firing. *Equine Veterinary Journal*, **13**, 81–84.

McIlwraith, CW (2010) The use of intra-articular corticosteroids in the horse: What is known on a scientific basis? *Equine Veterinary Journal*, **42**, 563–571.

Mesoly, J. (2002) Endurance tragedies draw scrutiny. *EQUUS*, December. Available at: http://www.equisearch.com/horses_riding_training/sports/endurance/endurancetragedies/ (accessed on 20 April 2012).

Murray, R.C., Walters, J.M., Snart, H., Dyson, S.J. & Parkin, T.D.H. (2010) Identification of risk factors for lameness in dressage horses. *The Veterinary Journal*, **184**, 27–36.

Parfit, D. (1984) *Reasons and Persons*. Oxford University Press, Oxford.

Qureshi, Y. (2010) 30 injured greyhounds put down at dog track. *Manchester Evening News*, April 27.

Reed, S.R., Jackson, B.F., Mc Ilwraith, C.W., *et al.* (2011) Descriptive epidemiology of joint injuries in Thoroughbred racehorses in training. *Equine Veterinary Journal*, Published online. doi: 10.1111/j.2042-3306.2010.00352.x.

Regan, T. & Singer, P. (1989) *Animal Rights and Human Obligations*. Prentice Hall, Englewood Cliffs, New Jersey.

Richardson, D. (2007) *Lessons from Barbaro*. Special lecture at the Annual Convention of the American Association of Equine Practitioners. Orlando, Florida.

Rollin, B.E. (1978) Updating veterinary ethics. *Journal of the American Veterinary Medical Association*, **173**, 1015–1018.

Rollin, B.E. (1981) *Animal Rights and Human Morality*. Prometheus Books, Buffalo, New York.

Rollin, B.E. (2006a) *An Introduction to Veterinary Medical Ethics*. Blackwell Publishing, Ames, Iowa.

Rollin, B.E. (2006b) Giving analgesics to mask pain in horses. In: *An Introduction to Veterinary Medical Ethics*, 2nd edn. Blackwell Publishing, Ames, Iowa.

Sandøe, P. & Christiansen, S. (2008) *Ethics of Animal Use*. Blackwell Publishing, Oxford.

Smith, R.K., Birch, H., Patterson-Kane, J., *et al.* (1999) Should equine athletes commence training during skeletal development?: Changes in tendon matrix associated with development, ageing, function and exercise. *Equine Veterinary Journal*, **31**, 201–209.

Taylor, S.E., Smith, R.K.W. & Clegg, P.D. (2007) Mesenchymal stem cell therapy in equine musculoskeletal disease: Scientific fact or clinical fiction? *Equine Veterinary Journal*, **39**, 172–180.

Verheyen, K.L.P., Henley, W.E., Price, J.S. & Wood, J.L.N. (2005) Training-related factors associated with dorsometacarpal disease in young Thoroughbred racehorses in the UK. *Equine Veterinary Journal*, **37**, 442–448.

van Weeren, P.R., Firth, E.C., Brommer, H., *et al.* (2008) Early exercise advances the maturation of glycosaminoglycans and collagen in the extracellular matrix of articular cartilage in the horse. *Equine Veterinary Journal*, **40**, 128–135.

Wilsher, S., Allen, W.R. & Wood, J.L.N. (2006) Factors associated with failure of Thoroughbred horses to train and race. *Equine Veterinary Journal*, **38**, 113–118.

Zebarth, B.J. & Sheard, R.W. (1985) Impact and shear resistance of turf grass racing surfaces for Thoroughbreds. *American Journal Veterinary Research*, **46**, 778–784.

Questions and Answers

Q: It sounds quite logical to say 'whatever might be natural for the animal is beneficial'. It would probably be ethnically justifiable. Naturally, an animal should be allowed to take its own decisions but this never happens. We define when and what an animal does, not only for sport animals but for companion, laboratory and farm animals. Are these practices just trying to make us feel better or do they really contribute to welfare or the ethical justification of the use of animals?

A: You are right: if animals were treated entirely naturally then we wouldn't be doing any of this. I was trying to find a way of drawing a line with which I was comfortable. If an animal can do something anatomically and physiologically and would do it naturally, then I would feel more comfortable. I agree that the animal would rather not be doing it at all.

Q: My question is about your utilitarian calculus of values. You said that there is so much economic gain from these sports. Suppose you stop the sports, what would happen? Your assumption is that the consequence of stopping the use of animals in sport is that people would spend money elsewhere. Take, for example, the people who are employed in the sport. There always will be a transition period when an economic activity is stopped; after a while employees will be employed doing something else.

Denmark is the world's largest pork producer. I have worked with economists to calculate the cost of closing down pork production in Denmark. If the closure is slow enough, then it doesn't cost anything because the workers would do something else.
A: There are a significant number of people employed in the British horse-racing industry. If they were to lose their jobs, this would have a significant impact on their welfare.

Q: Why are animals motivated to do what we want them to do? How ethical is it to 'trade' on their vulnerability because we make them so very dependent on us? I was thinking particularly about the trainer–animal relationship, for example search and rescue dogs, or sporting animals.
A: The relationship between people and animals is asymmetrical. Recently, I was teaching a new puppy to sit and thought why am I making him sit when he doesn't want to? Is that ethically justified? You could argue that a puppy needs to know when he has to sit so that he doesn't get run over by a horse as it walks past him, for example. Man's relationship to dogs is dominant, which is kind of evolutionary.

Q: Do you think the Grand National should be banned?
A: Only this last week, there's been another report from the British Horseracing Authority on the Grand National. It took much advice from various charities.

Q: Around the time of the Grand National, I saw a quote in a paper, '*Horse racing is the only time that the great British public would condone someone publically beating an animal with a stick*'.
A: There's currently a debate around the use of the whip in racing, particularly amongst the equine veterinary profession. It cannot be justified to use the whip simply in an attempt to incite a horse to go faster. Some studies have shown that those horses that are whipped most are those that run slowest. It's difficult to know whether horses don't like being whipped and so slow down, or whether they are whipped because they are running slowly. There is also a valid argument that jockeys need to carry a whip to keep a horse straight. For example, if a horse suddenly swerves as it comes into a fence, then this can create a dangerous situation with welfare implications. There's a series of races being run at Towcester called 'hands and heels'; jockeys aren't allowed to use whips, other than in an emergency.

Q: You drew a parallel between elite human athletes, who take performance-enhancing drugs or use other strategies to mask their injuries and thereby improve their chance of success, and animal sporting elite, creatures that might have similar strategies imposed by others and might not actually choose to have those things done were they given the choice. Is there an ethical difference?

A: All elite athletes carry injuries. There is a difference between a human athlete choosing to have a treatment which he/she knows may be detrimental in the long run versus an animal having one imposed upon it. There's an ethical difference.

Q: If animals carry injuries into later life after the end of their sporting life, is that part of the burden which they have to pay for their position at the top of the sporting tree? Is this often under the welfare radar?

A: I'm sure we ought to think about it more. What's the alternative? If an animal with a tendon injury isn't treated, what's going to happen to it?

Q: You could argue that fighting is natural behaviour for animals. Should we focus on our motives for using animals in particular ways rather than the end results?

A: It's a fact of life that humans use animals. We should do so in an ethical way.

Q: We have a choice to either view the argument in terms of ends or means. This is often overlooked.

Q: When I was a stud veterinarian, I was asked to treat racehorses. The common practice was to inject steroids into inflamed joints. I became very distressed because the outcome was for these horses to race and then retiring when they were only three years old.

   Now, I look after laboratory animals. At least we are trying our best to look at animal use from an ethical view, that is to balance the costs to the animals against the benefit, however difficult that may be. Is there a way to do an ethical assessment on the use of animals for sport? Would it help if the veterinary profession looked at this?

A: Yes. Veterinarians in practice are under these pressures every day. Perhaps we should look at the idea of the ethical matrix? If veterinarians knew more generally about ethical tools which are available, then that could only help.

Author's Commentary

The weeks surrounding the ICVAE [September 2011] saw significant media coverage in the UK of horse fatalities in the Grand National, the banning of the winning jockey for overuse of the whip, a subsequent review of the whip rules by the British Horseracing Authority (BHA), the imposition of new whip rules, a threatened strike by jockeys when the first fines were imposed under the new rules and a sudden backtracking and alteration of the new whip rules by the BHA. Public interest in and disquiet about these events was reflected in and anticipated by the questions at the ICVAE, which focused upon whether we are ever justified in using animals in sport, and the essentially unequal nature of man's relationship with animals.

My opinion is that it is a fact of life that man does use animals, whether for food, transport, as companions or for sport. That we have, for centuries, been able to impose our will upon animals and to force or persuade them to do as we please is an evolutionary fact. One could argue that this will and ability is part of man's *telos*. Man's use of animals for sport is nothing new, but what is new is our developing understanding of animal behaviour, welfare and physiology. The challenge in the twenty-first century is to devise methods of analysis, which will enable us to determine what it is ethically acceptable to use animals competitively, given this new knowledge. Academics from many disciplines will have contributions to make to this discussion. I share the view expressed by one questioner about the need for veterinarians to find a way to make such ethical assessments. Veterinarians are uniquely placed to provide scientific information on the benefits, harms and welfare implications of animal treatments. It is necessary for the veterinary profession to stick its collective head above the parapet and to contribute to the development of practical methods for assessing which treatments of competitive animals are and are not ethical in the twenty-first century.

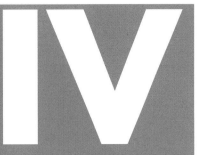

Cultural, Political, Legal and Economic Considerations

JOHN WEBSTER
University of Bristol

The title of this final session on *Veterinary and Animal Ethics* was 'Cultural, political, legal and economic considerations'. This, to paraphrase Bernard Rollins, puts Descartes before the horse. These things are not considerations to be pondered by moral philosophers; they are facts of life within which ethics must operate. The five papers in this session examined how attitudes and actions towards animals have been shaped by culture, driven by economics, enforced by laws and steered by government regulations and incentives. The continuing evolution of cultural beliefs and legal definitions of what is a right calls for a 'bottom-up' approach to practical ethics, which first identifies real issues of the day, then applies the eternal moral principles of beneficence and autonomy to seek justice for all concerned parties: the moral agents, animal owners and society at large, and the moral patients, sentient animals, both domestic and wild. We, the moral agents, have responsibilities to them: they owe us nothing.

Prescriptive law is necessary to set absolute standards of acceptability in our treatment of animals. However, it is not a mechanism for achieving standards that improve upon the baseline. Legislation by incentives, for example through the use of subsidies within the European Common Agriculture Policy, can encourage improvements in the husbandry of animals and the living environment. However, this approach has, to date, been promoted with only moderate enthusiasm and limited funding. More impressive improvements to the welfare of the food animals have come through the apparently amoral operation of the free market. Major retailers, very aware that there is no such thing as the standard consumer, have

Veterinary & Animal Ethics: Proceedings of the First International Conference on Veterinary and Animal Ethics, September 2011, First Edition. Edited by Christopher M. Wathes, Sandra A. Corr, Stephen A. May, Steven P. McCulloch and Martin C. Whiting.
© 2013 Universities Federation for Animal Welfare. Published 2013 by Blackwell Publishing Ltd.

explored the market potential of increasing product range for foods once regarded simply as commodities, for example free-range eggs, organic milk and 'Label Rouge' poultry. Products perceived as 'high welfare' are becoming increasingly popular, the most conspicuous example being free-range eggs, now over 50% of the market in England.

It is clear that the evolving value (ethical) judgments of society are having a greater impact on our attitudes and actions towards animals than the deliberations of our welfare scientists or the regulations set down by our legislators. This is entirely healthy. However scientists, educators and legislators still have essential roles to play. Our responsibility is to ensure that public perception of what defines ethical treatment of sentient animals is as close as possible to the animal's own perception of what makes a life worth living.

Global Cultural Considerations of Animal Ethics

15

MICHAEL C. APPLEBY

World Society for the Protection of Animals

Abstract: There is wide variation in attitudes to animals. Within cultures and countries, there are differences in ethical approaches, concepts of welfare and stakeholder involvement. Between countries, there are differences with historical and social origins, for example the degree of industrialisation and urbanisation. Between continents, there are deeper differences, for example the different emphasis placed on animal welfare versus animal killing in Asian countries compared with Europe. Between cultures, including religious cultures, there is variation with effects on attitudes and on practices affecting animal welfare, sometimes positive and sometimes negative. It is important to stress the need for sensitivity in dealing with these issues, but many or most religions have traditions or laws requiring humane treatment of animals. Much progress has therefore been made by accentuating positive areas of agreement and achieving cooperation in measures to improve welfare, including elimination of worst practices.

Keywords: culture, concern, ethics, globalisation, husbandry, killing, law, religion, slaughter, welfare

15.1 Introduction

Animals are a hugely important part of our world, and people depend on them for income, social status, food, clothing, comfort and cultural identification. So it is not surprising that the opinions about animals and how they should be treated are often strongly held or that there is considerable variation in attitudes about these

Veterinary & Animal Ethics: Proceedings of the First International Conference on Veterinary and Animal Ethics, September 2011, First Edition. Edited by Christopher M. Wathes, Sandra A. Corr, Stephen A. May, Steven P. McCulloch and Martin C. Whiting.
© 2013 Universities Federation for Animal Welfare. Published 2013 by Blackwell Publishing Ltd.

matters – within and between cultures, within and between countries. Much of this concerns animal ethics, and this paper describes some of this variation, considers some of the factors that affect it and discusses some appropriate responses.

15.2 Variation within a Culture

Even within a country and among people who in most respects can be regarded as having a common culture, there is great diversity in attitudes to animals. This includes the fact that many people rarely think about animals at all, or, when they do, regard them as someone else's responsibility. This may either take the form of expecting someone else (e.g. farmers, retailers or government) to ensure that animals are appropriately cared for, or more broadly that someone else should take the decisions on what level of care is appropriate. To take food animals as an example, a recent survey in the USA (Prickett et al. 2008) found three categories of consumers. 'Naturalists' (46% of the population) believe farm animals should be able to exercise outdoors and exhibit normal behaviours. 'Price seekers' (14%) would sacrifice animal welfare in exchange for lower prices. 'Basic Welfarists' (40%) are willing to pay higher prices to ensure welfare, but believe welfare can be ensured simply by providing ample food and health care.

There are at least three other reasons for variation in attitudes to animals within a culture (Appleby 1999). First, there are different ethical approaches, as outlined elsewhere in this volume, and these have different implications for the treatment of animals (Table 15.1). Most people adopt a mixed approach, but the weight they place on the different elements affects their attitudes. For example, those who think animal rights and human duties to animals are most important ethically are least likely to approve of killing animals for human purposes.

Second, people do not all have the same concept of animal welfare. They may believe one of the following or a mixture of two or three (Duncan & Fraser 1997; Fraser et al. 1997). Animal welfare may concern mental aspects such as feelings and preferences. It may concern physical aspects such as health and fitness. Or welfare may concern the ability of animals to express their 'nature', for example by living in natural conditions.

Third, there is variation between stakeholders. For example, how farm animals are housed will always be affected by monetary considerations, and the importance of this to producers, processors, retailers and consumers will differ. In most of our interactions with animals, there is at least some overlap between our interests and theirs; for instance, it is to the benefit of both farmers and their stock if the latter are healthy. However, the overlap between human and animal interests is not complete. The farmer is in general concerned with animals as a group rather than as individuals. So even if a particular practice leads to decreased performance of an individual, it may increase financial performance overall. Thus increasing stocking density of laying hens often reduces the food

Table 15.1 Some approaches to ethics, and possible associations with attitudes to animals.

Ethical approach	Emphasis	Examples	Emphasis for animals
Consequentialism	Consequences or outcomes of actions	Cost-benefit analysis	Animal welfare
Deontology	Morality of the actions themselves	Rights and duties	Animal rights
Agent-centred	Moral agents, usually people	Virtue ethics	Animal protection

conversion efficiency of individual birds – and probably also their welfare – but increases financial output of the house.

The reasons for variation in attitudes to animals just listed, that is differences in ethical approaches, concepts of welfare and stakeholder involvement, may all interact and are not randomly associated. For example, farmers and veterinarians put more emphasis on physical aspects of welfare than on mental or natural aspects, whereas other citizens concerned for animals commonly emphasise the importance of animal feelings and natural living conditions.

These factors doubtless also differ between cultures and countries. There has been little systematic review of this, but we can nevertheless describe some of the larger scale variation in attitudes to animals that exists.

15.3 Variation between European Countries

It is well recognised that interest in animal welfare varies between European countries. Concern has historically been stronger in the north of Europe, particularly the UK, the Netherlands, Germany and Scandinavia, and weaker in the south. Reasons are complex. Several factors correlate with this variation, including temperature (hotter in the south, which affects how animals are kept) and religion (Catholicism is commoner in the south, Protestantism in the north, with many effects on attitudes). The most persuasive explanation, though, is that concern has largely developed in urban people whose involvement with animals differed from that in rural areas – people who kept pets more often than farm animals. The UK and the Netherlands, for example, have become more industrialised than many other countries, particularly in the south, with 2% or less of the population involved in agriculture (Ludvigsen *et al.* 1982).

Despite this variation, there has been considerable legislative activity and other policy measures at the European level. Indeed, the variation may be seen to have encouraged or necessitated such activity, partly for convergence of values and partly to promote a 'level playing field' for trade and other commercial purposes. The Council of Europe (founded in 1949 and now with 47 member countries including those of the EU) has played an important role in putting forward and influencing animal welfare policy, much of which has been developed further by the EU and northern European countries such as Switzerland. Perhaps most notably, the EU's 1997 Treaty of Amsterdam (EUR-Lex 1997) states that:

> *'The High Contracting Parties, desiring to ensure improved protection and respect for the welfare of animals as sentient beings, have agreed [that] in formulating and implementing its agriculture, transport, internal market and research policies, the EU and the Member States shall pay full regard to the welfare requirements of animals, while respecting the legislative or administrative provisions and customs of the Member States relating in particular to religious rites, cultural traditions and regional heritage.'*

It is striking, though, that protection of animal welfare remains subject to many considerations within Member States, including cultural and religious. The effect of such considerations may be positive or negative for animal welfare. For example, France puts emphasis on food quality, which has some positive effects – it is more common to keep free-range, slow-growing broiler chickens than in other countries – and some negative, such as the force-feeding of ducks and geese for *foie gras* production.

15.4 Variation between Continents

Concern for animal welfare is also relatively strong in areas such as North America (particularly Canada) and Australasia, presumably because emigration from Europe led to cultural similarities. However, there are also marked differences between countries. One contrast that is often noted is between the USA and Europe, illustrated by the paucity of animal protection legislation in the USA compared with Europe. Many factors contribute to this, but an important one must be that in the USA there is less acceptance of actions by government that restrict individual liberties (including on treatment of animals) and less emphasis on the role of government in supporting individual people, which may also affect views on the appropriateness of government action for animals. These differences may further cause, or be partly mediated by, differences in language, including quite subtle differences in how language is used. Thus while 'animal welfare' is interpreted in Europe as the *state* of the animal, in the USA it more commonly refers to *animal care*. This is analogous to the use of 'welfare' to mean aid or payment given to people in need, and 'animal well-being' is closer to the European meaning.

In many Asian countries, there is less concern for animal welfare than in Europe, but more concern for the killing of animals. So in Japan, for example, many families have their own rice paddies, but few rear animals such as ducks that they themselves would have to kill. Sick animals are sometimes allowed to die slowly rather than being culled, because people are reluctant actually to kill them. Some of this is religious, part of the attitudes to life and death of Asian religions, but that is not a full explanation.

People in countries where concern for animals is high must be careful when commenting on others with different priorities. Herscovici (1985) censured a lack of such care in those who criticise Canadian native people for trapping animals. If trapping were stopped, it would end a lifestyle that has been traditional for generations and the response of the people involved is often forthright:

> 'The Inuit say that the philosophy of animal rights is merely the latest outburst of the cultural and economic imperialism they've come to expect from Europe and the South. Bringing aboriginal trappers off their hunting territories is a crucial step towards 'clearing the land' for pipelines, power dams and other high-tech frontier 'development' projects, and all the disruption of wildlife habitat that they bring with them. For this reason, many wildlife biologists question whether the demands of the animal rights groups are even really in the interests of wildlife.'

Even more persuasively, countries that have difficulty feeding their people understandably put more emphasis on food availability than on animal welfare. Concern for animals is often less active in developing than in developed countries. However, this is not always so, as many of the world's poorest people depend on animals for income, social status and security as well as food and clothing. The welfare of their animals is important to them, and many measures to improve animal welfare also benefit their owners (McCrindle 1998).

15.5 Variation between Specific Cultures

It has already been noted that many specific cultural factors, including religion, have effects on attitudes to animals and on practices affecting animal welfare, sometimes benign and sometimes adverse. The most common issue discussed in this context is slaughter, especially the question of whether animals should or should not be stunned beforehand. This will not be discussed in detail here, but it is important to note that many methods of religious slaughter have their origin in avoidance of previous, inhumane practices. For example, one of the factors in the objection to stunning prior to slaughter for Halal food is the principle that animals killed for such food should be uninjured. Indeed, most religions have traditions or laws requiring humane treatment of animals (Raj 2004). If these are followed, there may be many benefits to welfare, including prior to and during slaughter. However, there has often been less attention given to animal treatment earlier in life. Islamic texts, including sayings of the Prophet Mohammad (*peace be unto him*), provide considerable support for the importance of animal welfare during handling and husbandry. It can therefore be argued that many commercial practices of animal rearing, feeding, handling and transport do not follow strict Islamic guidelines, and that meat produced by such practices (e.g. from animals housed intensively) cannot properly be described as Halal. For this reason, the International Halal Integrity Alliance has adopted a draft standard for welfare of livestock, drawn up in collaboration with the World Society for the Protection of Animals (Rahman *et al.* 2009).

It remains true that treatment of animals by people of different culture, including religion, often gives rise to concern. How should such concern be addressed?

15.6 Working Together

It is first important to stress the need for sensitivity. It is always best to tread softly among other people's sensibilities.

It is possible, for example, that the groups who offended the Canadian native trappers, mentioned above, could instead have engaged in dialogue with them and persuaded them to use traps that are more humane than the old-fashioned gin traps (Care for the Wild 1994). This might be regarded as, at least, better than continuation of existing practices.

The issue of stunning without slaughter is another on which there has often been confrontation rather than communication. It is understandable that the British Veterinary Association (2011) described a decision by the EU Council not to require meat from animals slaughtered without stunning to be labelled as a disappointing 'backwards step'. However, it may also be anomalous, as much Halal meat in the UK is from animals that are actually stunned before killing. It is even possible that labelling non-stunned meat would increase its incidence, as some Moslems would preferentially purchase it.

Sensitivity may sometimes involve careful use of language. In some fora, more progress may be made by discussing animal care or animal management rather than by insisting on consideration of animal welfare.

More generally, it is usually most appropriate to 'accentuate the positive'. This may do more to eliminate the negative than a more aggressive approach. Thus, while it often causes resentment and resistance to criticise people for cruelty or for causing poor animal welfare, it is often possible to agree on the desirability of good welfare. This may then achieve cooperation in measures to improve welfare, including elimination of the worst practices.

This sort of positive approach has been crucial in the major areas of agreement that have already been discussed, including accords between the diverse countries of Europe and emphasis on the importance of welfare by the International Halal Integrity Alliance. Similarly, positive discussions with groups including the World Society for the Protection of Animals led to the following declaration at the World Halal Forum in The Hague in 2009 (Appleby, personal observation):

'This forum recognises the importance of animal welfare in the production of Halal food, and resolves that organisations and communities involved in halal food production should explore ways to reduce pain, distress and other welfare problems in their sourcing and treatment of animals during rearing, transport and slaughter. This forum

should collaborate with academic researchers and other experts in investigating the welfare implications and acceptability of different treatments including slaughter methods, to benefit both animals and humans.'

Another important example is the adoption of global animal welfare standards by the World Organisation for Animal Health (OIE). These were initiated because the OIE (2011) recognises that animal health is affected by other aspects of animal welfare, and in 2005 the first standards on transport and slaughter were agreed unanimously by the member countries. These currently number 174, including many developing countries. Implementation of these standards, which is starting in a number of countries, has the potential to lead to improved animal welfare in the majority of OIE members.

There is strong reason to believe that increased attention to animal ethics and animal welfare worldwide, and communication and collaboration within and between cultures, is leading not to a 'levelling down' effect, as was feared by some people, but to 'levelling up'.

References

Appleby, M.C. (1999) Tower of Babel: Variation in ethical approaches, concepts of welfare and attitudes to genetic manipulation. *Animal Welfare*, **8**, 381–390.

British Veterinary Association. (2011) Press release: Disappointment at backwards step on religious slaughter labelling. British Veterinary Association, London.

Care for the Wild/European Federation for Nature and Animals. (1994) Trapping animals for Fur. Care for the Wild, West Sussex.

Duncan, I.J.H. & Fraser, D. (1997) Understanding animal welfare. In: *Animal Welfare* (eds M.C. Appleby & B.O. Hughes), pp. 19–31. CAB International, Oxfordshire.

EUR-Lex. (1997) Treaty of Amsterdam amending the treaty on European Union, the treaties establishing the European Communities and related Acts: Protocol on protection and welfare of animals. Available at: http://eur-lex.europa.eu/en/treaties/dat/11997D/htm/11997D. html#0110010013 (accessed on 19 April 2011).

Fraser, D., Weary, D.M., Pajor, E.A. & Milligan, B.M. (1997) A scientific conception of animal welfare that reflects ethical concerns. *Animal Welfare*, **6**, 187–205.

Herscovici, A. (1985) *Second Nature: The Animal Rights Controversy*. CBC Enterprises, Toronto, Ontario, Canada.

Ludvigsen, J.B., Empel, J., Kovacs, F., Manfredini, M., Unshelm, J. & Viso, M. (1982) Animal health and welfare. *Livestock Production Science*, **9**, 65–87.

McCrindle, C. (1998) The community development approach to animal welfare: An African perspective. *Applied Animal Behaviour Science*, **59**, 227–233.

OIE (World Organisation for Animal Health). (2011) The OIE's objectives and achievements in animal welfare. http://www.oie.int/animal-welfare/animal-welfare-key-themes (accessed on 4 May 2011).

Prickett, R., Norwood, F.B. & Lusk, J.L. (2008) *Consumer Preferences for Farm Animal Welfare: Results from a Telephone Survey of U.S. Households*. Department of Agricultural Economics Seminar Series, Oklahoma State University, Stillwater, Oklahoma.

Rahman, S.A., Appleby, M.C., Kolesar, R. & Parente, S. (2009) Draft international Halal integrity alliance standard for animal welfare. World Halal Forum, Kuala Lumpur.

Raj, A.B.M. (2004) Cultural, religious and ethical issues associated with animal welfare. In: *Global Conference on Animal Welfare: An OIE Initiative*, pp. 235–247. OIE, Paris.

Questions and Answers

Q: Having worked both in the UK and overseas, I'm often challenged with the assertion by non-veterinarians that the veterinary profession in a number of countries doesn't do enough for animal welfare, doesn't act as advocates for animals in many fora and doesn't facilitate and empower people who work in other industries to act as advocates for animals.

We've had a lot of discussion about the declaration that (UK) veterinarians make to uphold the welfare of animals under their care but what about animals that aren't under their care, those farmed in the USA, or dogs with rabies, which are potentially managed inappropriately in India, for example? Do veterinarians have a responsibility for these global issues?

A: Yes. Nobody lives with an declaration sitting on their desk but both training and declarations affect our attitude. These vary a lot between different countries; we shouldn't forget that the status of veterinarians differs hugely too. Veterinarians are generally of high status in the countries we're working with here, but do not always have such high status elsewhere.

I'm greatly encouraged by the activity of intergovernmental organisations, including the OIE which took what, at the time, seemed a radical stance, that animal health is affected by other aspects of animal welfare and that if anybody was going to develop global guidelines on animal welfare it would have to be them. The OIE has made good progress on this.

Encouraging and enabling the OIE to move forward, including implementing their guidelines worldwide, is a sign of hope for the future. It's piecemeal, it's small, there are many negatives and some things are getting worse but, in my view, things are, in general, getting better. There is the threat of competition round the world but a levelling down of standards is not happening, instead standards are levelling up.

Q: You've concluded on the positive note that if we work with people then things can move forward. There are a number of papers on appreciative enquiry in which people try to find evidence of good practice. Appreciative enquiry can be compared with the critical approach, which has failed historically. Why does the critical approach persist when there's so much evidence that appreciative enquiry should be the way forward?

A: Sometimes it's ignorance. Sometimes it's because we really don't understand what's going on, the underlying reasons and how best to move forward. One reason for religious slaughter methods was that they were developed to replace earlier inhumane methods. It's one reason we've been able to make progress on Halal slaughter, because killing without stunning was part of the ideal that an animal should be killed without blemish or injury. Quite large sectors of the Muslim community have come to accept that the stunning is not itself an injury and indeed reduces the injury of pain and harm that killing without stunning causes. Increased communication and understanding has meant that quite a large proportion of Halal slaughter is now done with pre-stunning.

One of the worst things about the animal welfare world is infighting. Some of this is caused by the facelessness of the enemy, the size of the problem and the fact that you cannot go to the owner of feedlots and deal with him so you criticise other people who, for example, aren't vegetarian or aren't doing it the best way they could, as you see it. Communication and collaboration help to accentuate the positive.

Q: It seems that some people with whom we might not work so closely have actually done much for animal welfare, for example, the radicals who make farmers talk because they're afraid of them. Isn't a division of labour needed? These are people who dare to say radical things using radical pictures. This opens minds and forces more pragmatic actors to act.
A: In a sense, one other aspect is diversity. Progress is piecemeal; some things are getting worse while others are getting better. I remain an optimist partly because of the value of the positive approach but the spoiler on the wing is also part of the picture.

Q: I like to draw a comparison between European school kids, who think that milk comes from a supermarket bottle and disassociate the animal and the end product, and Islamic countries in which family members do the slaughtering themselves and are therefore immediately engaged with the slaughtering process. If slaughter becomes mechanised and is done behind closed doors, what will be the effect on the value systems of these communities, which generally think that they have an innate respect for individual animals?
A: The situation is complex. Millions of sheep every year go from Australia to the Middle East. Most are killed in abattoirs rather than within the family, which can get a token to say that a sheep has been slaughtered on its behalf. Trying to kill 100 000 sheep during the week of the Hajj is chaotic and horrible. In a sense, over-efficiency has caused problems rather than the reverse. Why can't a family get a token saying a sheep has been slaughtered in Australia on its behalf?

Involvement is generally a positive. But it can also lead to problems where people don't have the right equipment and methods for killing or dealing with animals. Small farms can have welfare problems as well as big ones. Individual slaughter of an animal by hand can cause problems on a large scale as well. There isn't a simple answer.

Author's Commentary

Both the number of animals suffering welfare problems around the world and the complexity of cultural and other factors that contribute to those problems often seem daunting. So it was interesting that this discussion covered the whole range of possible approaches to understanding and addressing such problems. Important points were whether people are involved with or disassociated from animals, and how this affects their attitudes to and treatment of animals. At the other end of the scale, how can we make more progress in tackling issues on a global scale? My view is that work is needed at all levels: hands-on work to understand and address specific problems and to inform higher-level discussions, in parallel with work in national and international forums that will have wider impacts. Such fora have indeed had considerable impact, influencing legislation, ending cruel practices and introducing humane alternatives, although a vast amount remains to be done. And in many, perhaps most cases, an important element in the success of these fora (both on a national and an international basis) is the inclusion of all key stakeholders. One striking development over several decades, in multi-stakeholder fora concerned with welfare, has been a decline in rancour and an increase in positive cooperation, with the appreciative identification of common ground emphasised here. It is right to say that such discussions may be prompted and accelerated by radicals whom the majority would not want to join the forum – and who might not want to join anyway, partly because they do not want compromise. The same may also be said of conservatives who do not want compromise either, or any change at all in the status quo. Yet I have known both radicals and conservatives participate in such forums who behave more moderately there than outside; confidentiality of the discussions is often vital (e.g. use of the Chatham House Rule), so that participants know that their comments are not on public record. Thus some individuals may fulfil both radical/conservative and pragmatist roles. As the adage says, it is better to have the camel inside the tent spitting out, than outside spitting in. Inclusion of a wide variety of stakeholders is valuable in finding conclusions that are both workable and acceptable to as many constituencies as possible. Further, those conclusions will be more credible and effective subsequently because of the involvement and ownership of diverse contributors.

Communication and collaboration within and between cultures, and between people who have different values and attitudes to animals, will not rapidly solve all the problems of poor welfare that exist worldwide. However, they have already contributed to ameliorating many of those and are the best hope for further progress in future.

Animal Ethics and the Government's Policy: 'To Guard and Protect'

16

SOPHIA HEPPLE AND NIGEL GIBBENS

Department for Environment, Food and Rural Affairs

Abstract: Historically, (British) Government policy affecting animals has been anthropocentric. By the mid-nineteenth century, the Government recognised that it had social responsibility for kept animals. Legislation was enacted and extended that shifted the focus from unacceptable actions by the perpetrator to unacceptable outcomes for the animal; a change that accounted for the animal's feelings. However, it was 150 years before animals were legally recognised as sentient by the European Community. It is often the differing values placed on animals that can lead to policy issues developing into wicked problems, such as bovine tuberculosis. Current Government policy assesses the potential impacts of policy change on a wide range of stakeholders, including animals, but the benefits to humans are the priority. The ideal is that Government policy benefits all; however, the reality is that there may be adverse consequences for some animals. Whilst society at large can take on responsibility towards animals, regulation is needed to guard and protect them. The Farm Animal Welfare Committee (FAWC) has suggested that society should aspire to give (farm) animals *a good life*. Whether Government policy can achieve such moral progress whilst fulfilling the needs of its other stakeholders remains an open question.

Keywords: a good life, animal ethics, consequence, European Commission, Government policy, kept animals, law, legislation, protection, religious slaughter, value, welfare

Veterinary & Animal Ethics: Proceedings of the First International Conference on Veterinary and Animal Ethics, September 2011, First Edition. Edited by Christopher M. Wathes, Sandra A. Corr, Stephen A. May, Steven P. McCulloch and Martin C. Whiting.

16.1 Historical Perspective on English Law and Its Regard for Animals

Government policy and law-making regarding animals have historically been anthropocentric. Early legislation in Great Britain and Ireland was not based on an animal's intrinsic worth, but rather such laws were passed to protect the interests of their owner. Thus Erskine (1809) commented, '*Animals are considered as property only: to destroy or abuse them, from malice to the proprieter, or with an intention injurious to his interest in them, is criminal; but the animals themselves are without protection; the law regards them not substantively; they have no rights!*'

From the eighteenth century onwards, advances in science confirmed long-held opinion that animals were sentient (it was not until the late twentieth century before sentience was established legally within Europe). A stumbling block in the legislative process for protecting animals in the UK was the fundamental issue of whether Government should interfere in areas of public morality, which generally was assumed to be more properly addressed by the Church, media, education, etc. This stumbling block not only concerned animal protection but the rights of children and other social issues such as working conditions and slavery. Whilst certain members of society sought to prevent cruelty to, and suffering of, animals, the man of the house could discipline his child to within a hair's breadth of death (permitted 'reasonable chastisement') without breaking the law. Early pioneers in animal protection sought to modify social attitude and behaviour through legislation, '*Rights of Beasts be formally acknowledged by the State, and that a law be framed upon that principle, to guard and protect them from flagrant and wanton cruelty, whether committed by their owners or others*' (Lawrence 1796).

This change in approach created problems with enforcement, since prosecutions were mostly brought by private individuals: who should pay for prosecutions on such moral issues as animal and child cruelty? In addition, just as children's legislation challenged the autonomy of the patriarch, animal welfare legislation challenged an owner's right to treat his/her property as he/she wished. The first attempts at introducing substantive law to protect animals were thus presented as ways of controlling public disorder rather than dealing with any effects on animals. They reflected Hogarth's approach towards alcoholism and debauchery through his stark caricatures such as Beer Street and Gin Lane. In 1751, he published his Four Stages of Cruelty, which were multiple copies of engravings and woodcuts, reproduced on cheap paper to ensure mass distribution. Hogarth was horrified by the routine treatment of animals and believed that wanton cruelty promoted the same action towards humans. However, in the early nineteenth century, the Government was firm that these matters were not a matter for the State: '*This House ought only to legislate when an act of legislature is gravely and generally called for; and not merely to gratify petty, personal and local motives, such as are infinitely beneath the deliberate dignity of parliament ... I can safely assert, that cruelty ... is not in the nature nor in the habits of English gentlemen*' (Windham 1800).

However, by the end of the nineteenth century, the Government had produced its first substantive animal protection laws (including amending, repealing and improving upon them several times over); the first officially recognised animal protection society was founded in 1824 (the Society for the Prevention of Cruelty to Animals receiving royal patronage, becoming the Royal Society for the Prevention of Cruety to Animals (RSPCA), in 1840); and Charles Darwin had devoted two chapters in his *Descent of Man* (Darwin 1871) to the 'comparison of the mental powers of man and lower animals' where he declared that the second chapter was '*solely to shew that there is no fundamental difference between man and the higher mammals in their mental faculties*'.

Darwin's discourse on animals' feelings of pleasure, pain, happiness and even loyalty is well known. However, his concluding remarks reflect these changes within society and Government over this period:

> '*The term, general good, may be defined as the means by which the greatest possible number of individuals can be reared in full vigour and health, with all their faculties perfect, under the conditions to which they are exposed. As the social instincts both of man and the lower animals have no doubt been developed by the same steps, it would be advisable, if found practicable, to use the same definition in both cases, and to take as the test of morality, the general good or welfare of the community, rather than the general happiness; but this definition would perhaps require some limitation on account of political ethics.*'

By the mid- to late nineteenth century, the Government had recognised that it had some form of social responsibility for the community under its jurisdiction, particularly vulnerable subjects who were less able to defend themselves: this community included animals. For them, legislation had been extended so that whilst early Acts focused on actions by the perpetrator (such as wanton cruelty), later amendments focused on the outcome for the animal (unnecessary pain and suffering). There was thus a shift in interpretation of what constituted an offence. This demonstrated an attitudinal change that accounted for the animal's feelings; similar legislation putting the child's interests first was not realised until 1925. The Prevention of Cruelty to Animals Act 1849 was the first legislation that describes a welfare outcome measure as the determinant of non-compliance; the continued use of the term 'unnecessary suffering' in law today demonstrates its importance and effectiveness.

Other welfare legislation enacted in the late nineteenth century cemented the State's acceptance of a clear responsibility for protecting animals at risk, irrespective of the owner's attitude or wishes. The Commission report on vivisection in 1876 (HMSO, Cardwell 1876) acknowledged the need for laws to protect animals against the 'inhumanity' found in even 'persons of very high position [such] as physiologists'. The Injured Animals Act 1894 similarly assumed a greater State responsibility for animal protection above that of the owner, permitting humane destruction of animals that were seriously injured without the owner's consent.

It was easiest to legislate and enforce issues which were in the public arena (e.g. treatment of working or experimental animals, remembering that there were public displays of vivisection) versus those kept privately (e.g. pets and pit ponies); the focus was on the extremes of poor welfare, that is cruelty, torture or suffering. In the UK, it was not until 2006 that the Animal Welfare Act imposed a legal duty of care upon responsible persons to provide the basic needs of their pets and other animals.

16.1.1 The role of lobbying in effecting change in UK Government policy

It was no coincidence that in the UK those 'eccentric' persons, who were instrumental in the first animal welfare legislation (Martin's Act) in 1822 (after over 20 years of unsuccessful Bills through Parliament) and who also took the first prosecutions under the new Act, were also instrumental in creating the Society for the Prevention of Cruelty to Animals (SPCA) in 1824. The Society's aim of 'mitigation of animal suffering, and the promotion and expansion of the practice of humanity towards the inferior class of animal beings' (HMSO 1932) was to be achieved by education and enforcement (including the employment of agents to take private prosecutions) and the lobbying of MPs. The SPCA (later to become the RSPCA) was instrumental in lobbying for numerous amendments, including a ban on bull-baiting, resulting in Pease's Act in 1835, the Cruelty to Animals Acts of 1849 and 1876, and the Protection of Animals Act 1911. All involved significant lobbying by the RSPCA. The fact that the RSPCA was proposing new bills and amendments did not go down well with some in Government; they suggested that improved regulation regarding the licensing of horse slaughterhouses in 1844 should be opposed just because (private) societies should not be seen to be encouraged to meddle in other people's business. However, such comments were in the minority and the amendment was enacted within just two months of its proposal.

Lobbying today is just as important in effecting change in Government policy, although Government now acts proactively to engage and consult principal stakeholders when formulating, implementing and reviewing new policy.

16.1.2 Council of Europe: Development of a European conscience

The Council of Europe (CoE) was established in 1949 to promote European unity with respect to human values, law and democracy. Membership is wider than that of the European Community (EC; currently 47 members); each country can decide to adopt and implement each convention. The voluntary nature means that there is more variation between countries in the degree of implementation compared with EU directives and regulations. However, the details of the conventions have often been used as a basis for EU directives and regulations. The treatment of animals was first addressed by the CoE in September 1961 (Council of Europe 1961). 'Considering that the humane treatment of animals is one of the hall-marks of Western civilisation, but that, even in member States of the Council of Europe, the necessary standards are not always observed', the CoE Assembly recommended 'that the Committee of Ministers should draft, and invite the member States to sign and ratify, a Convention for the regulation of the international transit of animals'.

The Council sits with invited observers; for example, the transport expert group included industry and animal health experts as well as non-Governmental organisations. Developing standards takes considerable time but once complete they are usually well accepted and comprehensive. Conventions now cover pets, farm animals, laboratory animals, slaughter and transport of animals. The CoE's work in the area of animal protection is currently suspended due to resource constraints and other priorities.

16.1.3 Development of modern animal welfare policy

'*The common people may ask with justice, why abolish bull-baiting, and protect hunting and shooting*' (opposition to the first Bill to ban bull-baiting, Windham, 1800).

In England, the recent Animal Welfare Act 2006 brought together over 25 separate pieces of UK animal protection legislation. Yet when guidance was issued on how to demonstrate a duty of care for a dog or cat, the Government was criticised as a 'nanny State' in some media. Similarly, Government-funded research on the farmed duck's requirements for water has been ridiculed. The EU banned the import of cat and dog fur in 2009 under Article XX of the WTO agreement (1947) to 'protect public morals' that yet continues to allow cultural traditions such as the force-feeding of ducks and geese to produce *pâté de foie gras*, bullfighting in certain Member States and religious traditions such as the slaughter of animals without prior stunning. This cultural relativity can be explained in part by the EC's legal position with respect to animals.

The first welfare legislation in 1974 (Council Directive 1974) adopted by the European Economic Community (EEC) concerned stunning before slaughter; its preamble stated:

> '*Whereas the Community should also take action to avoid in general all forms of cruelty to animals; whereas it appears desirable, as a first step, that this action should consist in laying down conditions such as to avoid all unnecessary suffering on the part of animals when being slaughtered. … Whereas, however, it is necessary to take account of the particular requirements of certain religious rites.*'

However, this was not legally binding. The original objectives of the EEC, and from 1993 the EC, were economic and focussed on the promotion of free trade (Council Directive 1993). There was nothing in the founding constitutions that set principles with regard to the status of animals other than that of agricultural products that could be freely traded. Whilst the first EC animal welfare law in 1993 continued the theme adopted by the EEC '*to pay full regard to the welfare requirement of animals*', this remained a statement within a directive preamble only.

It was not until 1999 and the Treaty of Amsterdam that animals were formally and legally recognised as sentient by the EC, and that the full regard to animal welfare became an enforceable part of the EC's Treaty:

> '*In formulating and implementing the Union's agriculture, fisheries, transport, internal market, research and technological development and space policies, the Union and*

the Member States shall, since animals are sentient beings, pay full regard to the welfare requirements of animals, while respecting the legislative or administrative provisions and customs of the Member States relating in particular to religious rites, cultural traditions and regional heritage.'

Where appropriate, European legislation (1998) (Council Directive (1998) on the protection of farmed animals focuses on the *'provision of housing, food, water and care appropriate to the physiological and ethological needs of the animals, in accordance with established experience and scientific knowledge'*. Minimum standards of basic welfare are set. Member States must make provision to ensure that the owners or keepers take all reasonable steps to ensure the welfare of animals under their care and that unnecessary pain, suffering or injury are not caused. There are various statutory requirements for all Member States (either directly or through industry-led initiatives) to provide farmers with appropriate guidance and training in order to ensure that they can meet the minimum welfare standards stipulated in European law.

However, the caveat in the Treaty of Amsterdam (1999) on provisions relating to *'religious rites, cultural traditions and regional heritage'* allows traditional food production methods whereby rearing and slaughter are at odds with positive welfare. For example, some Member States (i.e. Belgium, Bulgaria, Spain, France and Hungary) permit fatty liver (disease) to be induced in geese and ducks by force-feeding. Many countries either specifically ban the procedure or it is considered inherently unlawful under national animal welfare rules. The CoE Convention for the protection of animals specifically prohibits the production of *foie gras* using traditional force-feeding methods except 'where it is current practice'. For the UK, production of *foie gras* is not a traditional practice, and banning its production is merely a simple policy issue. More difficult to manage and to decide policy are those areas where opposing views can never (or rarely) achieve a compromise. These include slaughter without prior stunning or those where owners have little or no control over the fate of their animals, for example decisions on mass culling of animals during a notifiable disease outbreak.

The impact of this caveat was experienced by Government policy-makers and enforcement bodies in the UK when a bovine tuberculosis (bTB) reactor, 'Shambo', was identified within a herd belonging to a Hindu community in 2007. However, whilst Hindus across the world prayed first for Shambo, then 'Bhakti' and 'Dakshini' (all of which were bTB reactors in the same herd), another prominent Hindu, Lakhani (2007), said that the opinion expressed at Skanda Vale in Wales was *'seriously wrong'* because it did not take into account the *'greater context in which we operate'* as do Hindu teachings: *'If the life of one animal may endanger other lives or human lives as well, then we must take into account the greater good and sacrifice the individual good.'* The Court of Appeal reached the same decision when upholding the decision to slaughter Shambo, notwithstanding that the decision interfered with the Hindus' religious rights, which are protected under the European Convention of Human Rights.

16.1.4 Development of Government policy on animal disease

We need to turn to the nineteenth century, the origins of animal health law and the establishment of the veterinary profession, to understand development of modern Government policy in relation to animals. Developments in veterinary science, particularly epidemiology, plus an endemic outbreak of sheep-pox, led the Government to enact the first legislation in 1848 to protect the nation's farm animals. The primary driver was financial but the consequential benefit was improved animal health and welfare. Compulsory mass slaughter and enforced movement restrictions were first introduced in the nineteenth century when cattle plague (rinderpest) killed half a million adult cattle. This outbreak introduced the concept of a national herd: its protection and treatment became a public – rather than a private – concern. Animal health and animal welfare became inextricably linked through the Contagious Diseases (Animals) Act 1869; cattle welfare during transport was addressed and requirements for the provision of feed and water during transport were stipulated. This legislation therefore introduced a responsibility for the consignor and transporter to provide for an animal's basic needs in an effort to prevent unnecessary suffering. The origins of the State Veterinary Service were in the creation of the Government's first veterinary department in 1889 as the concept of public responsibility towards the nation's flocks and herds of farm animals took shape. Lawrence's vision in 1796 of a State that would guard and protect vulnerable animals was being realised, not only by preventing acts of wanton cruelty and unnecessary suffering but also widespread suffering caused by uncontrolled diseases, '*Their strict enforcement has alleviated an immense amount of suffering amongst animals: the spread of disease was usually due to culpable negligence, and the measures taken to prevent such negligence are not the least important laws for the prevention of cruelty to animals*' (de Montmorency 1902).

16.2 Development of Government Policy on bTB: A Wicked Problem

A 'wicked' problem is most simply defined as one that is highly resistant to resolution (Briggs 2007). First described by Rittel in 1967 (Churchman 1967), and later defined in more detail by Rittel and Webber (1973), a wicked problem can be difficult to define and has a number of common features. They are often multi-causal and attempts to address them often lead to unforeseen consequences. They are rarely stable and may have no simple solution. Importantly, from a government's perspective, responsibility for resolution does not sit with a single organisation or stakeholder. Solutions can be socially complex and involve modifying stakeholder attitudes and behaviours. Often policy may focus on a partial solution that may lead to further problems. Lazarus (2009) reviewing super wicked problems, such as climate change, quoted Ackoff, as saying '*Every problem interacts with other problems and is therefore part of a set of interrelated problems, a system of problems...*

I choose to call such a system a mess.' Some policy issues concerning animals can also be identified as wicked problems. It is often the differing values of the animals involved that can lead to issues developing into wicked problems. It becomes an even greater mess when different species with different values to different sectors of society are intimately involved in the same wicked problem.

In developing Government policy where animals are affected, consideration of society's interest in those animals and the interests of the animals in their own right is only part of the policy-making process. In the case of bTB, wildlife – particularly the badger population – is a source of (disease) risk for the national herd. Government policy has had to take account of the trade-offs between potentially conflicting objectives for public health, farm animal welfare and productivity, international trade, wildlife conservation, wildlife welfare and stakeholder opinion or belief.

The principal public driver for animal health control has been, and remains, anthropocentric, prioritising the health, well-being and property of human society. The public health function of Government was developed in response to zoonotic diseases that posed a risk to human health. The State's concern with bTB began in the late nineteenth and early twentieth century, when it was realised that the consumption of raw milk caused tuberculosis, sometimes fatally, in the human population. Consumption of infected cows' milk is thought to have led to over 2500 deaths and cause over 50000 human cases of tuberculosis annually in the early 1930s. During this period, 40% of cattle herds tested positive and 40% of cattle carcasses in public abattoirs had visible bTB lesions (Macdonald 1984). Pasteurisation, meat inspection at slaughterhouses and a cattle testing and slaughter programme were instituted and became effective safeguards for public health. However, whilst bTB was significantly reduced in the national herd, it was not eradicated; the prevalence always remained high in south-west England, and the badger was identified as the wildlife reservoir responsible. Subsequently, a number of culling strategies were used in an attempt to reduce the wildlife reservoir of bTB. At the same time, there was a concomitant shift in public attitude towards Government intervention in matters of public and animal health without clear evidence and justification. '*Anger is growing in the scientific community over Lord Zuckerman's report "Badgers cattle and tuberculosis" that has nothing to do with sentiment and much to do with the scientific quality of Zuckerman's evidence and argument ... TB kills badgers – one way or another – but the evidence for gassing is shaky*' (*New Scientist* 1980).

Debate has continued since (Macdonald 1984; Grant 2009; Swarbrick *et al.* 2010), but the Chief Scientist's report to Government (King 2007) summarised that '*TB control will require interventions that reduce the prevalence of disease in both cattle and wildlife and thus any removal of badgers must take place alongside current or future cattle controls*'.

When considering the ethics of bTB control and its impact on animals, cattle have benefited from the voluntary and then statutory bTB testing policies if the aim was to reduce disease in these populations. From an individual cow's perspective, testing positive for bTB, her life will be cut short by slaughter. However, the slaughter policy is for the benefit of the health of the national herd as a whole. Moreover, because the infected animal might in time develop symptoms of bTB, it could be argued that on balance she would prefer not to experience her future life (not considering false-positives for simplicity). For the badger, the benefits of culling are less clear. There are no detailed data on disease prevalence to assess the impact of any control strategies on the health of the badger population. We cannot easily trap and test badgers; in any case, trapping and holding a wild animal *per se* is a welfare issue. Therefore, differentiating infected from healthy badgers is not as simple as for cattle, which means that badger-culling policies have resulted in the deaths of healthy badgers as well as infected. The humane culling of infected badgers could be justified as being in the best interests of that badger as it is for the infected cow. However, the Government's position on wildlife disease is generally not to intervene, letting disease take its course if such animals are found in the wild. This position, mirrored in the Animal Welfare Act 2006, determines that society assumes no responsibility for the suffering of wild animals affected by 'natural' causes whilst they are living in the wild. Therefore, the decision to cull badgers in the wild is an anthropocentric priority; it is action deemed necessary to control a public and domestic animal health risk when there seems to be no other realistic policy alternative, such as vaccination (King 2007). The outcome is that infected badgers are culled in their best interests whilst the culling of healthy badgers is an unavoidable corollary.

The current debate tends to focus on the ethics of badger culling and its impact on the badger population, with less focus on the thousands of cattle that are slaughtered annually in the UK as part of the current control strategy. Nevertheless, bTB in the cattle population is a problem that is getting worse, not better. The challenge to Government is to develop robust, evidence-based policy, which balances interests. In the bTB debate, the interests of cattle and badgers are in opposition. There is no simple answer and deciding on the best course of action is ultimately a political judgement. bTB is most certainly a wicked problem.

16.3 Animal Ethics, Animal Welfare and Government Policy-making Today

With regard to animals, legal recognition of sentience does not mean that the public and its Government must recognise any rights (Regan 1983) or that their interests must be considered equally (Singer 1993). However, Government (and even European) policy is required to provide transparent evidence of the ethical basis for policy decisions that impact on animal welfare.

The legal recognition of animal sentience is reflected in the explanatory notes to the Animal Welfare Act 2006. They set out the considerations that courts should regard when determining whether suffering is unnecessary:

'Considerations focus on the necessity, proportionality, humanity and competence of the conduct. The court should take all relevant considerations into account, weighing

them against each other as appropriate. Where, for example, a horse suffers while being used for the purpose of riot control, this may well be considered necessary for the purposes of protecting persons or property (one of the considerations specified in the section). Or, where legitimate pest control activities entail an animal suffering, a court may consider whether this was in compliance with a relevant enactment, for a legitimate purpose, and proportionate to that purpose. The court would also consider the extent to which the suffering could reasonably have been avoided or reduced (another of the considerations specified in the section). Where suffering inevitably occurs in the course of complying with any regulations, licence or code of practice an offence would not normally be committed.'

However, this detailed explanation also infers a policy position with respect to the higher regard for human interest over that of animal. For example, the suffering of a police horse is deemed acceptable for protecting property. Government policy therefore does not exclusively respect animal interests, even within the Animal Welfare Act 2006.

Government policy on the consideration of animal interests through the 'animal welfare' concept is described (but not advocated) by Garner (2008):

'Animal welfare has reached such a degree of acceptability in Britain, as in many other countries, that it can be regarded as the moral orthodoxy. The recognition that animals are sentient is held to mean that we have direct moral obligations towards them, and not to their owners or those seeking to represent their interests. While having moral standing, however, the animal welfare position further holds the principle that humans are morally superior to animals. As a result, since animals have some moral worth, we are not entitled to inflict suffering on them unless the human benefit thereby resulting is deemed to be necessary.'

Consideration of the animal's interest is only part of the policy-making process, even when developing an animal welfare–specific policy. Government policy is fundamentally about producing or modifying rules that represent (and also influence) society's opinions and moral principles. Any law and guidance that accompanies such agreed policy ensures that society is clear about what is acceptable. The law goes further in that it provides for judgement and punishment of those who break the rules. These are selected on the basis of a (human) judgement of what is considered right at the time of making them, together with the consequences of those rules, which may not necessarily confer any benefit for animals. Current policy development therefore carefully considers potential consequences of change, assessing a wide range of potential impacts (e.g. on people, animals and the environment) before a final decision is made.

The Green Book (HM Treasury 2003) (as amended 2011) is the (UK) Treasury's guidance on policy development for central Government. It sets out the key stages in the development of a policy proposal, including the rationale for intervention, setting of objectives, options' appraisal, implementation and evaluation. It provides a framework for economic, financial, social and environmental impact assessments (IAs) and their relative weighting; it aims to ensure consistency and transparency in the appraisal process throughout Government.

IA is critical to Government policy. An IA should provide evidence for the policy's rationale, demonstrate transparency of decision-making and influence policy design. Critically, it identifies the expected impacts of policy options on public, private or civil society organisations, as far as possible quantifying and monetising the impacts for each affected group. An additional current requirement for policy-makers in England is that they must follow the Principles of Regulation in the Coalition Government (HM Government 2011), which require that Government will regulate to achieve objectives only *'having demonstrated that satisfactory outcomes cannot be achieved by alternative, self-regulatory, or non-regulatory approaches'* and that *'the regulatory approach is superior by a clear margin [to possible alternatives]'*.

The basis of the economic approach, as set out in *The Green Book*, is that humans decide trade-offs between policies. In doing this, they implicitly balance some impacts that are well understood and easily valued in financial terms against those that are less well understood and less easily valued. IAs seek to represent these trade-offs, make them explicit and show where the balance of costs and benefits lie. The responsible Minister is required to sign off the final IA document with the declaration *'I have read the Impact Assessment and I am satisfied that (a) it represents a fair and reasonable view of the expected costs, benefits and impact of the policy, and (b) that the benefits justify the costs'*. Considerable effort goes into the cost benefit appraisal to provide this assurance, allowing a thorough appraisal of the rationale for State intervention.

In developing policy specifically for animals or policy that affects animals incidentally, the expected impacts on animals should be identified, quantified and valued as far as is possible and reasonable. Animal welfare impacts are typically quite difficult to quantify and value, and sometimes appear in an IA as 'non-monetised benefits' that are set against fully quantified and monetised costs. Here again, the Minister should be satisfied that the benefits are great enough to justify the costs. Common – but difficult – examples include qualified rights and religious freedom. Another impact is sustainability, which aims to ensure that the (human) quality of life is improved without compromising the natural resources of future generations. For instance, impact on environmental sustainability is applicable to Government policy on food productivity and agricultural intensification. Whilst the Government can improve methods for quantifying and monetising animal impacts, there is always likely to be an element of political judgement in reaching the final decision.

16.4 Conclusions

The ideal is that Government policy benefits all; however, the reality is that a policy is likely to have adverse consequences for some parties, whether they are people, business, the environment or animals. The Government accounts for the views of and impacts on relevant stakeholders, but must also guard and protect sentient beings, including animals, who cannot speak for themselves. In this sense, the Government is acting as a guardian (Wathes 2010). Whilst deregulation and self-regulation are important factors in demonstrating that society can take responsibility for itself, there will always be a need for regulatory protection for animals. Kept animals are property; without regulation, people can treat or destroy their own property as they wish, as long as their action causes no harm to other persons or property. However, an owner is responsible for his animal and can be held accountable for its welfare. Government policy and regulation clearly reflects society's current concerns, whilst any change in Government policy can also influence society's thinking. These are fluid: over the last 200 years, Government policy has evolved from basic protection against wanton cruelty and unnecessary suffering to species-specific minimum standards. In the twenty-first century, as we understand animal feelings better through advances in cognitive neuroscience and affective states, society can push these standards even higher. The Farm Animal Welfare Council suggested that whilst the Five Freedoms can avoid suffering and provide for a life worth living, we also need to look beyond this and focus on how we can give animals a good life. This would represent a vision of 'moral progress' (Wynne-Tyson 1985). Whether Government policy can fulfil such a vision, together with fulfilling the needs of all its other stakeholders, remains an open question.

'It cannot seriously be disputed that the development of law, at all times and places, has in fact been profoundly influenced both by conventional morality and ideals of particular social groups, and also by forms of enlightened moral criticism urged by individuals, whose moral horizon has transcended the morality currently accepted. (Hart 1961)'

References

Animal Welfare Act (2006) Available at: http://www.legislation.gov.uk/ukpga/2006/45/data.pdf. Accessed on 10th July 2012

Animal Welfare Act (2006) Explanatory Notes to the Animal Welfare Act. Available at: http://www.legislation.gov.uk/ukpga/2006/45/notes/data.pdf. Accessed on 10th July 2012

Briggs, L. (2007) Tackling wicked problems: A public policy perspective. Barton ACT, Australian Public Service Commission, Commonwealth of Australia.

Cardwell, E. (1876) Report of the Royal commission on the practice of subjecting live animals to experiments for scientific purposes; with minutes of evidence and appendix [also Digest of evidence, and General analytical index], HMSO, London.

Churchman, C.W. (1967) Wicked problems. *Management Science*, **14**, 141–142.

Council Directive (1974) 74/577/EEC OJ L 316, 26.11.1974, p. 10–11. Available at: http://eur-lex.europa.eu/smartapi/cgi/sga_doc?smartapi!celexplus!prod!DocNumberandlg=enandtype_doc=Directiveandan_doc=1974andnu_doc=577. Accessed on 10th July 2012

Council Directive (1993) 93/119/EC OJ L 340, 31.12.1993, p. 21–34. Available at: http://eur-lex.europa.eu/LexUriServ/LexUriServ.do?uri=CELEX:31993L0119:EN:NOT. Accessed on 10th July 2012

Council Directive (1998) 98/58/EC Concerning the protection of animals kept for farming purposes OJ No. L 221 08.08.1998, p. 23. Available at: http://eur-lex.europa.eu/LexUriServ/LexUriServ.do?uri=CELEX:31998L0058:EN:NOT. Accessed on 10th July 2012

Council of Europe (1961) Parliamentary Assembly RECOMMENDATION 287 (1961)[1] on the international transit of animals. Available at: http://assembly.coe.int/Main.asp?link=/Documents/AdoptedText/ta61/EREC287.htm. Accessed on 10th July 2012

Darwin, C. (1871) *The Descent of Man and Selection in Relation to Sex*, p. 35 and 98. John Murray, London.

de Montmorency, J.E.G. (1902) State protection of animals at home and abroad, 18 Law Quarterly Rev. 31.

Erskine, J. (1809) Parliamentary debates (Lords) HL Deb 15 May 1809, vol. 14 cc553-71. Available at: http://hansard.millbanksystems.com/lords/1809/may/15/cruelty-to-animals-bill#S1V0014P0_18090515_HOL_2. Accessed on 10th July 2012

Garner, R. (2008) The politics of animal rights. *British Politics*, 3, 110–119.

Grant, W. (2009) Intractable policy failure: The case of bovine TB and badgers. *The British Journal of Politics and International Relations*, 11, 557–573.

Hart, H.L.A. (1961) *The Concept of Law*. Clarendon Press, Oxford.

HM Government (2011) Impact assessment guidance when to do an impact assessment; Annex A: Principles of regulation in the coalition government. Available at: http://www.bis.gov.uk/assets/BISCore/better-regulation/docs/I/11-1111-impact-assessment-guidance.pdf. Accessed on 10th July 2012

HMSO (1932) Royal Society for the Prevention of Cruelty to Animals Act, 1932, Chapter XXXIX. Preamble to: An Act to incorporate and confer powers upon the Royal Society for the Prevention of Cruelty to Animals, London.

HM Treasury (2003) (amended 2011) *The Green Book Appraisal and Evaluation in Central Government*, London. Available at: http://www.hm-treasury.gov.uk/d/green_book_complete.pdf. Accessed on 10th July 2012

Hogarth, W. (1751) *Engravings and Woodcuts* (two woodcuts plates III and IV by J Bell 1750).

King, D. (2007) Bovine tuberculosis in cattle and badgers. Report to the Secretary of State, July 2007. Available at: http://www.bis.gov.uk/assets/biscore/corporate/migratedD/ec_group/44-07-S_I_on. Accessed on 10th July 2012

Lakhani, J. (2007) Radio Wales interview, 26 July 2007. Available at: http://news.bbc.co.uk/1/hi/6917226.stm. Accessed on 10th July 2012

Lawrence, J. (1796) *A Philosophical Treatise on Horses, and on the Moral duties of Man towards the Brute Creation*, Volume 1 of 2. Longman, London.

Lazarus, R.J. (2009) Super wicked problems and climate change: Restraining the present to liberate the future Georgetown law faculty publications and other works. Paper 159.

Macdonald, D. (1984) Badgers and bovine tuberculosis – Case not proven. *New Scientist*, 25 October 1984, pp. 17–20.

Regan, T. (1983) The Case for Animal Rights. University of California press, Berkeley.

Rittel, H.W.J. & Webber, M.W. (1973) Dilemmas in a general theory of planning. *Policy Sciences*, 4, 155–169.

Singer, P. (1993) *Practical Ethics*. Cambridge University Press, Cambridge.

Swarbrick, O., Walsby, J. & Wicks, B. (2010) Controlling bovine TB. *Veterinary Record*, 167, 715–716.

Treaty of Amsterdam (1999) Treaty on the functioning of the European Union, Title II, Article 13. Official Journal C 115, 09/05/2008, pp. 0001–0388. Available at: http://eur-lex.

europa.eu/LexUriServ/LexUriServ.do?uri=OJ:C:2008:115:0001:01:EN:HTML. Accessed on 10th July 2012

Wathes, C. (2010) Guarding the welfare of farm animals. *Veterinary Record*, **167**, 583–584.

Windham, W. (1800) Parliamentary history of England from the earliest period to the year 1803, Volume 35, col 204 and 206.

World Trade Organization (1947) *The General Agreement on Tariffs and Trade (GATT 1947)*, 1999 Treaty on the Functioning of the European Union (Treaty of Amsterdam), Article 13.

Wynne-Tyson, J. (1985) *Extended Circle: A Dictionary of Humane Thought*. Centaur Press, Fontwell, Sussex.

Questions and Answers

Q: If it then is true that Governmental actions reflect in one way or the other what society wants, then how far is it then the duty of the Government to educate society in the way that society wants the right things?
A: That's absolutely right. How does one educate society? We're engaged in a debate. If you see improving animal welfare as a journey, that journey is constant. Government, every time it makes an incremental change, has to underpin that by gaining understanding for what it's doing. You push the barrier with the dog or rabbit code and you might get into trouble but there's a constant effort. Getting[school] education in at the earliest possible stage is very important and something that this Government is looking at amongst many others. If society is going to change, it needs to be helped to change.

Q: You talk very optimistically about the role of Government bringing in polarised views, trying to get them together, except for TB of course. For an issue like the mega dairies where the debate is polarised, some organisations take different positions. There's the issue of sustainable intensification too. Is Government's role to facilitate a consensus view on the mega dairies or are you going to sit and watch?
A: Government needs to take a position on these issues. There's a tension about sustainable intensification. We're on this welfare journey and know where we're going. There's nothing wrong with intensive production; if done well and with good management, you can deal with animal welfare concerns but if the future does avoid climate change, how are we going to achieve increased food security with good welfare outcomes? Mega big farms is another polarised debate. Some say, this isn't a good system for various reasons, not all of which are welfare. Others say, '*But we need to be effective. We need to be productive. We can apply greater management controls if we do it this way than if we've got smaller.*' Government can only put forward a balanced reflection of those arguments and it's not for me to say whether, ultimately, there would be an intervention. The debate is very active of course.

Q: You mentioned taking account of animal welfare in policy-making. When you're carrying out a cost benefit analysis or an impact assessment, how is animal welfare measured? The only mechanism which I've seen used is 'willingness to pay', which is not measuring animal welfare *per se*, but what the general public values or perceives as good animal welfare. Intrinsically, I would have thought that they would value animals that they value, like badgers or kittens over rats. How we can get closer to an absolute measure of good welfare rather than what the public thinks is good welfare?

A: That's a very good point. We need to understand where society is and what people might value. If you ask a consumer before they go into the supermarket what is their buying preference and then let them complete their purchases, then their buying preference isn't what they told you it was. Their deeds don't reflect their aspirations. We also have to marshal hard evidence about welfare impacts. Scientific understanding of an animal's perspective, as opposed to physiological impacts, is important evidence to place in the mix that we put before ministers.

Q: We've known in relation to our own motivation and pleasures for over 50 years that there's a distinction between hygiene factors and motivators in the sense that an absence of dissatisfaction does not automatically mean satisfaction. Shouldn't we go for the good life?

A: My reflection was, of course, from an animal-centric point of view: *a good life* is better than *a life worth living*. From a consumer's point of view, if asked, without any financial impact of that decision, the same applies. However, how do you achieve that goal in a way where policy doesn't lead to an unintended outcome? The debate is not whether to advance animal welfare over time – provided you can bring society with you – but how to do it effectively? If we do it just in the UK, what will the impact be and have we advanced welfare for the greater number of animals? It's a numbers game. If we export our industry, we haven't achieved that.

C: There are very good robust measurements of bad welfare and abuses to welfare, which have been accepted throughout Europe. The indicators of positive welfare are very fuzzy indeed.

Q: Do you think there's a moral problem between cutting across human rights for animal disease control but not for purposes of non-disease based on poor welfare. Which cultural or traditional heritage arguments are invoked?

A: There's a moral challenge. The courts do a very good job of reflecting the environment in which decisions are made. In the case of disease control, the evidence was very strong unlike the individual's religious rights. A Hindu cleric's interpretation of the euthanasia of TB-infected cattle would suggest a strong case, that is sacrificing the individual for the sake of the population was worth doing. The difficult issue of religious slaughter is that society has accepted that religion is something that you don't mess with lightly. The weight of the argument is very different; it's not just a UK or EU issue but is a global one. Is there a moral problem? Yes, of course: things don't work in the same way in both issues. Is it amenable to quick solutions? No.

Authors' Commentary

Many of the questions focussed on the Government's role with respect to responsibility towards animals and educating citizens about animal needs. The paper's conclusion summarises these issues with a quote by Hart (1961) which, in discussing the development of law, incorporates the various influences on Government policy, that is conventional morality, social ideals and enlightened moral criticism by those who choose to question current accepted norms. It is from such criticism that we continue to ask more questions, develop and test new hypotheses so that we can better understand the needs of animals and transfer that knowledge to society as best we can. How society chooses to interpret and act on such education and knowledge transfer however is yet another challenge for the Government.

The Government is committed to ensuring that minimum standards of animal welfare are maintained during day-to-day animal care and, where appropriate, at the time of killing. Animals are sentient beings and, as such, must be given, at the minimum, their basic needs; any suffering should be avoided as far as is possible. These requirements are enshrined within current law in the Animal Welfare Act 2006. Whilst good self-regulation can be acknowledged and/or rewarded, this cannot completely absolve the need for continued regulation in certain areas of Government policy.

The Government's commitment to a welfare research and development programme reflects the areas of welfare concern highlighted during the discussion. Such projects have already and will in future look at issues that include evaluating the impacts of both extremes of livestock intensification and extensification, including fish, to ensure that both welfare and profit can be maximised in the sustainable environments to which farmed animals are exposed. We are evaluating the best ways to influence behavioural change in stockmen as well as a future focus on looking at developing and measuring positive welfare indicators, not just negative ones, in order to advance the concept of. We are also funding further work on education in schools. We will continue to push the frontier on welfare research where there is a clear policy need for this.

Veterinary Ethics and Law

17

MARIE FOX

University of Birmingham

Abstract: This paper addresses the governance of veterinary practice. I argue that the existing self-regulatory framework is outdated and contrasts sharply with the close legal governance of the practice of human medicine. Specifically, I contend that the current regime is too reactive and that mechanisms for dealing with complaints raise concerns about the independence and transparency of decision-making. Furthermore, the limited options open to the disciplinary committee, and the limited rights of appeal for those subject to complaints give rise to further concern. In short, the current model, established 45 years ago, continues to display all the traditional shortcomings of the self-regulatory paradigm. For dissatisfied clients, the only alternative is litigation on the basis of either professional negligence or breach of contract, but there are formidable obstacles to success in litigation. I conclude that the Veterinary Surgeons Act 1966 is no longer fit for regulatory purpose and that, notwithstanding various practical and economic barriers to reform, the veterinary profession should heed the lessons of human medicine and take the initiative in promoting legislative change. While the regulatory body, the Royal College of Veterinary Surgeons, favours legislative reform, there seems little political will for new legislation. However, unless this occurs there is a real risk that future reforms will be forced upon the profession in response to scandal or breaches of human rights, which will do nothing to promote public trust and confidence in the veterinary profession.

Keywords: complaint, concern, conduct, ethics, governance, law, legislation, litigation, medicine, negligence, professional regulation, RCVS, rights, veterinarians, veterinary ethics, Veterinary Surgeons Act

Veterinary & Animal Ethics: Proceedings of the First International Conference on Veterinary and Animal Ethics, September 2011, First Edition. Edited by Christopher M. Wathes, Sandra A. Corr, Stephen A. May, Steven P. McCulloch and Martin C. Whiting.
© 2013 Universities Federation for Animal Welfare. Published 2013 by Blackwell Publishing Ltd.

17.1 Introduction

This paper examines the ethico-legal governance of the veterinary profession in the UK. Veterinarians are subject to a self-regulatory regime similar to that which regulated other professions, notably medicine, in the past. Self-regulation is justified by an ideology of professionalism that proposes that professionals have the requisite integrity to be trusted to work free from external scrutiny, combined with possession of specialist skills or knowledge that render regulation by non-professionals inappropriate (Saks 1995; De Prez 2002). Additionally, self-regulatory models are more cost-effective than public regulatory regimes, since monitoring and enforcement costs, as well as costs of amending standards, are lower (Ogus 1995, 98). Under such models, law's role is limited to providing a framework for professional regulation. Thus, the legislation governing the profession – the Veterinary Surgeons Act 1966 – contains little substance about the regulation of veterinarians. It is concerned principally with the maintenance of the veterinary register,[1] oversight of veterinary education and elections to office and to council. It does place the regulatory body, the Royal College of Veterinary Surgeons (RCVS), on a statutory footing and outlines the mechanisms by which it exercises its disciplinary powers. However, the RCVS lacks power to monitor or investigate the profession, and details of ethical governance are provided by professional guidance, which lacks a statutory basis (RCVS 2010, 2011a). Moreover, since the 1960s, the landscape of professional regulation has radically altered, prompted by an erosion of trust in many professions and sceptical social attitudes which perceive self-regulation as fuelled by protectionism and self-interest (Allsop & Mulcahy 1996; Ogus 1995). The upshot for the medical and legal professions has been more onerous statutory regulation,[2] while for the veterinary profession, as Radford noted a decade ago, 'legislation fails to reflect the developments that have lately taken place in regulation of comparable professions' (Radford 2001, 316). These regulatory shifts have also been accompanied by social changes within the profession. Since 1966, the number of registered veterinarians has risen significantly;[3] and many now operate out of large practices, a growing number of which are corporate-owned. Additionally, the veterinary profession is characterised by a much higher degree of specialism, increased use of technologies (and thus treatment options) and an orientation towards small animal practice. Changes have also occurred in our beliefs about the

---

[1] Legislative amendments too have focused on registration – see, *inter alia*, Veterinary Surgeons' Qualifications (European Recognition) Order 2007, Veterinary Surgeons (Registration Appeals) Rules Order of Council 2009.

[2] For instance, Courts and Legal Services Act 1990, Legal Services Act 2007, Francis 2011; National Health Service Reform and Health Care Professions Act 2002, Health and Social Care Act 2008, Secretary of State for Health 2006, Davies 2006.

[3] A 2008 Report of a House of Commons Committee noted that only 8143 vets were registered with the RCVS in 1966 (House of Commons 2008) but by 2011 the figure had grown to 24575 (RCVS 2011c, 4).

moral (Donovan & Adams 1996; Calarco 2008) and legal (Francione 1995; Radford 2001; Fox 2004) status of animals, while our relationship with companion animals has become particularly complex, since they have been rendered simultaneously more akin to family members and more commodified.[4] Against this backdrop, and as veterinary medicine faces increasingly complex challenges, the growth of veterinary ethics is no surprise (Tannenbaum 1995; Rollin 2006). Although veterinary law has attracted little academic attention in the UK (Radford 2000; Glynn & Gomez 2005; on the USA see Wilson & Garbe 1990; Soave 2000; Hemenway 2010), I argue that, given the importance of the profession to human and animal health, its legal governance merits greater scrutiny. Although it is widely accepted that the 1966 statute is outdated, there is little political or professional will to effect necessary reforms. Thus in March 2008 Lord Rooker, Minister for Sustainable Food, Farming and Animal Health, indicated that Defra lacked the necessary funds for a White Paper on reform at least until 2011 (House of Commons 2008, para 24), thereby placing the onus on the veterinary profession, which in turn was criticised in a House of Commons Committee Report into the operation of the 1966 Act for not having made greater progress with reform proposals in the wake of consultations held with the profession in 2003 and 2005 (House of Commons 2008, para 21).[5] While the veterinary profession has been subject to proportionately fewer complaints and less litigation than the medical profession,[6] I suggest that any complacency is misplaced and that it is crucial to frame reforms that better fit the regulatory challenges of the twenty-first century.

17.2 Disciplinary Proceedings against Veterinarians

The key features of the 1966 Act regarding professional regulation are the provisions which govern disciplinary proceedings in ss. 15–19. Three grounds are stipulated in s. 16 for removal or suspension from the veterinary register: conviction 'of a criminal offence, which in the opinion of the disciplinary committee renders him unfit to practice veterinary medicine' (s. 16(1)(a)); a finding that a veterinarian has been guilty of 'disgraceful conduct in a professional respect' (s. 16(1)(b)); or a finding that entry on the veterinary register is fraudulent 16(1) (c)). Additionally, a new Health Protocol has now been added to the RCVS Code of Conduct. This provides that veterinarians who experience health problems

---

[4] Haraway charts how we increasingly view 'pets' as 'companion animals' (Haraway 2008, 134) and spend significant amounts on their care, including veterinary fees. Thus, in 2006 in the USA, approximately $9.4 billion was spent on veterinary care for pets (2008, 50).

[5] The report also noted the low level of response to both consultations from individual veterinarians (House of Commons 2008, para 10).

[6] In its evidence to the House of Common's Committee, the British Veterinary Association (BVA) stated that '*there is a high level of public confidence in the veterinary profession, and on this basis it could be argued that substantial changes to the 1966 Act are neither justified nor necessary*' (House of Commons 2008, para 15).

should be supported in a structured programme overseen by the Preliminary Investigation Committee (PIC) rather than being referred to the Disciplinary Committee (DC). While it is true, as the protocol acknowledges, that the complaints procedure can be an inappropriate mechanism in such cases, health problems may be relevant to complaints and it is problematic that the determination of veterinary fitness to practice is not considered holistically as is the case with doctors. Under Rule 18.4(c) of the Veterinary Surgeons and Veterinary Practitioners (Disciplinary Committee (Procedure and Evidence) Rules 2004), the DC also has the option of reprimanding or warning a respondent as to future conduct.

In this paper, I will concentrate on ground 16(1)(b), where the College's jurisdiction stems from complaints against veterinarians. However, it is important to note at the outset that the wording limits the College's jurisdiction by its focus on 'behaviour', so that complaints about negligence or fees, for instance, are outwith its remit unless they are sufficiently serious to amount to 'disgraceful conduct'. Thus, many dissatisfied clients are left with no alternative but to seek redress through the courts for negligence or breach of contract. Space precludes a consideration of legal remedies against veterinarians, but there are significant difficulties in demonstrating both breach of the standard of care (implied in contracts or necessary to establish negligence), and that any breach caused the harm suffered (McHale & Fox 2007, Ch 3; Soave 2000, Ch 3). Since low success rates are compounded by well documented obstacles to litigation, principally huge costs and delay (Cane 2006), significant disincentives to legal actions against professionals exist. Yet, as the House of Commons Committee, in its review of the 1966 legislation, concluded:

> 'It is not satisfactory for the customer who has a genuine case for complaint about the professional standards of a vet to only have recourse to the civil law without any appeal to a regulatory body.' (House of Commons 2008, para 42)

The Committee also concurred with Defra's submission that the RCVS should be empowered to investigate lesser complaints of 'unsatisfactory professional misconduct'.

17.3 Handling Complaints

According to the RCVS, 700–800 complaints are received annually. These are assessed by a legally qualified case manager to determine whether they potentially constitute *'disgraceful conduct in a professional respect'*. The manager is advised by case examiners (one a veterinarian and member of the PIC and the other a lay observer). If they conclude that an arguable case exists, the complaint is referred to the PIC (in about 30% of cases); otherwise the case is closed, although advice may be given to the veterinarian concerned (RCVS 2011b). Under s.15, the PIC's role is to investigate whether the case should be referred to the DC. The PIC is composed of the President and Vice Presidents of the RCVS and three elected members of Council. It sits in private (with three lay assessors present) to determine whether there is a realistic prospect that the veterinarian concerned is guilty of disgraceful conduct, which according to the RCVS means 'not a probability but rather a genuine (not remote or fanciful) possibility' of guilt (RCVS 2007, 10). The meaning of 'disgraceful conduct' (*vide infra*) is unacceptably vague, but the RCVS's illustrative list of actions that may come within its scope includes serious departure from standards in its Guide to Professional Conduct; causing serious harm (or a risk thereof) to animals or the public; committing violent offences; evidence of a harmful deep-seated personality or attitude problem; and dishonesty (RCVS 2007, 10). In its deliberations, the PIC must balance protection of the public and maintenance of the profession's reputation against legitimate safeguards for the veterinarian (RCVS 2007, 10). If the PIC concludes there is no real prospect that the veterinarian was guilty of disgraceful conduct, the complaint is closed, although the veterinarian may again be given advice, either in person or in writing.

The DC is comprised of a Chairperson and 11 other members of Council, elected by Council, at least one of whom must be a Privy Council appointee. No member of the PIC may serve on the DC, which is a properly constituted judicial tribunal and must comply with the Veterinary Surgeons and Veterinary Practitioners (DC) (Procedure and Evidence) Rules 2004. The DC is advised on procedure by a legal adviser and the burden of proof is stated by the RCVS to be '*the highest civil standard i.e. so that it is sure (tantamount to the criminal standard)*' (RCVS 2007, 11).

A veterinarian removed under s. 16 may apply to have his/her name restored once 10 months have elapsed. He/she will be required to reappear before the DC to satisfy it that he/she is fit to return to practice. If suspended, the veterinarian is debarred from veterinary activity until the period of suspension has expired, at which time his/her name will be automatically restored. Appeals against a decision of the DC lie to the Privy Council (s. 17).

17.4 Defects in the Complaints Procedure

Although the complaints procedure has been revised by secondary legislation and the RCVS to flesh out the skeletal framework offered by the 1966 legislation, a number of fundamental problems with the disciplinary procedures persist.

First, for any scheme of regulation to command public confidence, it is crucial that justice is seen to be done. Yet the 1966 Act vests prosecutorial and adjudicative functions in the same body, which is antithetical to client interests, to transparency and to accountability (Freckleton 2006). Potentially it also leaves the DC open to challenge for infringing the human rights of veterinarians subject to its procedures, as this arguably infringes Article 6 of the European Convention on Human Rights. Furthermore, aside from the right of veterinarians, who are struck off or suspended, to appeal to the Privy Council, the DC is not accountable for its decisions to any independent body, such as an Ombudsman.

Secondly, the system is concerned to discipline veterinarians when things go wrong, rather than seeking to prevent things going wrong in the first place. As was the case in medicine, the 1966 statute was premised on the assumption that '*mere possession of tertiary qualifications is sufficient for a lifetime license to practice*' (Freckleton 2006, 55). In the wake of the Bristol and Shipman Inquiries, reforms to how doctors are regulated have done much to foster a culture of professionalism, which employs professional and clinical standards, routine assessment and monitoring coupled with support mechanisms for doctors. The Bristol Inquiry Report stressed the necessity for '*appraisal, continuing professional development and revalidation to ensure that all healthcare professionals remain competent to do their job*' (Kennedy 2001, para 15). Implementation of such measures has been controversial, with proposals for revalidation of doctors' fitness to practice and for oversight by an independent body proving especially contested. The GMC's original proposals for revalidation attracted robust criticism in the Shipman Inquiry Report, where Dame Janet Smith stressed the need for a revalidation process to carry real consequences if a doctor's performance was unsatisfactory (Smith 2004, Ch 26). The GMC has now designated revalidation its 'number one priority' to be implemented by the end of 2012 (GMC 2010). It presents this as a new way to regulate, focused on maintaining and improving practitioner competence, offering support and encouraging patient feedback. It is envisaged that doctors will be revalidated every 5 years, provided the GMC is satisfied (based on annual appraisals and other evidence) that the doctor is fit to practice. In other respects, however, the recommendations of the Bristol and Shipman Inquires have been significantly watered down, so that the predicted demise of self-regulation has proven somewhat misplaced. Thus, the current Government's decision to scrap the independent Office of the Health Professions Adjudicator, established by the Health and Social Care Act 2008, means that determinations of fitness to practice will, after all, remain within the jurisdiction of the GMC. Nevertheless, so far as regulation is concerned, the medical profession is light years ahead of the veterinary profession, where revalidation continues to be implacably opposed (BVA 2007, 2009). However, the British Veterinary Association's (BVA) stance on Continuing Professional Development (CPD) has softened, and regulations that came into force in 2010[7] provide that veterinarians '*may be requested to complete and return an annual CPD declaration*' while the draft Code of Conduct requires that they '*must maintain and develop the knowledge and skills relevant to their professional practice and ... undertake a minimum of 105 hours of CPD over any consecutive three year period*'. Yet, there is still evidence of considerable resistance in the body of the profession (House of Commons 2008, para 64), suggesting the need for strong leadership by the profession on these issues.

[7] Veterinary Surgeons and Veterinary Practitioners (Registration) Regulations Order of Council 2010.

Thirdly, as noted above, the scope of the complaints procedure is limited, and its boundaries uncertain. The phrase 'disgraceful conduct in any professional respect' is antiquated, dating from the 1881 Veterinary Surgeons Act. Although the RCVS appear to treat it as synonymous with the commonplace 'serious professional misconduct' used in the GMC guidance and elsewhere, it is arguable that the wording of the 1966 Act sets a lower standard of acceptable professional conduct for veterinarians than that applicable to doctors. And, as Brazier and Case point out, critics complain that for doctors *'the threshold of what constituted misconduct was set too high, and when such a finding was made, penalties were too lenient'* (Brazier & Cave 2007, 8). In the case of veterinarians, penalties are yet more lenient, particularly given the high burden of proof to be satisfied. Indeed, it is questionable whether there is a meaningful difference between suspension and removal, given that a veterinarian struck off may apply for readmission to the register within 10 months,[8] whereas doctors may not apply for readmission until 5 years have elapsed. Aside from removal and suspension, there is no provision in the complaints structure for formal warnings, the imposition of restrictions on practice or interim suspensions (RCVS 2005, para 42–43). Given this, it is impossible to dissent from the House of Commons Committee's conclusion that *'there ought to be a wider range of sanctions available … to give flexibility and proportionality to the operation of the complaints process'* (House of Commons 2008, para 44).

Finally, I would argue that the appeals procedure is unsatisfactory since the Privy Council's jurisdiction is limited and it has taken a non-interventionist stance in reviewing disciplinary proceedings. In the case of doctors, this prompted legislative reform under s. 30 National Health Service Reform and Health Care Professions Act 2002, which substituted a right of appeal to the High Court. According to one commentator, the High Court has *'shown an inclination to intervene more often'* than the Privy Council did (Heppinstall 2006, 278). In the case of veterinarians, the Privy Council has consistently reiterated its reluctance to interfere since *Marten v RCVS's Disciplinary Committee* (1966) where the Court of Criminal Appeal held, in a case decided under the 1881 statute, that *'an appellate tribunal should be slow to interfere with a professional body's exercise of discretion as to sentence'* (per Lord Parker CJ at para 10 A).

17.5 Disciplinary Appeals

A review of some of the reported cases heard by the Privy Council offers an indication both of those rare cases where an appeal may succeed and of how judges have interpreted the key phrase 'disgraceful conduct in a professional respect'. In practice, the Court has reversed the DC's direction only when it has found that a merely

[8] In *Walker* (below), the Court observed that the penalties differed in the eyes of the public and that in practice re-registration may take longer than ten months.

technical breach of the legislation or Code of Conduct supported a finding of 'disgraceful conduct' or where there has been a procedural breach of the appellant's due process rights. For instance, in *Tait v RCVS* (2003), notwithstanding the seriousness of the charges against the appellant which had led to the deaths of two dogs, the Privy Council upheld his contention that the DC had erred in refusing an adjournment when he was unable to attend the hearing due to illness.

In other cases, the Court has overturned a direction to suspend or remove a veterinarian because little or no potential for harm to humans or animals existed. Thus, in *Plenderleith v RCVS*, it ordered the reinstatement of a veterinarian whose registration was suspended for 4 months when he permitted two veterinarians in his employment, who were EU nationals but whose registration had yet to be approved by the RCVS, to administer procedures to animals. While accepting that the appellant's conduct constituted a breach of s. 19 of the 1966 Act, Lord Slynn ruled that not '*every breach of the disciplinary code or of the statute or every commission of a criminal offence is necessarily to be regarded as "disgraceful conduct in a professional respect" … there must be a line below which conduct does not satisfy this test*' (at para 229, G). The court concluded that on all the evidence the appellant could not be regarded as guilty of disgraceful conduct, but cautioned that it was a 'special case' (at para 230, B). Nevertheless, a similar approach was adopted in *Walker v RCVS* (2008) where a specialist equine veterinarian had been removed from the register when the DC found that two charges of falsely certifying that racehorses had received booster vaccinations against equine influenza within a year of their last vaccination amounted to disgraceful professional conduct. The Privy Council substituted a 6 month suspension for removal from the register. While emphasising the importance of correct veterinary certificates, the Court was critical of the reasoning of the DC, which served to '*group all cases of false certification together in one bracket*' (per Lord Mance at para 14). Having surveyed the outcomes of earlier wrongful certification decisions by the DC, it concluded that in the instant case '*the nature and circumstance of Dr Walker's offending place it in a significantly lower category of seriousness than any of the cases where removal from the Register was directed*' (at para 22). The Court concluded that given Dr Walker's frankness and remorse, and the fact that he was satisfied that the horses were fully protected since there was no medical rationale for the yearly vaccinations required by the Jockey Club, a 6 month suspension was appropriate.

However, cases which jeopardise animal welfare have been regarded more severely, and later the same year in *Williams v RCVS*, the Court upheld the DC's decision to remove from the register a veterinarian who had falsely certified for export purposes that horses were free from Contagious Equine Metritis and that the requisite tests had been undertaken at a Defra-approved laboratory. The Court highlighted the slight risk that an unfit horse could have been exported due to the appellant's actions, which combined with his prior history of suspensions and warnings in respect of inappropriately signed export certificates, warranted removal.

Similarly, in *Archbold v. Disciplinary Committee of the RCVS* (2004), the appellant was removed from the register having falsely certified that two cows were fit for human consumption under a scheme designed to control Bovine Spongiform Encephalopathy (BSE). He had also falsely stated that he had administered lethal injections to the animals, whereas in fact he had merely provided barbiturates in hypodermic needles to the owner. In this case, the Privy Council highlighted the appellant's dishonesty and its possible consequences, since '*it could have led to undue animal suffering, put public health at risk and provided a vehicle for fraud*' (per Sir Kenneth Keith, at para 7). In these circumstances, the court rejected the contention that removal from the register was excessive punishment, noting that the *Tait* case (above) had ruled that '*proven dishonesty comes at the top end of the spectrum for gravity for misconduct*' (per Sir Keith, at para 14).

Two years later in *Macleod v the RCVS*, an experienced veterinarian working in a small animal veterinary practice established a separate clinic 7 miles away. This was staffed wholly by veterinary nurses and advertised vaccinations, routine pet checks, worming treatments, etc. It was not disputed that the clinic aimed to provide vaccinations at a lower cost than fees charged at clinics where vaccinations were administered by veterinarians. Local veterinarians complained and the appellant was found guilty of disgraceful conduct in relation to five animals which were administered prescription-only medicine by veterinary nurses in breach of s. 58 of the Medicines Act 1968. The veterinarian contended that the actions of her staff fell within exemptions in s. 58(3) of the Medicines Act and schedule 3 para 6(a) of the Veterinary Surgeons Act, which permit veterinary nurses to carry out certain treatment provided that the animal is '*under the care of a registered veterinary surgeon ... and the medical treatment ... is carried out by the veterinary nurse at his direction*'. This interpretation was rejected by Lord Carswell, who stated that while the circumstances in which treatment is carried out under the direction of a veterinarian could vary widely, '*[t]he concept does, however, connote an element of immediacy and potential control of the treatment which was wholly lacking in the carrying out of the vaccination at the [appellant's] clinics*' (para 18). The court also upheld the DC's ruling that the system in place for providing 24 h cover was inadequate, with insufficient checks on messages left on an answering machine. Yet, while conceding that her actions were capable of jeopardising animal welfare, the Court concluded that suspending the appellant's registration for 8 months was disproportionate given the absence of dishonesty and the fact that she was '*labouring under a misapprehension*' (para 27), and substituted a reprimand and warning.

Finally, so far as the scope of 'disgraceful' conduct is concerned, *Kirk v RCVS* (2003) offers a rare example of how behaviour which is not dishonest and which causes no harm to animals can nevertheless support a finding of unfitness to practice. Here the Privy Council upheld the DC's decision to remove the appellant from the register following four convictions for assault and two for public health offences. Having outlined the appellant's chequered disciplinary history, entailing '*literally dozens of prosecutions and at least two previous disciplinary proceedings*', Lord

Hoffman concluded that notwithstanding the considerable loss that his services would represent to the public, nevertheless veterinarians '*are expected to conduct themselves generally in accordance with the standards of professional men and women and...their Lordships find it difficult to say that violent or antisocial behaviour of the kind involved in Mr. Kirk's convictions cannot in principle be a ground for a finding that he is unfit to practice*' (para 33).

17.6 The Case for Reform

This paper has questioned the adequacy of the current legislation for governance of the veterinary profession. While it is true that there has been no public outcry, the likelihood is that many clients dissatisfied with veterinary performance lack remedies, while veterinarians are given scant incentive to improve and courts are left to grapple with outmoded legal concepts. Unsurprisingly, legislative reform has been mooted for some years, with Defra reiterating to the House of Commons Committee in 2008 that the Act was in '*urgent need of updating to bring it in line with modern concepts of professional regulation*' (House of Commons Committee 2008, para 17, Ev51). Yet Defra's decision to abandon a planned White Paper on legislative reform, combined with resistance or apathy within the profession (House of Commons 2008, paras 14, 85), has hampered the framing of concrete proposals for reform. Given the various criticisms levelled at the 1966 Act, the BVA's position that only minor tinkering with the current legislative regime is required is untenable (BVA 2007, 2009). The problems, as we have seen, are manifest, ranging from the overly narrow and unclear grounds for complaint, limited lay involvement in adjudication, the lack of investigative powers, the inadequate range of penalties and the absence of incentives to improve professional practice. Significant changes within the profession, coupled with extensive reforms to regulation of human medicine since the late 1990s, reinforce arguments that legislation governing the veterinary profession is no longer fit for purpose. Clearly the responsibility for reform should rest with Defra. However, since it has displayed no further inclination to legislate, I would argue that this represents an opportunity for the RCVS and BVA to demonstrate leadership and frame concrete reform proposals, including the draft bill, which the House of Commons Committee report advocated (House of Commons 2008, para 22). It is notable that other professions such as dentistry and pharmacy have been considerably more proactive in initiating reform, and unless the veterinary profession adopts a similar approach, it risks undermining its claim to professionalism. Taking the initiative in framing real change is infinitely preferable to having change forced upon the profession as occurred with regulation of doctors (McHale & Fox 2007, Ch 4). The veterinary profession's tentative embrace of CPD and greater lay representation is simply not enough when compared with measures introduced by other health professions. Furthermore, the growth in numbers of ancillary and complementary professionals entails that all forms of veterinary care should be comprehensively regulated by statute in order for adequate protection to be given to clients and their animals. While measures such as the establishment of the Veterinary Nurses Council by the RCVS are a step in the right direction, they do not go far enough.

Against this backdrop even a position motivated purely by self-interest would suggest the logic of supporting reform proposals to jettison outdated and vague concepts such as 'conduct disgraceful in a professional respect', to introduce proper monitoring and investigation, to improve lay participation and to implement external review.[9] Such measures may well serve to avert the likelihood that otherwise at some future point self-regulation will have to be sacrificed. Of course, significant obstacles to legislative reform exist, in particular as regards funding. And it is undoubtedly true that measures to ensure professional fitness to practice in the field of human medicine have in some cases proven burdensome and overly bureaucratic (Freckleton 2006, 57). Yet to at least some extent, such problems were a consequence of having reforms imposed upon it. Consequently, I would argue that a failure to embrace reform leaves the veterinary profession in a potentially vulnerable position due to its continued dependence on individuals fulfilling ill-defined professional obligations. The worst-case scenario would be for the profession to resist change, only to have it forced upon it in the wake of a scandal, such as those which ultimately prompted changes to the regulation of the medical profession, or a human rights challenge to outdated disciplinary procedures.

Cases Cited

Martin v RCVS's Disciplinary Committee [1966] 1 Q.B. 1.
Plenderleith v the RCVS [1996] 1 W.L.R 224.
Tait v the RCVS (2003) UKPC 34.
Kirk v RCVS [2004] (unreported).
Archbold v. Disciplinary Committee of the RCVS [2004] UKPC 1.
Macleod v the RCVS [2006] UKPC 39.
Walker v. the RCVS [2008] UKPC 20.
Williams v. The RCVS [2008] UKPC 39.

References

Allsop, J. & Mulcahy, L. (1996) *Regulating Medical Work*. Oxford University Press, Oxford.
Brazier, M. & Cave, E. (2007) *Medicine, Patients and the Law*. Penguin, London.
BVA. (2007) *Review of the Veterinary Surgeons Act: Report and Recommendations*. British Veterinary Association, London.

[9] As De Prez argues 'the threat of forfeiture of self regulation will [often] hone the regulator's instinct for survival' (De Prez 2002, 44; see also Diver 1980).

BVA. (2009) *Response to the RCVS Review of the Veterinary Surgeons Act*. British Veterinary Association, London.

Calarco, M. (2008) *Zoographies: The Question of the Animal from Heidegger to Derrida*. Columbia University Press, New York.

Cane, P. (2006) *Atiyah's Accidents, Compensation and the Law*, 7th edn. Cambridge University Press, Cambridge.

Davies, M. (2006) *Medical Self Regulation: Crisis and Change*. Ashgate, Aldershot.

De Prez, P. (2002) Self-regulation and paragons of virtue: The case of "fitness to practice". *Medical Law Review*, **10**, 28–56.

Diver, C. (1980) *A Theory of Regulatory Enforcement*. Public Policy, **28**, 257–301.

Donovan, J. & Adams, C.J. (1996) *Beyond Animal Rights: A Feminist Caring Ethics for the Treatment of Animals*. Continuum, New York.

Fox, M. (2004) Re-thinking Kinship: Law's construction of the animal body. *Current Legal Problems*, **57**, 464–486.

Francione, G.L. (1995) *Animals, Property and the Law*. Temple University Press, Philadelphia, Pennsylvania.

Francis, A. (2011) At the Edge of Law *Emergent and Divergent Models of Legal Professionalism*. Ashgate, Aldershot.

Freckleton, I. (2006) Contemporary challenges in the regulation of health practitioners. In: *First Do No Harm: Law, Ethics sand Healthcare* (ed. S. McLean), pp. 39–58. Ashgate, Aldershot.

Glynne, J. & Gomez, D. (2005) *Fitness to Practise: Health Care Regulatory Law, Principle, and Process*. Sweet & Maxwell, London.

GMC. (2010) *Revalidation: A Statement of Intent*. General Medical Council, London.

Haraway, D.J. (2008) *When Species Meet*. University of Minnesota Press, Minneapolis, Minnesota.

Hemenway, H.B. (2010) (reprint) *Essentials of Veterinary Law*. American Journal of Veterinary Medicine Publication, Chicago, Illinois.

Heppinstall, A. (2006) Review of Glynne and Gomez, fitness to practice. *Medical Law Review*, **14**, 277–284.

House of Commons Environment, Food and Rural Affairs Committee. (2008) *Veterinary Surgeons Act 1966: Sixth Report of Session 2007–2008*. The Stationary Office, London.

Kennedy, I. (2001) *Learning from Bristol: The Report of the Public Inquiry into Children's Heart Surgery at Bristol Royal Infirmary 1984–1995* (Command 5702). Bristol Royal Infirmary, Bristol.

McHale, J. & Fox, M. (2007) *Health Care Law: Cases and Materials*, 2nd edn. Sweet & Maxwell, London.

Ogus, A. (1995) Re-thinking self-regulation. *Oxford Journal of Legal Studies*, **15**, 97–108.

Radford, M. (2000) Towards a better understanding of animal protection legislation. In: *Veterinary Ethics: An Introduction* (ed. G. Legood), pp. 33–48. Continuum, London.

Radford, M. (2001) *Animal Welfare Law in Britain: Regulation and Responsibility*. Oxford University Press, Oxford.

RCVS. (2005) *Review of the Veterinary Surgeons Act*. Royal College of Veterinary Surgeons, London.

RCVS. (2007) *Processing a Complaint*. Royal College of Veterinary Surgeons, London.

RCVS. (2010) *Code of Professional Conduct*. Royal College of Veterinary Surgeons, London.

RCVS. (2011a) *Draft Code of Professional Conduct for Veterinary Surgeons*. Royal College of Veterinary Surgeons, London.

RCVS. (2011b) *How We Investigate Complaints*. Royal College of Veterinary Surgeons, London.

RCVS. (2011c) *Annual Report Part II*. Royal College of Veterinary Surgeons, London.

Rollin, B.E. (2006) *Veterinary Medical Ethics: Theory and Cases*, 2nd edn. Blackwell, Ames, Iowa.

Saks, M. (1995) *Professions and the Public Interest*. Routledge, London.

Secretary of State for Health. (2006) *Trust, Assurance and Safety – The Regulation of Health Professionals* (White Paper Command 7013). Secretary of State for Health, London.

Smith, J. (2004) *The Fifth Report of the Shipman Inquiry, Safeguarding Patients: Lessons from the Past, Proposals for the Future* (Command 6394). Stationery Office Books, London.

Soave, O. (2000) *Animals, the Law and Veterinary Medicine*, 4th edn. Austin & winfield, San Francisco, US.

Tannenbaum, J. (1995) *Veterinary Ethics*, 2nd edn. St Louis, Missouri.

Wilson, J.F. & Garbe, J.L. (1990) *Law and Ethics of the Veterinary Profession*. Priority Press, Indianapolis, Indiana.

Questions and Answers

Q: Can you comment on whether overtreatment and the resultant overcharging of clients should be viewed as disgraceful professional conduct?

A: Interpretation of disgraceful conduct in both the medical and veterinary professions has focused more on the moral connotations of the phrase rather than economic ones, even though they can't be divorced. I suspect that most complaints are screened out. One of the most significant differences between the medical and veterinary professions is that there's still implicit trust in doctors because of the NHS: people feel generally quite well disposed to health professionals, notwithstanding the fact that some of them have behaved appallingly. This implicit trust is absent in the case of veterinary profession, where transactions are more commercial: many are horrified at some of the charges. The issue of insurance is interesting. Clients should query, '*Why do you want to know that? How relevant is it?*' I'm not sure that the fees question should necessarily be incorporated into how we interpret disgraceful professional misconduct but one argument would be to jettison the phrase. It could be replaced with a list of behaviours that are unacceptable that might include overcharging. The RCVS has a list of indicative conduct.

Q: It's rather a question of where to start. These issues have been debated internally at the RCVS and have perhaps not had the oxygen of publicity that the debate requires.

You're quite right in saying that the Veterinary Surgeons Act is old: the RCVS interprets it as best it can. Indeed, the way in which the profession has used and modified the Act has been praised. I have, indeed, just received a QC's opinion on how much further we might interpret the Act: finding the time, money and the driver for Parliament to need to change is the key issue. Therefore it is unlikely, given all the other things that Government is required to deal with, that it will find that driver.

Interpreting the Act can be done within certain limitations and this will be tested in the courts, as you rightly imply. The veterinary profession is the only one that still goes to the Privy Council on appeal: for all other professions, appeal is to the High Court.

The RCVS is trying to separate the disciplinary process from the investigative one. It has embraced the 'separation of powers'. Between 15 months and 2 years is needed to achieve the very small parliamentary change that's required.

A: There are practical constraints but governments do find the time and money once something goes wrong. Defra has been underfunded but it will address these issues if something goes wrong. The debate has been going on since 2003. We need to find about 2 years to reform the Act: this was also the case 10 years ago and the delay makes the impasse striking. There is now a mass of legislation, for example exemption orders and rules, which can be difficult to interpret. One thing that this and the previous Government have been guilty of is that when they reform legislation, they don't just abolish the Act and replace it with something that's well drafted and simple, but add other legislation on top of it. This is a failure of the way that we're drafting legislation at the moment.

Q1: The last time that this issue came before ministers, it was looked at by the Defra select committee, which said effectively, '*Sort yourselves out and come back with a proposition*'. The current minister has reiterated this offer and awaits the profession's call.

Q2: The reality of the current situation with the government is reasonable. However, until you put something before ministers, who weigh up the checks and balances or risks associated with doing or not doing something, then you don't know the outcome. We aren't in a regulatory climate. The RCVS continues to work on reform of the Act; until it puts something before the Government, we won't know whether they're prepared to take it forward.

A: In terms of Defra's challenge to the RCVS, I have been thinking of bills drafted by the Law Commission, which is the Law Reform Body for England and Wales. The Commission produces draft bills in areas in need of statutory reform where they have appointed Commissioners. Their legal scholars are capable of good legislative drafting. I was wondering if there are ways to persuade a body like this to take up regulation of the professions and come up with a bill which might usefully be put before Government. Obviously you need to find the time, but I can't imagine that it would be contentious.

Q: As veterinarians are involved in diverse activities, I want to focus on clinical activity and ask if there is any information on clinical audit, clinical governance and the review of clinical case management. My impression from doctors and medical students is that veterinarians lag quite far behind. There's a spectrum from doing what you're doing without any review to something so spectacularly wrong that you would be struck off. Veterinarians are defensive about having their clinical work reviewed. There is a lot to be said, therefore, for seeing if veterinarians could introduce within their profession a more proactive stance in terms of improving clinical governance and clinical audit and understanding that what we do is not always the right thing.

A: Or that what veterinarians are doing is a good thing.

Q: Has clinical review had any impact in medical law, for example the number of doctors sued, or is it a separate issue?

A: It's hard to know why people don't sue, for example whether that is due to an unworkable system or reforms. The number of negligence actions seems to be falling but it's hard to trace a correlation between this and reforms. There are better complaints procedures and there is also more of an audit trail. Some health service managers say that having audits helps, but the cost is high and it is bureaucratic. This is another reason why it's better if there is a dialogue between regulators and the profession rather than it being something which is imposed from outwith the profession. There are lessons to be learnt, but you might not need or want to go as far as the medical profession. Good things are being done and good practice being observed by veterinarians, but these aren't always recorded.

Author's Commentary

The issue of reform to professional regulation of veterinarians, and in particular whether this should be achieved through primary legislation as opposed to continuing to work within the parameters of the 1966 Act, clearly divides the veterinary profession. At a time when the economic deficit and Comprehensive Spending Review entails that all budgets are stretched and when Defra lacks both the budget and the necessary political will to drive through reform, it is perhaps unsurprising that there is little incentive for the veterinary profession to take action. In such a context, advocating wide-scale statutory reform is readily perceived as politically naive. Nevertheless, it is also clear that, in practice, veterinarians are increasingly faced with difficult ethical choices as new technologies enhance their ability to push the boundaries of animal 'therapy', as genetic knowledge raises new questions of what procedures clients can consent to on behalf of 'their' animals, as insurance of companion animals becomes normalised and as commercial practices proliferate. While law is certainly limited in its ability to supply answers to such questions, I would argue that as veterinarians stray onto increasingly treacherous ethical terrain, while simultaneously operating within commercial constraints, it is important that the regulatory framework within which they operate is based on sound and transparent principles and that mechanisms for ensuring their fitness to practice conform to human rights norms. Moreover, legislation must encompass the expanding ambit of 'veterinary' practice, as veterinary nurses and complementary practitioners become more numerous. Faced with these challenges, I argue that the interests of veterinarians, as well as their patients and clients, would be better served by a modern statute which grapples with the issue of how to define best professional practice and a framework for implementing measures, which ensure as far as possible that veterinarians conform to such practices and are supported in doing so. Where complaints are received, they should be handled in a way that ensures that due process is observed, the human rights of veterinarians are respected and confidence in the profession is retained. Notwithstanding the good faith efforts to tinker with the current statutory scheme, it is now time for Defra, the RCVS and the BVA to accept their responsibility for ensuring that professional regulation of veterinarians is fit for the twenty-first century.

Ethical Citizenship

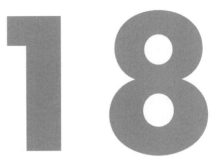

BJÖRN FORKMAN

University of Copenhagen

Abstract: The resources to treat animal welfare problems are limited, yet many of the problems with animal use are caused by the way people treat or perceive animals. Complaints against poor farming practices, poor husbandry and against animal testing show there is a concern from a select public against treating animals in certain ways. This paper addresses possible explanations for why this concern is not more influential in changing production systems.

Keywords: animal welfare, concern, consumer, information, intensification, production

18.1 Introduction

Farm animal production in Europe has become ever more intensified and specialised, especially over the last 50 years. Production systems have been intensified by increasing farm size, decreasing space per animal and reducing the time spent on each animal, especially by automation. It is not only the production system that has intensified; animals themselves have also changed and have become more specialised. A meat animal may be very different from its commercial ancestor of 50 years ago or of its non-meat selected conspecific. The most drastic example is perhaps the broiler chicken, but it is also true for other farm animals, for example beef cattle. In many cases, selection for yield has been accompanied by an increase in production-related diseases or animal welfare-related problems (Webster 1994).

Veterinary & Animal Ethics: Proceedings of the First International Conference on Veterinary and Animal Ethics, September 2011, First Edition. Edited by Christopher M. Wathes, Sandra A. Corr, Stephen A. May, Steven P. McCulloch and Martin C. Whiting.
© 2013 Universities Federation for Animal Welfare. Published 2013 by Blackwell Publishing Ltd.

In Europe, there is a high level of concern about animal welfare (Verbeke 2009). In a recent Eurobarometer survey, one third of respondents considered that animal welfare was important (ten on a scale of one to ten; European Commission 2007). The mean score was 7.8, with only a small difference between the original 15 countries and the 10 most recent member states (7.8 vs. 7.5). Although there are a number of regional differences, the overall impression is that animal welfare is top of the agenda for many citizens in Europe.

18.2 Citizens Want More Ethical Treatment of Animals

There are many different aspects of animal welfare, and there can be a contrast in the way different interest groups view it (Lassen *et al.* 2006; Bock & van Huik 2007). Whereas organic producers and many consumers emphasise the importance of natural behaviours and a natural environment, many scientists working in the field of animal welfare instead emphasise an animal's feelings (De Greef *et al.* 2006; Miele & Kjærnes *et al.* 2009).

Irrespective of the ethical standpoint or theory to which the individual citizen adheres, there are indications that the standard of farm animal welfare is inadequate for most citizens. For instance, 55% of EU citizens believe that farm animal welfare should receive more importance in their country's agricultural policy, whereas only 7% believe that it receives too much attention (European Commission 2007; see also Kjærnes & Lavik 2007). Similarly, in a Europe-wide poll, 82% agreed that humanity has a duty to protect the rights of animals, whatever the costs (European Commission 2005).

That consumers put a value on animal welfare that is transferred to the product *per se* is shown by the fact that when they are told that a product is animal welfare friendly, then its sensory properties are more highly rated than if no such information is available (e.g. Napolitano *et al.* 2007, 2010). Therefore when questionnaire or focus group studies find that consumers put more emphasis on flavour for example, than on animal welfare (e.g. Meuwissen *et al.* 2007), the result might be seriously flawed. Flavour is only independent of the animal's rearing conditions if the conditions are not known to the consumer.

While these investigations have primarily focused on production animals, it is not unreasonable to suppose that there are similar concerns for other animals, for example laboratory animals or other captive animals.

18.3 Problems for Citizens and Consumers

Farm animal welfare is thus something that is deemed to be highly important, but which some think that standards of are too low. The conundrum is why production systems that cause obvious welfare problems are still in use, with, for example, gestation crates still allowed in most countries and conventional cages for laying hens only now being phased out in the EU.

18.3.1 Increased cost

There are several possible explanations why there have not been more dramatic improvements in animal welfare; one often cited is the increased cost (e.g. Hjelmar 2011). Many of the alternative systems that could yield higher animal welfare would increase the cost of meat and other animal products, in some cases to such an extent that they would become more luxury products than they are today.

While many EU citizens state that they would be prepared to pay for more animal welfare (62%, with 39% indicating 'considerable enthusiasm'; European Commission 2007) in practice, preparedness to pay for 'additional' welfare is rather low (Vanhonacker & Verbeke 2009; Hjelmar 2011). Retailers and farmers know this and may therefore lobby governments not to introduce stricter legislation. At the same time, there is a widespread acceptance of the idea that farmers should be compensated for the increased cost of improving welfare standards, both among those citizens who believe that such an improvement is necessary and those who do not (European Commission 2007).

There is also a widespread concern that increased costs will selectively affect production in the citizen's own country, and thus the sale of that country's animal products; the same holds true on a European level. Approximately nine out of every ten EU citizens therefore believe that similar animal welfare standards should be applied to food products imported from outwith the EU as those that are, in effect, within the EU (European Commission 2007).

18.3.2 Alienation and lack of information

The roles of a consumer and a citizen are more divided than in some other cases when it comes to animal products (Vanhonacker & Verbeke 2009). In many countries, consumers do not consider animal welfare when buying food, perhaps because the current tendency is to separate the meat from the animal, buying pork and not swine meat, for example. In some cases, there is an explicit tendency to not want to think of the meat as coming from an animal, and therefore not be faced with the question of welfare, at least not at the moment of purchase. This poses a major problem for retailers since a majority of European citizens state that they want more information on animal welfare (European Commission 2007).

Almost a third of EU citizens have never visited a farm, with some countries having a much higher proportion of non-farm visits (e.g. Greece, 66%). With such low proportions, it is not surprising that 85% of citizens state that they possess little or no knowledge of the conditions under which animals are farmed in their own countries.

In many countries, there is no tradition of specific animal welfare labels. Eggs, however, are a notable exception. In EU law, they have to be labelled by production system, for example as coming from conventional cages, furnished cages, loose housed hens or organic hens (with minor local differences; e.g. conventional cages are banned in Sweden). Despite being more expensive, alternative systems of husbandry have gained acceptance and a fair number of the eggs sold through retail outlets come from alternative systems. A possible reason for this is that the welfare aspect is very clear and unambiguous. If this is the case, then the 'egg-story' is highly relevant, showing that clear animal welfare labelling can affect the habits of the consumers.

Welfare, finally, is a complex concept, and although it is sometimes very obvious when welfare is compromised (e.g. broken legs), it can be harder at other times. So, for example, organic farmers and many consumers place a high value on the naturalness of the life of the animals and their behaviour, whereas others, for example veterinarians, place a higher value on health (Christiansen & Forkman 2007). These values may conflict with each other, not least when it comes to factors such as access to an outdoor run. At present this and other similar conflicts, for example that animal welfare-friendly products are seen as being healthier and of better quality (European Commission 2007), have not yet played a big role in the public discussion.

As discussed previously, management practices and the ability of farm managers have major roles to play in preventing poor welfare. In addition, the ability of a farmer to detect a sick or lame animal does not carry large environmental costs. Therefore, at least a concern for some aspects of animal welfare does not impose additional costs for environmental pollution and other important areas.

However, one of the reasons for intensification is that resources are used more efficiently; a fast-growing broiler that is slaughtered at 40 days of age will use less energy, kg for kg, than an organic broiler that is slaughtered at twice that age. If more extensive systems are used, then they will require more resources that may have adverse consequences for the CO_2 footprint. This will force the consumer and citizen to compromise between two ethical considerations, minimising environmental costs or maximising animal welfare. There is a risk that the message gets ever more complex as it becomes ever more difficult to choose between different options, and that the consumer finally gives up and chooses a product based on either habit or price (Vanhonacker & Verbeke 2009).

18.4 Responsibility of the Citizen/Consumer

In the following discussion, I will assume that the consumer/citizen does want to improve the welfare of the animals. This is not necessarily true, either because the individual believes that the question of animal welfare is not important or because he believes that the welfare is good as it is. This is an opinion expressed by slightly less than one-third of Finnish, UK, Irish and Swedish respondents in a Eurobarometer survey (European Commission 2007), and similar results have been found for Swedes and Norwegians in a separate study (Kjærnes & Lavik 2007). At the other end of the scale, almost all Greeks (96%) interviewed in the Eurobarometer were of the opinion that (farm) animal welfare should be improved in Greece. However, it is noteworthy that in all countries a majority of the respondents answered that animal welfare needs to be improved in their own country.

18.4.1 Gathering information

Information is needed to make an informed choice, whether it is as a consumer or as a voter. There are many definitions of animal welfare (Appleby & Sandøe 2002), but, irrespective of the one chosen, information is necessary if the consumer is to use it. If the absence of pain is an important aspect of animal welfare, then the citizen needs to know what management procedures are routinely done and whether they cause pain. This is not a trivial point. For a very long time, it was commonly believed that the new born, whether animal or human, could not feel pain (Anand & Hickey, 1987). As late as 1985, a young infant '*had holes cut on both sides of his neck, another cut in his right chest, an incision from his breastbone around to his backbone, his ribs pried apart, and an extra artery near his heart tied off*'. The infant was awake throughout and only paralyzed with a curare compound. He died a month later (Lee 2002). In the light of this, it is not surprising that castration of animals at a very young age is generally allowed without anaesthesia or analgesics. The current evidence is, however, that although neonates, such as piglets, may heal faster (Heinritzi *et al.* 2006), there is no reason to suppose that the feeling of pain is less in neonatal than in older animals (Carroll *et al.* 2006). While there are today few who doubt that even young animals feel pain, there is still fierce discussion of other topics, for example if fish can feel pain (see Braithwaite 2010).

A majority of Europeans seem to agree on the need for greater understanding; approximately six out of every ten EU citizens say they would like to receive more information about farming conditions in their country (the question was not directly related to animal welfare, European Commission 2007). Interestingly enough, the need for more information was not correlated with the respondent's knowledge.

The question that arises is to what extent should it be the responsibility of citizens to search for information and to what extent should stakeholders present it? The most preferred method for getting information is via the television, perhaps indicating that citizens think that information should be actively presented rather than merely being made available (European Commission 2007).

18.4.2 Acting on the information

Citizens want more information about animal welfare and consider that the standard of farm animal welfare is less than it should be. Despite this, only 11% of Eurobarometer respondents thought that consumers have the power to ensure animal welfare and only 25% thought that the government could ensure it (approximately the same for veterinarians and animal welfare organisations).

Responsibility for better animal welfare is instead placed primarily on the shoulders of the farmers themselves (European Commission 2007).

It is hard to know how to interpret these results. It seems likely that although citizens are concerned about farm animal welfare and believe that something should be done about it, they are not prepared to act on their beliefs as consumers, possibly because they do not believe that it will make a difference.

18.5 Conclusion

An ethical citizen has to act on his or her convictions. There are two major ways of affecting animal welfare. One is by means of legislation and the other through market forces. In both cases, the citizen/consumer can make a difference, either through a change of purchases or by voting. At present, however, the consumer/citizen does not seem to be prepared to use that power.

References

Anand, K.J.S. & Hickey, P.R. (1987) Pain and its effects in the human neonate and fetus. *New England Journal of Medicine*, **317**, 1321–1329.

Appleby, M.C. & Sandøe, P. (2002) Philosophical debate on the nature of well-being: Implications for animal welfare. *Animal Welfare*, **11**, 283–294.

Bock, B.B. & van Huik, M.M. (2007) Animal welfare: The attitudes and behaviour of European pig farmers. *British Food Journal*, **109**, 931–944.

Braithwaite, V. (2010) *Do Fish Feel Pain?* Oxford University Press, Oxford.

Carroll, J.A., Berg, E.L., Strauch, T.A., Roberts, M.P. & Kattesh, H.G. (2006) Hormonal profiles, behavioral responses, and short-term growth performance after castration of pigs at three, six, nine, or twelve days of age. *Journal of Animal Science*, **84**, 1271–1278.

Christiansen, S.B. & Forkman, B. (2007) Assessment of animal welfare in a veterinary context – A call for ethologists. *Applied Animal Behaviour Science*, **106**, 203–220.

De Greef, K., Stafleu, F. & De Lauwere, C. (2006) A simple value-distinction approach aids transparency in farm animal welfare debate. *Journal of Agricultural and Environmental Ethics*, **19**, 57–66.

European Commission. (2005) Attitudes of EU citizens towards Animal Welfare. Special Eurobarometer 229/Wave 63.2.

European Commission (2007) Attitudes of EU citizens towards Animal Welfare. Special Eurobarometer 270/Wave 66.1.

Heinritzi, K., Ritzmann, M. & Otten, W. (2006) Alternatives for castration of suckling piglets, determination of catecholamines and woundhealing after castration of suckling piglets at different points of time (Alternativen zur Kastration von Saugferkeln, Bestimmung von Katecholaminen sowie Wundheilung nach Kastration von Saugferkeln zu unterschiedlichen Zeitpunkten). *Deutsche Tierärztliche Wochenschrift*, **113**, 94–97.

Hjelmar, U. (2011) Consumers' purchase of organic food products. A matter of convenience and reflexive practices. *Appetite*, **56**, 336–344.

Kjærnes, U. & Lavik, R. (2007) Farm animal welfare and food consumption practices: Results from surveys in seven countries. In: *Attitudes of Consumers, Retailers and Producers to Farm Animal Welfare* (eds U. Kjærnes, M. Miele & J. Roex). Welfare Quality® Reports No. 2., Welfare Quality®, Cardiff.

Lassen, J., Sandøe, P. & Forkman, B. (2006) Happy pigs are dirty! – Conflicting perspectives on animal welfare. *Livestock Science*, 103, 221–230.

Lee, B.H. (2002) Managing pain in human neonates – Applications for animals. *Journal of the American Veterinary Medical Association*, 221, 233–237.

Meuwissen, M.P.M., van der Lans, I.A. & Huirne, R.B.M. (2007) A synthesis of consumer behavior and chain design. *NJAS*, 54-3, 293–312.

Miele, M. & Kjærnes, U. (2009) Investigating societal values on farm animal welfare: The example of Welfare Quality®. In: *An Overview of the Development of the Welfare Quality® Project Assessment Systems* (ed. L. Keeling), pp. 43–55. Welfare Quality® Reports No. 12., Welfare Quality®, Cardiff.

Napolitano, F., Braghieri, A., Caroprese, M., Marino, R., Girolami, A. & Sevi, A. (2007) Effect of information about animal welfare, expressed in terms of rearing conditions, on lamb acceptability. *Meat Science*, 77, 431–436.

Napolitano, F., Braghieri, A., Piasentier, E., Favotto, S., Naspetti, S. & Zanoli, R. (2010) Effect of information about organic production on beef liking and consumer willingness to pay. *Food Quality and Preference*, 21, 207–212.

Vanhonacker, F. & Verbeke, W. (2009) Buying higher welfare poultry products? Profiling Flemish consumers who do and do not. *Poultry Science*, 88, 2702–2711.

Verbeke, W. (2009) Stakeholder, citizen and consumer interests in farm animal welfare. *Animal Welfare*, 18, 325–333.

Webster, J. (1994) *Animal Welfare: A Cool Eye towards Eden*. Blackwell Science, Oxford.

Questions and Answers

Q: Research shows that British consumers are thoroughly confused about welfare labels and that supermarkets have no interest in rationalising third-party schemes, for example Freedom Food or Red Tractor, because each is trying to gain market share. Are such schemes the answer?
A: At least these schemes exist in Britain. In most countries, there's no alternative and it is very hard to actively choose an animal welfare–friendly product. The only exception in most countries is eggs. Even so, there can be much discussion about the level of animal welfare in the different production systems. There is usually just information about the production system and not whether the eggs come from farms with good or bad welfare.

Q: You use the label 'consumer'. Is not the consumer a mixture of retailer and consumer? What responsibility do retailers have as the surrogate for the consumer?
A: My preference would be to put much more emphasis on retailers. UK retailers have done a good job in demanding higher welfare standards from Danish exporters of pig meat to the UK, for example. Swedish importers, who pride themselves on being very animal welfare friendly, haven't made the same demands, despite the

fact that the scheme for the UK market is already up and running in Denmark. Of course this means that they wouldn't be able to sell Danish meat at premium price, as in many Swedish supermarkets. Retailers ought to take a bigger responsibility but I don't know whether you can persuade them to do it.

Q: I've been involved in several studies of consumers and don't think they are as rational as you think. You assume that the only problem is that if consumers had a bit more information and felt a bit more secure, then they'd choose more welfare-friendly products. However, in the studies with which I've been involved, when consumers go into a supermarket they have a different agenda, for example to feed their children. If they're concerned about problems then they're concerned about primarily health. We also did qualitative studies. There's a very small minority of consumers who have a drive to be very rational. If you talk to European retailers, apart from those in the UK, they say, 'We want to move but don't believe in welfare brands; we believe in quality brands'. What is moving are brands with a combined message, for example about climate, poverty, food safety, health and animal welfare. If you can, you should link animal welfare to a story about what are people concerned about when they enter a shop. If you want ethical citizens, you should find a common agenda in which consumers and citizens meet.

A: We agree more than you think. While I was preparing this talk, I was reading a study that showed that organic meat tastes better than commercial meat. Apparently, you can show that animal welfare-friendly meat tastes better. Unfortunately blind tests don't show the same result. If you tell people, 'This is animal welfare-friendly, this is not' then taste is going to be better in the former. Taste is not independent of context. Studies of blind tests so far are erroneous. You shouldn't be doing blind tests; instead you should be telling people, 'Yes this is animal welfare-friendly and this is not'. This is not cheating. You taste with your eyes, nose, and experience that type of meat, and the knowledge of where it came from.

Q: But others can also sell products with a story of good animal welfare; it's not only the good ones who do so.

A: You need someone to control the storytelling. You can't just have a picture of cow in a field and say, 'Look, this is like the California cow'. To do so is to lose the competitive advantage that animal welfare can bring; you need regulation of claims.

C: In the context of the argument that welfare can only be sold as part of an overall high quality package, particularly in the UK, the price of high welfare eggs has remained robust while that of organic eggs has dropped. The price differential between the conventional cage and organic eggs was about 60%. The price differential between conventional cage and free range and high welfare non-organic eggs is only 8%. One of the reasons is that it's not just that welfare is considered a good thing by the public but you can achieve significant improvements in welfare at a small cost.

Q: You could perhaps have made more about the distinction between citizens and consumers. We are all citizens, we are all consumers but behave differently as the two. The difference between what people say when they enter a supermarket and what they do is often portrayed as hypocrisy. It is not hypocrisy; it is the different sides of participation in the process. People would vote for a law which put up food prices for everybody. That is quite different from asking them to make the decision in the supermarket when those before and behind them in the queue have bought cheaper food. This is another reason to involve sociologists and social scientists, including economists.

A: I agree. You can either vote for a change in law or you can take a stand as a consumer. People do seem to make this distinction, saying, for example, *'We are prepared to pay more but it's important that there's a level playing field, at least within the EU. The same regulations should be introduced so that we don't lose market shares. We want to continue buying British beef, Danish bacon or Swedish pigs, and we don't want to lose our own production.'*

Q: How should welfare friendliness be assessed? There is welfare-friendly milk and also welfare-friendly eggs. Assessment of the welfare of cows and hens focuses on rearing and production, but is different for meat where people worry about rearing methods as well as slaughter. The meat could come from the cow that produced the milk. What do consumers think about when they consider welfare friendliness?

A: It seems that most consumers and citizens know very little about how meat or milk is produced. If you ask *'What do you want us to do with the calf that has been born?'* they might answer, *'What calf? I just want to drink the milk'*. In the same way, many consumers will ask, *'Why are male chicks from layers slaughtered? Can't they be raised for meat?'* Generally, consumers have very little knowledge about food and farming. The eurobarometer shows that they are keen to have more information about production methods. Most feel that they don't have enough information with some exceptions, for example Denmark. Elsewhere in the EU, there is a hunger for more knowledge and information about the way animals are treated and reared.

C: Welfare-friendly retailers first have to define very precisely what they mean by welfare-friendly. Secondly, they have to guarantee provenance by independent audit. Information must be available on demand: only in this way can trust be built.

Author's Reflection

A conclusion from the questions of the session and the conference is that there is a general scepticism about the consumers' willingness to pay for animal welfare. Within Europe, there are few examples where a purely animal welfare label has acquired a large part of the market, the possible exception being eggs. One conclusion is that the way forward is by legislation, preferably at a European level.

There are, however, two aspects that I believe are important. The first relates to the egg story mentioned previously. A likely reason for the success is that the alternatives are very clear and intuitive, and standardised between retailers. By comparison, the relatively few animal welfare labels in Europe are often either retailer-specific and/or complex: this may be one reason for their relatively low impact. We may learn from the egg story however, for example when addressing other welfare problems, such as crated sows. A prohibition of the use of farrowing crates would be costly, and is therefore not likely within a foreseeable future. An alternative could be legislation that focuses on labelling meat from piglets of crated and non-crated sows, thereby facilitating the consumer's choice.

The second aspect that makes me hopeful of more animal welfare-friendly production is the relatively low cost of some welfare-friendly production systems, not just as a percentage of the production costs but in real terms. This means that if there is a way for the consumer to only pay the actual increase in production cost, the price difference in the shop would be comparatively small. The challenge is how to implement this.

Principles, Preference and Profit: Animal Ethics in a Market Economy

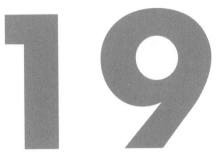

JOHN McINERNEY

University of Exeter

Abstract: Although human behaviour is structured within a framework of ethical principles and moral codes they have very little prominence in economic analysis, except insofar as they may influence individual people's preferences or the collectively accepted constraints on economic activity. Economics sees animals primarily as capital resources in processes designed to generate human benefit, and in this role they are susceptible to exploitation and valuation based entirely on their productivity. In societies where markets represent the coordinating mechanism for production and consumption, the reflection of ethical principles and moral values is dependent on the decisions made by individual economic agents, each pursuing their own self-interest. Ethics can influence the behaviour of livestock producers, but economic survival is ultimately dependent on making sufficient operating profits and this results in obvious conflicts with the animals' welfare; this is especially true in low-income situations. 'The market' is not, in general, able to resolve these conflicts. Food consumers could exercise significant ethical influence on the way livestock farming is conducted, but the preferences they express in the market are generally too diffuse

Veterinary & Animal Ethics: Proceedings of the First International Conference on Veterinary and Animal Ethics, September 2011, First Edition. Edited by Christopher M. Wathes, Sandra A. Corr, Stephen A. May, Steven P. McCulloch and Martin C. Whiting.
© 2013 Universities Federation for Animal Welfare. Published 2013 by Blackwell Publishing Ltd.

and ill-informed to have great effect in practice. It requires intervention by regulation and legally enforced codes to ensure that free market incentives do not lead to socially unacceptable treatment of animals; economists would presume only to analyse their impact and not to declare what those codes should be. Ethical concerns doubtlessly place a lower bound on the way we treat animals, but beyond this there would appear to be a wide range in what is accepted as 'right' (and implicitly in attributed value) across different species.

Keywords: economics, ethics, markets, value, welfare

19.1 Introduction

Although both are centred on human behaviour, economics and ethics are in many respects unlikely bedfellows. Ethics is essentially concerned with explorations of how we, as individuals and societies, ought to live our lives. By contrast, economics attempts to explain how we actually do manage our lives. Furthermore, ethics is seen to occupy a kind of intellectual high ground, whereas economics seems more associated with base motives of people's self-interest and personal gain.

This dichotomy is, to a large extent, valid. For the last 75 years economics has emphasised its credentials as a scientific approach to human behaviour, avoiding value judgements and concentrating on observation, explanation and empirical testing. This has been built on the seminal publication by Robbins (1935), which declared the essence of economics to be the study of the choices individuals and society collectively make in attempting to meet a variety of ends using scarce available means. Robbins was insistent that economics was in this context ethically neutral. It had nothing to say about whether the ends were good, bad or indifferent – they were simply the motivations for observed economic activity, our analyses being concerned solely with how best to mobilise and employ the scarce means in pursuing them. Economics, therefore, is about resource allocation, irrespective of what it is we seek to obtain. The flight from any suggestion of normative economics was further reinforced by the emergence of textbooks on 'positive economics' (see Lipsey 1963 and subsequent editions) where the subject is presented as a framework of axioms, hypotheses and relationships whose validity is judged by their consistency with observation and by their explanatory power and predictive capability.

Whether economics can ever really be ethically neutral is still subject to constant discussion (Cowell & Witzum 2007), many siding with Keynes in declaring it to be a 'moral science' (Atkinson 2007). Certainly the way it becomes confused with politics, and its analyses used as a basis for justifying what are essentially political decisions, leaves many people disputing that economics is value-free. Indeed, implicit in all the underpinnings of economic analysis, whether at the level of macro policy or the individual firm/consumer, are a variety of statements about how things 'ought' to be done. These, however, are not normative statements but rather the technical conditions that need to be satisfied if the scarce means are to be used to best effect. This, of course, immediately introduces an assumption as to the interpretation of 'best', leading to an overriding focus on 'efficiency' along with the assumption that everyone's motivation in making choices is to maximise their satisfaction/benefit and, by the same token, minimise the cost. Some would argue that this is clearly a value judgement, others that it is no more than the character-istic of rational behaviour as being a self-evident objective in meeting their ends.[1] Hausman and McPherson (1993) see it as 'a useful caricature' while Sen (1987) regards this 'engineering' approach to human behaviour as a major failing of modern economics.

All these issues represent productive material for academic discussion amongst economists but have little practical effect on the way economic analyses are conducted.

19.2 The Basic Model of Economic Activity

The essence of economics in its 'scarce-means-to-meet-competing-ends' framework is illuminated in Figure 19.1. The means are represented as *resources*, the source of all wealth and the basis of all economic activity. They are identified as being land (including all natural resources), labour or capital. The ends that drive the use of these resources are those complex dimensions of *human benefit* that people, as individuals and as a society, aim to achieve. Economics conventionally has encapsulated these in the generic term 'utility' but it is better understood as all the subjective satisfactions and well-being that people seek in life. Resources do not yield human benefit directly but do so only by being transformed into *goods and services*, viewed as the functional outputs of economic activity and the objects of human desire. So economics sees human behaviour as consisting of two linked processes, the technical one of production followed by the really worthwhile one of consumption, in both of which choices always have to be made. It is relevant to note here that the human benefit driving economic activity is not to be seen in monetary terms. While the benefits of some economic activities are captured in financial form – as income or profit, say – a large proportion of the goods and services that are valued in society are not traded, therefore have no obvious price and are experienced and enjoyed without ever appearing in monetary form. They are, nevertheless, still an integral component of economic value.

In outline, the economic model is analogous to an ecological model representing how a jungle works; the actors are different, but there are no intrinsic moral values, no self-evident rules about how the system should operate. Economic theory gives

---

[1] The corollary being that if we assumed irrational behaviour, actions would be essentially random and there would be no basis for constructing any system of explanatory relationships.

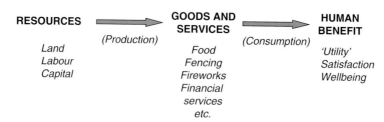

Figure 19.1 The basic model of economic activity.

a lot of attention to explaining how, under different assumptions and conditions, the system does operate, the nature of any equilibrium and the processes by which it might be reached. In this, it recognises that economic activity is driven entirely by human preferences (constrained by technical and natural forces); and while these preferences *may* have explicit ethical underpinnings in the case of some people and in some contexts, they may equally be ill-informed, misguided, unsavoury, selfish and devoid of any moral content. Economics has nothing particularly to say about any of this.

19.3 Animals in Economic Activity

Consider the role of animals in our economic processes and how moral precepts and ethical values may influence decisions in production and consumption. As seen in Figure 19.2, animals are a subset of capital resources with the role of producing goods and services of some sort. They include: breeding animals, producing further capital inputs; directly productive animals, yielding milk, meat and other products in the food chain; functional animals, producing draft power or transport; companion animals, yielding household pet or recreational services; or 'wildlife', offering a broadly defined environmental service. In this context, the value attached to an animal is determined solely by its productivity. The more goods and services, of whatever type, it produces the greater the animal's worth or 'use value'. In a market economy, this worth may be quantified via a price if the outputs are traded, but in many cases the values are external to the market and, although reflecting real benefits, do not automatically have a price label (they are 'unpriced values'). This productivist view of animals' value, reflected in their ability to satisfy some material need, is comparable to what Callicott (1986), in distinguishing between 'economic' and 'philosophical' value, refers to as their instrumental value, i.e., their utility as a means to some end.

However, it is evident that, independent of their productivity, some animals can carry what Regan (1983) refers to as, 'inherent value', – an attribute clearly recognisable from a moral/philosophical standpoint but one that at first sight is not easily captured in the means–end framework of economic analysis. Callicott (1986)

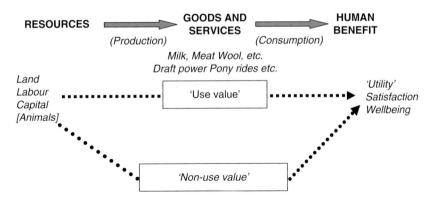

Figure 19.2 The economic model of livestock keeping.

is now well out of date, though, in saying that non-material utilities are usually excluded by the term economic value. Modern economics, led by its excursions into environmental issues, recognises that people are not solely maximisers of their consumption utility but may quite reasonably associate, 'non-use values', with resources, independent of their productivity (Krutilla & Fisher 1975). Those who contribute to the conservation of wildlife or natural features they will never personally experience – the blue whale, for example – are reflecting what is termed an 'existence value', a benefit derived from simply knowing it is there.[2] The willingness of people to incur cost in the cause of better farm animal welfare is an example of valuation that is nothing to do with economic productivity but reflects an additional non-use value associated with the animal itself. None of this need imply a moral value outwith normal economic behaviour, however; it is simply part of the complex manner in which people seek to gain the greatest benefit from the way they use their resources. Indeed, given the variety of human perceptions and motivations, such 'moral' behaviour may just as likely stem from misconceptions, Walt Disney images, propaganda or anthropomorphic sentiments as from any particular moral standards or ethical precepts.

A logical extension of this argument (McInerney 1991) is that when people show concern about the well-being of animals they are simply reacting to their own unease and discomfort about the way that animals are treated, and feel this as a loss of personal benefit. Animal welfare in this sense then becomes a subset of human welfare, rather than necessarily the independent phenomenon that animal scientists would claim to be studying. We don't know what the animals themselves would choose (and if their preferences conflict with ours, we always win anyway), we define their 'welfare' to be what we think it is, and make our production and purchase decisions perhaps naively feeling good about production conditions perceived as 'kind' to the animals (organic, free range,

---

[2] Other variants are identified in the literature as 'option value' and 'bequest' value.

small scale) and troubled about husbandry methods perceived as 'harsh' (intensity, factory farming and similar images). These perceptions and attitudes may be derived from some recognised ethical framework about our relationship to animals – and probably are at the boundaries where conditions are perceived as cruel or inhumane-but ethics does not then provide a very clear guide in evaluating choices at different points along the scale from very bad to very good perceived welfare. But in analysing economic behaviour, it is sufficient to include all this as part of observed human preferences with no need to enquire deeply into where they came from.

19.4 Ethics and Market Behaviour

The jungle is driven entirely by the innate animal instincts of its occupants, whereas the economy is driven by conscious decisions taken by the numerous human agents – resource owners, firms, consumers, institutions and governments. Maximisers they all may be, but the context in which they operate is structured by socially accepted ethical principles and moral codes. How might these influence economic behaviour towards animals?[3]

19.4.1 'Supply side' ethics

Commercial livestock farmers confront most directly the issue of animals as productive economic resources. As in all competitive market situations (and agriculture most closely approximates these conditions), the pressure for survival demands efficiency in the use of all resources, with profits being the criterion of success. This implies working the land hard, working the machinery hard, working themselves hard and, inevitably, working the animals hard. Modern livestock farming is now well beyond the point where it could claim that welfare and productivity go hand in hand, and there is an undeniable conflict between the farmer's economic interest and the welfare of his animals (McInerney 1993). The pursuit of profits can lead (and with the help of modern technology very easily does so) to excessive exploitation of the animals' biological productive capacity, and because the cost to the animal does not appear in the farm's business accounts, there is no financial incentive to forego its output potential. Furthermore ignorance, insensitivity, carelessness and lack of awareness about animals' well-being can all lead to exploitation of animals in the worst sense of that word.

But this is far from saying that livestock farmers are rampant profit maximisers. First, they have their own preferences, as well as financial imperatives, as to how they treat their resources and this is manifested in the observed pursuit of non-income (but utility maximising) objectives. Furthermore, the traditional

---

[3] For brevity, we consider only animals in the food chain, but the arguments can be generalised to all contexts where humans manage animals.

tenets of 'good husbandry' define practices that protect animals from the excesses of exploitation and represent an inbuilt (if unrecognised) ethical approach to livestock management. Most farmers would object vehemently to the thought they were in any way cruel or inhumane in their farming methods, and many take a positive pride in the way they keep their stock. All this *may* derive from a considered ethical stance – but equally may reflect just an image of 'good livestock farming', personal preferences, peer pressure and learned behaviour.

Nevertheless, animal ethics are very clearly in the domain of livestock farmers' decisions, and the pressures of market economics confront them with the financial cost (or benefits, see later) attached to ethical principles. One cannot generalise across the diversity of individuals, but it is not surprising that those principles might be interpreted somewhat elastically by many farmers in many situations. For although the concept of 'principles' implies something absolute and non-negotiable, one has to recognise that they must vary across different economic contexts. The poor subsistence farmer in Northern Pakistan treats his donkeys and goats in ways we would undoubtedly reject as cruel and violating all reasonable concepts of respect for animals; but the fact is he cannot afford our ethical principles when his own living conditions are pretty cruel too.[4] Economists are accustomed to dealing in 'trade-offs', but how do we handle the trade-off between principles and profits at the margins of economic survival?

19.4.2 'Demand side' ethics

If markets are the means by which product preferences are expressed, then in theory consumer demand represents a powerful way in which the ethical views people have can be directed back down the economic system to influence how animals are treated in livestock farming. This is because the way food (or any product) is produced becomes embodied in the final product as an inherent 'quality' characteristic. The increasing tendency to brand food products, to offer quality assurance and traceability, and to provide information labels allows these endogenous attributes to be presented for explicit choice by purchasers, alongside the other more visible characteristics that guide their decisions. So the more that consumer preferences explicitly focus on such things as the origin, environmental, welfare or other credentials of a product's provenance, the stronger are the economic messages to suppliers to cater for these values. The ethics of the consumer can in this way become the ethics of production.

This is reflected in the modest growth of a market for clearly labelled and assured animal products produced under defined 'higher welfare' conditions. They are more expensive (because they require higher cost structures at farm level) but that is no deterrent to the consumers who specifically want this aspect of quality

---

[4] This brings with it troubling ethical questions for affluent Westerners. If we import livestock products from the poor developing countries, are we underwriting the harsh conditions of their livestock husbandry or supporting the income aspirations of their people?

and for whom the standard commodity is inconsistent with their preferences. For farmers, they represent a commercial opportunity whereby they can combine what might be their own ethical preferences for 'kinder' treatment of animals with a segment of the market associated with a distinct moral code and to some extent exploit the notion that higher welfare *can* mean higher returns – a rare example of where principles, preference and profit can come together.

Unfortunately, although the prospects may improve, there are severe constraints on how effectively this can work more generally to influence the ethical treatment of animals in farming. For most people, their food preferences have very weak ethical underpinnings. Many simply don't think, or don't particularly care, about how farm animals are kept – and their stance is entirely acceptable in the market place. Even those who do care may not do so enough to pay the higher costs of products with a clear ethical label. Perhaps everyone would express opposition to 'cruelty' in farming, but the views on what that constitutes will vary so widely as to make it pretty non-functional as an influential principle (how can battery cages be cruel if they are legal? Slaughter without stunning can't be cruel if it's required practice in certain faiths). An even greater constraint is information. The separation between food consumer and agricultural producer is so great in the modern world that most of us have no clue about livestock production conditions – what they are like or how they should be – so even strong ethical concerns may find no means of expression in purchasing decisions (how many of us know the welfare background of imported New Zealand lamb, or the lifestyles of those who assembled our flat screen TV, or the pay and conditions of those who produced our 'been there, done that' T-shirt?). In terms of affecting the market, 'the ethical consumer' is a very variable animal.

This further raises the question as to who 'the consumer' actually is. The supermarket chains largely represent 'demand' for the agricultural producer and 'supply' for the household purchaser; they specify to farmers the conditions their livestock production must satisfy and to food processors how and from where they will source their product constituents, while presenting to domestic food consumers the array of products from which they can choose. In this setting, individuals with strong ethically based preferences have little real opportunity to turn them into a major economic force in the marketplace. The obvious place where ethical standards relating to animal treatment could influence the food supply chain is in the purchasing decisions of the supermarkets – and they have singularly failed to adopt a principled stance on this issue (FAWC 2005). Those that do claim to do so have been selective in their efforts, focussing just on specific products, carrying 'high end' brands for one segment of the market while offering across the range down to budget brands of ill-described and minimal quality characteristics. This, of course, is an entirely rational commercial strategy in a competitive market; supermarkets, too, realise they need to have principles but can't afford them to be universal.

A further constraint on consumer ethics influencing the conditions under which livestock are kept is the modern global nature of the market. As well as obscuring the production conditions of imported products,[5] World Trade Organisation regulations prohibit countries discriminating against imports on animal welfare criteria (on the spurious grounds that this would represent protectionism for domestic producers or imposing unreasonable conditions on overseas producers). The real power for ethical decision making in the modern marketplace lies with multinational corporations and international trading structures – and they, as Ryder (1998) points out, exhibit a complete moral blindness when it comes to the fates of animals.

19.4.3 The 'public ethic'

A third major influence in the model of market economies is that of the market regulator, often a public institution of some sort and best captured by the notion of 'the government'. Whatever preferences, values and moral standards may motivate the behaviour of individuals, they are not allowed totally free rein, even in the most extreme of 'free' markets, but are contained within a framework of principles that reflect a collective social view of what should and should not be allowed to happen. The choices of individual economic agents that might violate these moral values are constrained by laws, regulations and codes imposed to ensure their behaviour conforms to the ethics of the society[6] – a necessary imposition since otherwise the activities of self-seeking maximisers in the impersonal market process can ride roughshod over the interests of vulnerable entities.

Such shared values are defined in economic terms as public goods – benefits that accrue to everyone but are external to the market – and are widespread. The enforcement of public ethics is important in relation to the welfare of animals, where otherwise through ignorance, insensitivity, economic greed or sheer malice individuals could (and in many cases do) treat animals in ways regarded as totally unacceptable in a civilised society. They play an essential role, too, in compensating for a major limitation of the market economy in reflecting social value, namely, that influence is restricted to those who actually produce or purchase, and is in direct proportion to how much they sell or buy. But in a democratic society, everyone has the same right to a share in the public morals, regardless of whether and to what extent they are active in a particular market. So in defining acceptable animal welfare standards, for example, the views of vegetarians, vegans and those totally unconnected with livestock farming are just as valid in the formulation of society's attitudes and preferences and need non-market means of representation. Governments and professional institutions tend to be very slow in responding to changing public attitudes and preferences in updating the codes defining acceptable/required behaviour, and in this context the role of advocates, pressure groups, activists and publicists for the emerging attitudes is crucial in the non-economic 'market' for social values.

---

[5] Supermarket assurance schemes on their supply chains could correct for this but fail to do so convincingly.
[6] This may also be embodied in the codes of conduct for professional groups such as veterinarians, doctors, lawyers, etc.

19.5 Moral versus Economic Value

Leaving aside philosophical discussions, there is a practical difficulty in blending ethical precepts and economic analysis. As reflected in statements about whether things are right or wrong, fair or unfair, just or unjust, cruel or acceptable, etc., ethical principles appear to be absolute and non-negotiable, as though actions and outcomes can be viewed in these simple binary terms. Economic analysis, by contrast, considers all action as choosing between a wider range of outcomes and thereby effectively confronting a continuum of rightness, fairness or acceptability. In relation to the way animals are treated, for example, the practical options range between the extremes from 'cruel and inhumane' to 'ridiculously pampered'. All moral considerations would reject the first of these, but once past this lower boundary the choice that farmers, consumers and societies generally have to face is how far towards the latter it is appropriate (or 'right') to go. Whether or not animal ethics can define guidelines for this choice, it is certainly a standard economic decision of the type that young economists cut their back teeth on – namely, balancing the benefits people feel they gain from the 'kinder' treatment of animals against the extra cost, a classic case of evaluation at the margin.

In reflecting their preferences and utility functions, people will distribute themselves along this implicit (ethical?) scale. We would expect everyone except the reprehensible minority to exhibit first-order ethical behaviour (Dietrich & Rowen 2005), doing what is 'right' without consideration of any benefit to themselves. But beyond this choices will vary widely, motivated by second-order ethical behaviour whereby people feel a direct personal benefit from doing the right thing and increasingly so depending on the extent to which their actions exceed the socially acceptable or legally minimum standards. Do they have higher moral values, or are they simply portraying varying levels of economic (non-use) values they associate with animals?

In addition to the variation in individual's perceptions and choices, there seems to exist equivalently some broad collective social view of what levels of animal care and concern are appropriate in different contexts. And judging by the things we accept in the way animals are treated and what we are prepared to pay for, even in an ethical society with well-developed moral values towards animals a differential scale of valuations seems to be portrayed across different species and situations. This seems to be at odds with declarations about the equal rights of all sentient beings, whether human or animal, and implies a scale of varying economic values attached to their basic well-being.

19.5.1 'Low' welfare concern (low economic value)

A tentative representation of this observation is given in Figure 19.3, showing (the author's perceptions of) these different implicit valuations in terms of their relative position on a scale from low to high welfare concern. At the lower end of this scale is a line reflecting a collective view of what would amount to cruel and

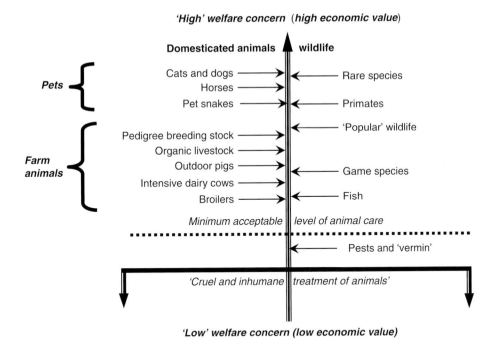

Figure 19.3 A conceptual scale of the social valuation of animals.

inhumane treatment of animals and totally rejected by all right-thinking people. The minimum levels of concern acceptable in society, as defined by moral codes, regulation and legislation, are somewhat higher than this ethical threshold. Beyond this, social choice is differentiated in terms of domesticated as against wild animals but there is a wide scale within each category. Amongst farm animals, we appear to be prepared to accept for broiler chicken what are regarded as quite harsh conditions, whereas we appear to think that outdoor pigs and organic livestock merit a somewhat better life. We act as though what is right for our pet animals in general far exceeds that which we consider acceptable for farm livestock, but even then there is a scale of values that we apply. This scale of values is equally evident in our attitudes to the well-being of wildlife, where fish don't seem to merit much concern compared to the generality of wildlife. The more 'intelligent' animals are, perhaps understandably, given more status in our perceptions, while we act as though it is ethically most important to consider the situation of those species of conservation concern. It is interesting that wherever we regard an animal as troublesome to our lives, whether as producers or consumers, and so define it as a pest it seems to allow people to treat its well-being in ways that would be ethically quite unacceptable otherwise. And those who remain unconvinced that ethics and morality should influence their personal attitudes towards animals can argue that Mother Nature is consistently far more harsh and cruel than even the most callous of humans.

References

Atkinson, A.B. (2007) Economics as a moral science. In: *Lionel Robbins's Essay on the Nature and Significance of Economic Science* (eds F. Cowell & A. Witzum), pp. 38–56. STICERD Monograph: London School of Economics, London.

Callicott, J.B. (1986) On the intrinsic value of non-human species. In: *The Preservation of Species* (ed. B. Norton), pp. 138–172. Princeton University Press, Princeton, New Jersey.

Cowell, F. & Witzum, A. (2007) *Lionel Robbins's Essay on the Nature and Significance of Economic Science*. STICERD Monograph: London School of Economics, London.

Dietrich, M. & Rowen, D. (2005) Ethical principles and economic analysis. *Journal of Interdisciplinary Economics*, **16**, 247–269.

FAWC. (2005) *Welfare Implications of Farm Assurance Schemes*. Farm Animal Welfare Council, Defra, London.

Hausman, D.M. & McPherson, M.S. (1993) Taking ethics seriously: Economics and contemporary moral philosophy. *Journal of Economic Literature*, **31**(2), 671–731.

Krutilla, J.V. & Fisher, A.C. (1975) *The Economics of Natural Environments*. Johns Hopkins University Press, Baltimore, Maryland.

Lipsey, R.G. (1963) *An Introduction to Positive Economics*. Weidenfeld and Nicholson, London.

McInerney, J.P. (1991) Assessing the benefits of farm animal welfare. In: *Farm Animals: It Pays to be Humane* (ed. S.P. Carruthers), pp. 15–31. CAS paper 21, Centre for Agricultural Strategy, University of Reading, Reading.

McInerney, J.P. (1993) Animal welfare: An economic perspective. *Agricultural Economics Society Conference*, Oxford. Reprinted in: Bennett, R.M. (1994) *Valuing Farm Animal Welfare*. Occasional Paper 3, Dept of Agricultural Economics and Management, University of Reading, Reading.

Regan, T. (1983) *The Case for Animal Rights*. University of California Press, Berkeley, California.

Robbins, R. (1935) *An Essay on the Nature and Significance of Economic Science*. Macmillan, London.

Ryder, R. (1998) *The Political Animal: The Conquest of Speciesism*. McFarland, Jefferson, North Carolina.

Sen, A. (1987) *On Ethics and Economics*. Blackwell, London.

Questions and Answers

Q: One of the lines which appeared to work for me when I was trying to tie together economics and ethics was to go to the leaders of the supermarkets and say, '*But you have a reputation*' because they were often saying, '*Yes we care about welfare*'. If you then examined their products, there'd be ones where they hadn't bothered to do the right thing. Is this a link between ethics and economics which we can use?

A: Supermarkets do care about their reputation but don't lose it by having bog standard, not welfare-friendly products. They cater for all market segments. If they said, '*We will not sell stuff that comes from low welfare source*', they could sustain that. They won't, because if Tesco does it, Asda might not, so they've all got to ensure they do the same things. If they came to an agreement and said, '*We will not sell this kind of rubbish food, we have minimum standards and we will adhere to them*' they could do it. There's no incentive for them to do it individually in a competitive market.

Q: FAWC is about to engage in more depth with retailers, who are important drivers of farm animal welfare. Many producers take great notice of their demands. Retailers will often invest, especially Sainsbury, Tesco and the Co-op, in direct supply chains, especially with milk producers and increasingly with sheep producers, for example they will place veterinarians on farms and advise on scientific and technological advances to produce welfare-friendly products. Their influence not only covers the UK but also New Zealand and South America.
A: The food retailers are getting there, but slowly. We could not get them to assert that their assurance schemes for imported products really insisted on the standards they claimed they were imposing on UK farmers. Until there is total transparency throughout their supply chain, their claims will not be convincing. They tend to impose welfare standards for fresh products but not for processed products; so much of unknown welfare standards is hidden in processed products.

Q: I was interested on your comment that [UK-produced] pigs in Denmark are more expensive. UK retailers pay higher prices for those pigs than they would if producers just abided by Danish law and regulations.
A: There is a higher cost to higher welfare but it's actually not that significant and is often exaggerated. It's an example of 'the toilet paper syndrome'. If an essential commodity had tripled in price, some would say '*that's terrible, the Government should do something*'. But if it was toilet paper, they'd say, '*Oh, well I only buy one roll every two weeks and they only cost 50p anyway so no big deal*'. An awful lot of the price increases that would occur through higher welfare production end up as no big deal in terms of the cost to the average household weekly expenditure. Doubling the price of eggs might on average amount to only an extra 15p a week per person in terms of expenditure on eggs. So many of these things are not actually the fundamental force that they're claimed to be. People throw their arms up at the idea of higher costs but don't get them in perspective.

Q: You appear to reduce everything to economics. There's a weak and a strong claim that can be made about the importance of economics. For example, a table can be explained philosophically, scientifically and economically. Your conclusion is that economics trumps ethics; it's more accurately interpreted as ethical egoism, trumps altruism.
A: I don't think it's as complicated as that. We live in an economic system, which is moderated by politics, sociology, circumstance, the weather, catastrophes, etc. It's not reducing things to economics, it's just recognising the environment in which we're living and working.

Q: Thank you for your honest treatment of economics and acknowledging the fact that the free market has incentives for unethical behaviour. Much Government thinking has been based on the idea that we're only motivated by money and human capital theory.

A: I disagree. Human capital theory is sound.

Q: It seems to me that there is hope that people are not just motivated by money and are motivated by other things. There is hope that ethics can triumph.

A: But people are also motivated by malice and jealousy and selfishness and all sorts of things – and at times those sentiments may triumph too. There is hope that some people, or even increasingly more people, may adopt an ethical approach to their economic activity but still the system overall is driven by the need to survive and prosper as a producer, the need to survive and bring up your family and feed your kids and lead the life you want to as a consumer. You don't override everything on monetary factors but that is underlying everything we do. We've all got to live within our income and so we don't give it all to charity. Sociology is also very important in the animal welfare debate but there is a tendency to think that only veterinarians understand that debate because it's about animals. The way society behaves and what Governments do determines what happens to animals.

Q: How is it that it seems to have worked for free-range eggs then? Consumers are buying many more free-range eggs and yet don't do the same with broilers or even milk that's better welfare oriented.

A: Eggs have a nice focus with pictures of free-range hens. Consumers can be misguided into thinking that free-range welfare is really a lot better than caged hen welfare. In relation to chicken meat it's more difficult; there's less public understanding of how broiler chickens are produced, there hasn't been enough testing of the market of producing non-broiler chicken and we've got very used in our consumption habits to very cheap chicken. You could actually get rid of broiler chicken if you banned them and people would then adjust to it. But it's really an information thing, and to get people realising it doesn't hurt them all that much to pay more for their chicken meat but they feel a lot better about consuming it. To get people to change their purchasing decisions, there's so much information to get to misguided consumers who have absolutely no idea of the background to the food system. But then, we are all ill-informed consumers. What do you know about the conditions of the guy who soldered together your DVD player or television set? You may know it was produced in China, but do you enquire about the welfare conditions of the labour? You don't even think about it, probably, and wouldn't know how to act on it if you do. Most people are like that when they buy food.

Author's Commentary

The core of my presentation was encapsulated in four statements: (1) there are no ethics in markets, which are simply impersonal arrangements for organising production and exchange; (2) there are no incentives for ethics in markets: incentives are built around pursuing individual self-interest; (3) indeed, there are incentives for *no* ethics in markets, because competitive pressures encourage gaining advantage over others in the market, including actions that would be considered unethical; and (4) ethical behaviour may be observed but, in the absence of external forces, it will be down to the choices, decisions and actions of the economics agents. My presentation looked at where those forces may come from, their potential influence and limitations in relation to the ethical treatment of animals. I believe its theme was a crucial perspective on the practical relevance of everything we were discussing. Throughout the conference, we had extended, diverse and frequently earnest presentations on how people ought to behave and how things ought to be done in relation to animals, but much of it seemed not to recognise – or at least take much account of – the fact that there is a real world out there which is driven by forces other than those subsumed in our professional, affluent, informed (and commendably ethical) western attitudes. If my 'economics overview' had been presented much earlier, I could have more usefully emphasised the point I made at the beginning of my talk – namely, that we had all been behaving like spectators at a football match, shouting at the players and the referee to tell them what they should be doing, whereas we weren't actually the ones who were playing the game. In the context of our discussions, those kicking the ball are the livestock producers, food sector companies, international traders, multinational corporations, international institutions, countless individual animal owners/keepers, etc., who either operate in commercial contexts having little direct contact with, or awareness of, how animals are treated or had a multitude of other concerns to deal with than animal ethics. To the extent that all their activities are driven and tied together within an economic system, then an overall economic view of the context in which 'veterinary and animal ethics' are manifested would have provided an informative backdrop to the conference discussions.

Postscript: There is a tendency for international conferences to be rather like multinational bombing raids. The various participants fly in from different directions at varying heights and speeds, drop their particular ordnance on what they believe is the target and then fly out again, having taken it all very seriously and professionally and believing they have done a good job. Whether the target was destroyed as intended, or just a big mess made on the ground, is inevitably uncertain and something that only becomes evident when the dust has cleared. Everyone feels it was an important thing to have been part of, however.

Debate: *'Is It Better to Have Lived and Lost than Never to Have Lived at All?'*

PATRICK BATESON

University of Cambridge

C:	Convenor, Pat Bateson	DM:	David Mellor	DMa:	David Main
JK:	James Kirkwood	SM:	Stephen May	RG:	Rebecca Garcia
BR:	Bernard Rollin	JH:	John Hellstrom	AS:	Anonymous speaker
JY:	James Yeates	HD:	Huw Davies	CB:	Caroline Bergmann
DS:	Douglas Stewart	SW:	Sophia Wiberg	NW:	Natalie Warran
MC:	Madeleine Campbell	AW:	Abigail Woods	SWO:	Sarah Wolfensohn
DW:	David Williams	HB:	Heather Bacon	NP:	Nathalie Parsy
MA:	Mike Appleby	JN:	Jo Nash	PJ:	Peter Jinman
MS:	Manuel Sant'Ana	JM:	John McInerney	CG:	Colin Gilbert
PS:	Peter Sandøe	GC:	Glen Cousquer		

Banner's principles of animal ethics mix the approaches of duties and consequences. This pragmatic solution is often used when humans have to make difficult moral choices about the treatment of animals in our care. Often we have to weigh up issues relating to an animal's quality and quantity of life. This balance lies at the heart of the moral – as well as the welfare – debate. During this debate, registrants considered a question, which can be interpreted variously, for example in terms of moral principles, specific issues such as population control or illustrative examples. The question was considered by James Kirkwood, Bernard Rollin and James Yeates before registrants were invited to speak.

Veterinary & Animal Ethics: Proceedings of the First International Conference on Veterinary and Animal Ethics, September 2011, First Edition. Edited by Christopher M. Wathes, Sandra A .Corr, Stephen A. May, Steven P. McCulloch and Martin C. Whiting.
© 2013 Universities Federation for Animal Welfare. Published 2013 by Blackwell Publishing Ltd.

C: If the question had been '*Is it better to have loved and lost than never to have loved at all?*', then I would have known how to vote, but I'm not sure that I know how to vote on this one. What I would like you to do now is secretly to vote yes, no or abstain and then, after the formal vote, I'll ask you to say whether or not you have changed your mind. We shall then see whether the debate has been so persuasive that we shall have a clear answer at the end.

James Kirkwood: '*It depends*'

Lost what, something trivial or something important? It also depends on what 'lived' means, as can be established by asking a professor of philosophy, a parrot and a carrot in turn. I'm going to leave aside 'lived' and 'lost' and focus on the word 'better'.

I was originally invited to argue one side of the question. With regret, I said that I couldn't accept the invitation; I couldn't make the case because I don't agree that life is always better no matter how bad its quality. Recently, I've been suggesting that it's better not to breed companion animals with serious genetic welfare problems, better that they are not born. But it doesn't follow that the opposite is right – that it is always better not to live than to live and lose.

Suppose a reptile that had an unremittingly bleak life in the Triassic period, laid one egg before then suffering a slow and miserable death from tuberculosis (which existed even back in those days) but its offspring hatched, and it turned out that that reptile was the direct ancestor of birds, including the swifts that have such fun racing round clock towers in the summer: would it have been better if that reptile hadn't lived? It all depends on what we mean by better. Better for whom and what, and better in what way and over what timescale? There's no general answer to our question. We must judge each case depending on its circumstances.

When do we find ourselves asking this question? The answer in my own case is rarely, or to be a bit more precise, never, except on the evening of 12 September 2011. It's too vague and blurry a question to spend time on (but it serves ideally tonight of course to give us freedom to prattle on about the bees in our bonnets). But we're all familiar with specific questions in this line of country; here are three examples:

1. Because of disease, Benji the dog is in pain. Treatment will take time and there's only a 25% chance it will work. Is it kinder to try treatment or to euthanise now? Is it better to let Benji live on with further 'loss' or not?
2. Rinderpest was a serious disease of cattle and wild ungulates with major welfare effects and high mortality. Research in the 1960s by Walter Plowright into the vaccine that led to the eradication of the disease globally, involved experimentally infecting and inducing the disease in some cattle. Was it better that these research cattle lived and lost or not? In an earlier attempt to control a terrible Rinderpest epidemic in the Netherlands in 1769, 15 November was made a national day of fasting and prayer. Unlike Walter Plowright's contribution, this didn't work but on the other hand no animals were harmed trying it.

3. Re-establishment of red kites in England involved taking nestlings from Spain for release. Although successful, some birds had major welfare challenges, that is they were shot and injured, and some were poisoned. No matter how carefully done, there's a risk that some animals in conservation programmes may live and lose. Would it be better if the risk had never been taken?

In all these examples, when considering whether welfare costs outweigh any benefits of living, we could focus only on the individuals that did the living and losing, that is the poisoned red kites, the cows given Rinderpest and so on, but this wouldn't be wise because, in such cases, whether or not these individuals lived was crucial also to the lives and welfare of many other animals. My point is that it's very important that we should always take a wider view, even in cases like the first example. The world is so big that it is easy to overlook that space and other essential resources are finite: it is like a big table at which, although there are many seats, their number is fixed. The seats are fully occupied, competition for them is hot, and there's no space to pull up extra chairs. Animals that don't have a seat at the table at best only get the crumbs that fall from it and, in time, will fail to thrive and die. They, in the jargon of this debate, lose.

There are always very many more animals than available seats, as Darwin pointed out, and only when seats are vacated can another animal get a chance to sit at the table. Each space may be occupied by one large animal or many little ones; the longer each animal retains its seat, the fewer will ever get the chance to sit there.

We humans now account for about 25% of the seating round that table; increasingly, we control which other animals get to sit at it and for how long. We, and our huge populations of farm animals, take up more space each year and our pet animals are occupying increasing numbers of seats also.

Now back to my starting point of genetic welfare problems in dogs. Should dogs be bred that are, for example, highly predisposed to chronic respiratory problems and birthing difficulties? We could debate this only from the dog's own point of view, as people frequently do, but it seems to me that we should step back and take a wider view *also*. We are trying to live and plan wisely to meet human needs, preserve biodiversity and protect the welfare of sentient animals. Shouldn't we take care that the earth's precious resources are used very carefully? For every animal at the table, another is denied a place. Breeding animals with genetic welfare problems denies life to those that could have been bred otherwise that would be more likely to enjoy it.

In considering 'better' in the context of welfare, I suggest we should encourage everyone involved in the breeding of new, and the maintenance of old, individuals to consider carefully not only the welfare of those animals but also the knock-on consequences for other animals. The solemn declaration by those becoming members of the Royal College of Veterinary Surgeons is that '*My constant endeavour will be to ensure the welfare of animals committed to my care*'. A few years ago,

I suggested that some words should be added to the effect '... *and in so doing be careful also of the welfare of those that are not*'. To my eye, that takes nothing away but adds an important dimension.

Bernard Rollin: '*The answer is maybe*'

Obviously a reasonable response to the question depends on how one interprets the notion of 'lost' or 'better' and some possible understanding of 'lost'. In order to unpack the claim, it is valuable to recall a well known quotation from Aristotle, which he derived from Solon, the law-giver of Athens, '*Count no man happy until he is dead*'. It's a profound quotation. As I understand this pronouncement, it means that however one has viewed one's life until a given moment in terms of happiness, there are certain events of sufficient profundity, which, for at least some people, cast a completely new and negative *gestalt* on everything that has hitherto transpired and could transpire in the future. In other words, there are possible events that would irrevocably colour a life in an irreversibly negative manner. Such is not the case with every life-altering catastrophic event.

One can, for example, easily imagine the crooked financier, Bernie Madoff, in his jail cell for his life sentence reminiscing and chuckling over his past pleasures and how long he was able to get away with his pyramid scheme. In real life, this case is impossible because, tragically, Madoff's son committed suicide because of his inability to live with the shame, thereby presumably creating a negative life colouring event. That's probably a bigger punishment for Madoff than anything else that happened.

There are catastrophes, however, which for many people are not compatible with any happiness saving interpretation. These events force one to re-evaluate the essential project or legitimating agents that give meaning and worth to a life.

Consider a Jewish parent in the midst of the Holocaust whose children were literally wrenched from his arms by an SS man and then their heads were dashed against the wall and whose wife was then gassed. For me, there exists no *gestalt* on this event that can buttress the claim that it was *a life worth living*. In such a circumstance, my only proper response is to wish I had never lived. In a similar vein, consider a person whose marriage and wife's love were the essential feature of his happiness. On his deathbed, he hears her say to his best friend, '*I wish the old bastard would hurry up and die so that you and I can run off with his money*'.

In the above situations, there is no consolation in saying at least I lived, something that only humans are capable of realising. Consider the question with regard to an animal, lacking language, syntax and the ability to think in distant future, abstract and counterfactual terms. It is extremely unlikely that an animal could even formulate the concept of life in itself or death, which Heidegger characterises as '*understanding the possibility of the impossibility of your being*'.

For an animal, whose life comprises a series of miserable news such as that experienced by a sow confined in a gestation crate or an animal in constant pain, there is no believing or hope for life to change, for hope requires the sort of non-proximal, future-directed mentation that animals lack. That's one of my arguments elsewhere why animal pain may be worse than human pain, because animals have no hope. Nor can the animal take solace in the proposition 'at least I lived' because it is not capable of grasping the abstract concept of life. Its life is no more than the sum total of its miserable experiences and memories thereof: an animal that is never able to express its *telos* cannot be said to have lived its life. In a real sense, a lion, which spends his entire life in a tiny cage is not a lion, it has lost its lion life. And I don't mean that poetically; I mean that quite literally.

It is for this reason I have argued elsewhere that one should not necessarily treat chronically ill animals for diseases such as cancer when such treatment entails a considerable period of suffering, whereas a person with a distant future or perspective can rationally choose to trade current pain entailed by a treatment for the prospect of living to see one's children graduate or visiting Tahiti again. An animal's mind cannot comprehend such a trade-off and future compensation for current suffering. The animal's life in such a case *is* its pain.

Thus in the case of a human life, the answer to the question surely depends on the individual's circumstances, since humans can selectively cherish valuable aspects of life. Only in circumstances such as those described above, where all of life is indelibly coloured negatively, is it better not to have lived. In the case of animal life, where one cannot hope to selectively stress positive aspects of life or cherish life itself, it is unequivocally better not to have lived when the preponderance of the being's experiences are negative. This is the source of our unequivocal belief in euthanasia as a gift for ending suffering, though there are challenges to that now.

Is there in animal life, a case analogous to the situation of which Solon and Aristotle remind us? Perhaps. Imagine a beloved family dog, which has been loved and well treated for its entire life. Suddenly, the owner goes mad and sadistically tortures the animal to death. It is possible to believe that even with an animal's limited mentation, such a case might indeed irrevocably colour the animal's memory so as to render all previous experience negative. I hope that's beyond animal thought because that kind of thing does happen.

Why do we disproportionately focus on the last few minutes of life when we slaughter an animal or euthanise it? That was a question that the *Canadian Veterinary Journal* asked me. Why, when the animal has some moments of misery, do we focus on that last incident of pain and suffering as against an entire life of misery? There is a nagging suspicion that the animal may in some sense grasp that this is it, this is all there is; that would be a disproportionate way to colour its experiential history.

James Yeates: 'No'

I want to focus on the idea of 'loss', specifically the obvious interpretation of loss of life as a deprivation. At first glance, loss of life appears to be a deprivation that is harmful insofar as it deprives an animal of enjoyable experiences or desires that might be fulfilled or beneficial, perhaps if it avoids negative events through euthanasia. But this runs into a classic Epicurean problem that when an animal is dead, it doesn't exist so it's quite hard to say that something is bad for a being that doesn't exist.

One way to solve this problem is to suggest that death harms an animal at the time that it's still alive, that is an animal has certain interests while it exists. In a way, death causes a retroactive change of those desires from those to be fulfilled to those that aren't going to be fulfilled and these occur while the animal exists.

Death therefore deprives an animal of positive interests, which are to be fulfilled. But what we can't do is create a similar account for animals that never existed. There's no point where we can say they've got these interests that are going to be fulfilled or not. They never have interests, certainly not desires, because they don't exist. Now if we can't say that an animal that does not exist has interests, then we struggle to say that it's lost anything or we struggle to say that it's been harmed by not existing. If we combine this argument with the account that death deprives an animal of the fulfilment of its interests, then the conjunction of these two arguments says, in part, that an animal is harmed by death, not harmed by never existing. Thus, it is better never to have lived than to have lived and lost.

DS: Who is asking the question, the person or the animal or somebody else? I can think of an eminent person who may have an uncomfortable life with his disease but who has nevertheless been successful and able to make a great contribution. He may feel – or not as the case may be – that he might not have liked to have lived at all, but what would we say? Would we think it was better that way? I'm sure that his contribution to science is something such that we would all agree that it was better for him to have lived and lost rather than not to have lived at all.

MC: If we think that animals probably can't have a concept of their life as a whole and they don't have this idea of hope and so forth, where does that leave the FAWC's principle of *a life worth living*? Because if the animal can't have such a concept, our idea about whether their whole life is worth living or not presumably doesn't coincide with their experience at any one moment, which is, I imagine, what's important to them.

BR: I don't believe that animals are aware of their life as a whole unit. Unity of apperception (self-awareness) means a unified consciousness clearly, animals have a unified consciousness and have short term, for example, future thoughts, otherwise the cat wouldn't wait outside the mouse hole, and they have memories. I don't think an animal has a meta-level notion of reflecting on its life. In spite of this, the FAWC principle works. It simply means giving animals successive experiences that are pleasant over a lifetime, even if it can't grasp the concept of its life as a whole unit.

MC: Is there any meaning to the concept of *a life worth living* from an animal's point of view?

BR: Yes, it would be a reflective judgement on your part of the animal's life rather than the animal's judgement.

DW: The original quote is by Tennyson. There's a big difference between losing in love and losing in life. The abortion of a fetus with a genetic deformity is, even for those who object to abortion, reasonably acceptable. If someone has Tay-Sachs disease and is going to be mentally retarded and handicapped to the extent that they're soon going to die, then some think that it's reasonable never to have existed and to have been aborted. From that perspective, there are incidences certainly, even in humans, where it's better to have never lived rather than to have lived and lost.

MA: In the area of animal welfare, I am passionately moderate. I want to illustrate this in relation to two quotations: one from Bernie Rollin from 30 years ago in Edinburgh and one from somebody to whom I spoke at teatime. I recall that Bernie said '*that the ideal is that we should not use animals*'. Clearly there was a strong element of negative use, which relates to our question. I discussed it with my brother, a veterinarian, who was against this idea. He mostly worked with small animals, but his picture was that a world without domestic animals would be a barren and strange world.

In relation to a specific example, would a world without cows be a better world? Would it be a better world for us? Would it be a better world for a neutral observer? Would it be a better world for cows? I come to the conclusion that it would not be a better world for cows, despite all the philosophical difficulties of addressing cows, which might or might not exist. The fact that a cow's life is not perfect still doesn't gainsay the fact that it may have many positives in life and much positive from us having brought it into existence.

The person to whom I spoke at tea had recently become a vegan. Her friends had said, '*if everybody was vegan wouldn't that mean that there wouldn't be any cows in the fields?*' This is going too far. Her responsibility as a vegan is not to get rid of all the cows in the world, it is her responsibility and her action; my passionate moderation comes from saying, rather than let's think of an unrealistic future in which there are no animals, let us think of a realistic future in which there are fewer animals but we look after them better. For me, it is better for those animals to have lived and lost a little; it is better for those animals as well.

MS: As a veterinarian, I'd like to put the emphasis on the veterinary context. I would like to see this question put within the context of, for example, stray dogs. This is a practical issue that veterinarians face every day. Is it better for those dogs to have lived and lost or just to euthanise them? This brings me back to the example of Kirkwood's Benji. Who is putting the question? How should the question be put to the owner? We don't just have responsibilities towards the dogs, but to the owner too, who may be suffering. We need to balance the suffering of the animal with the suffering of the owner, of course, and our own suffering as veterinarians.

C: In Moscow, there are packs of stray dogs which live in the centre of the City. They use the Metro to go out to the markets in the periphery of Moscow and then they go back to their packs at the end of the day. Nobody knows how they ever came to do this but they do. Maybe those stray dogs do not do such a bad job and have a reasonable life.

PS: As chairman of the Danish equivalent of FAWC, I have a broader way of dealing with all sorts of animals. One case concerns feral cats. People concerned about animals divide into two kinds. I like cats being out there, even though some of them are miserable, many have happy lives. Alternatively, others believe that if a cat is not owned, then it should be got rid of. That's a horrible vision which, in a way, implies one answer to this question. In Denmark, since the Iron Age there have been cats which just live close to humans. Even though there's a risk they'll lose, there's also a risk that they'll gain and the fact that they're there contributes to the world. I think there's something dangerous about us being such control freaks, that just to avoid a few animals losing that we wipe them out.

What makes this complicated for me as a philosopher is something personal. The first half of the question is really about value to someone. The second half is certainly not value to anyone because if you never lived, there's no one who's the carrier of that value but still there can be an impersonal value in these animals being there. That's a very deep philosophical issue, what do we think about living creatures being there? These are deep thought experiments; if we could either choose a very tidy world with no living being, no suffering or we could choose a dirty world with a lot of suffering but also a lot of all the good things, what would you choose? I would probably choose the dirty world.

DM: One of the conundras is the question of neonatal mortality. Is it better to have had a life without it being even remotely *a good life* or is it better not to have had life at all? There will be, almost inevitably, with any group of animals giving birth, a significant number that die, having been in relatively miserable circumstances before they die. Now given that that's inevitable, the proportion is small, we hope, but can be as many as 25% or in the wild it can be as many as 50%. In order to get any survival at all, it would appear that there's an irreducible minimum of animals that are going to be born, live a brief period and die in miserable circumstance. Is that the cost of being alive? Is that a burden we have to carry for being able to have lives that we enjoy?

SM: I want to look at this from another perspective. If we disagree with the implied answer, we're essentially saying that we don't agree with the existence of life or indeed the human race because in terms of natural selection and the processes that have been involved in the creation of life on this planet, then many have lived and lost. This is the point about natural selection. In terms of all of us, if they'd never lived at all we wouldn't be here. So in terms of life as a whole, it is better to have lived and lost than to have never lived at all.

JY: The argument that it is better for others to have lived so that others can live is predicated on the idea that to live is, in some way, good if it's not good that we live then it wasn't therefore good that other people lived in order for us to live.

JH: It's a very interesting question. Are we talking or is it the animal talking? We keep trying to tease that out because it has quite different outcomes. An example of the power of animals to shape many lives is a penguin, Happy Feet, which recently came ashore in New Zealand, a penguin which was about 5000 km from where it should have been. The New Zealand conservation organisation took the Darwinian approach that this animal had got there, should sort itself out and go back or perish. It quickly became apparent that the world thought this was a terrible way of dealing with this penguin, and as a result, through philanthropy and some government money too, about 150 000 NZ$ were spent looking after Happy Feet. A few days ago, he was released back into the Southern Ocean. I just heard that Happy Feet has vanished; the current theory is that he's probably been consumed by an orca whale. So Happy Feet lived and lost but in the process enriched the lives of hundreds of thousands of people, who probably would reflect that that wasn't a bad outcome.

HD: As a practicing sheep farmer and member of FAWC, I have to take ethical decisions every day, such as whether to tail-dock and castrate lambs or cast the one ewe that is lame in the middle of 300 ewes for the sake of helping her but still disturbing the other sheep. But the question really ties into a decision we have to make at lambing. This year our ewes were scanned at 190% with 90 triplets, 90 singles and twins. Ninety triplets sounds great but you can't rear three lambs on one ewe. We made the decision to raise the third triplet lamb as a pet. Each lamb was put on a bottle and then moved onto a machine, weaned and then sent to slaughter. Should we have euthanised those lambs at birth or should we have kept them on for 12 weeks in good condition but with the ultimate destination of the slaughterhouse?

FAWC uses *a good life, a life worth living* and *a life not worth living*. I have spent many hours watching my pet lambs this year; I'm absolutely convinced that they have not only *a life worth living* but *a good life*. We put in straw bales. It's got to the point where my wife had to drag me away from watching them because I had so much fun. I have made no money out of those lambs. Was it better that those lambs lived and lost or should I have euthanised them at birth, because the option to leave them on the mother wasn't there?

Next year, we will do the same as we did this year. I'm convinced that because the mother had two lambs left, the distress to her was minimal and the third lamb took to the bottle immediately. I don't think there was much stress either and I'm absolutely convinced that they had *a good life*, not just a *life worth living*. A stockman knows if his stock is happy; the triplets were happy and that made me happy as well.

SW: My concern is with farm animals regarding intensive food production. We make them live and we make them lose. Losing is not by death necessarily, it's the miserable life that the animals have.

AW: In *Animal Machines* (1964), Ruth Harrison's key claim about intensive farming was that the animal did not have a chance to live before it died. From that, we can surmise that, for her, it was better for an animal to have never lived at all. However, the Brambell Committee decided that it was better if these animals had lived. Our efforts should be directed to making sure that animals lived a little bit better before they lost; that approach has framed welfare goals ever since.

HB: In China, bears are farmed industrially and intensively for their bile I was heavily involved with an NGO that rescued bears from bear-bile farms. A lot of those animals had lived for 10 years and longer, in one case for 30 years, in a cage with an abdominal fistula, wearing metal jackets in conditions that can only be described as miserable for any sentient animal. In many of these cases, if you could choose between euthanasia before the process started then I, as a clinician, would have advocated mass euthanasia.

There are 10 000 bears on farms in China now and I still think that they would be better off dead. However, having dealt with those animals clinically and seen their capability to enjoy life, they go through a rehabilitation process. I've seen bears that have been in tiny cages for 30 years with severe health problems swimming, playing and running around. Is that *a life worth living*? Was it worth spending 30 years in a cage? It's really difficult to make those decisions but often if you give an animal the opportunity and the choices and monitor its behaviour, it will often make the decision for itself as to whether *its life was worth living or not*.

C: So your answer is yes, is it?

HB: It probably depends on the circumstances. It can be made worth living, depending on the individual.

JN: I visit farms every day and visit intensive units occasionally. I would quite happily euthanise intensively farmed pigs, for example because they do not have *a life worth living*. I also go to free farms where the pigs are happily wallowing and have a great life.

I also visit markets and abattoirs. A lot of sheep or cattle that go to markets and abattoirs have had *a good life*, they have had *a life worth living* up until that point. They then get extremely stressed and fearful going through the markets and to the abattoirs; up until then, they've had *a good life*.

JM: We cannot discuss the question from the standpoint of 'is it better for us' or 'what's a world like without cows?' It is not an ethical position to discuss whether or not it suits our preferences. Ethics is presumably something to do with principles other than simple preferences. We can't discuss something that never happened; something never having lived at all is a non-event. There's an infinity of non-events. You can't discuss whether this non-event is better or worse than that non-event. They are non-events. They have no qualitative characteristics.

What does this mean from the standpoint of the animal? If you say it is better to have lived and lost than not to have lived at all, then you have to say that for the male chick that is hatched and is almost instantaneously macerated because it has no economic value, it's better for it to have been hatched than not to have been hatched at all. That's hard to accept.

Is a bobby calf that only lives for 2 days before it is slaughtered not a lot different from the newly hatched chick, except by 2 days?

Think of a pheasant that is hatched for game shooting. Is it better for it to have been hatched so that it can be shot at 3 months old? If you go down this line you say, well that's only a matter of time. What about a pig that gets to bacon weight and is then killed at 6 months old? What's the difference between the pig, the game bird or the male chick? We have to conclude that we hadn't better keep any animals whose life we terminate because we will be violating the idea that it's better to have lived and lost. We'll end up stopping animal agriculture.

DM: Is the question about lambs, not really a question about whether or not quantity of life is relevant to animals? Because assuming that your lambs are as well looked after on their first day of life as they are for the next 12 weeks and, assuming that they have a humane death either on the first day of life or 12 weeks later, maybe there is no better life, maybe it's equally the same to the lambs. Whose life is better?

GC: I got the impression there was a value judgement associated with the word feral. It would be easy to argue that a free-living cat has elements of its life that are far better than the sloth for life of some of the domestic cats, particularly in the Western world.

Have you read Victor Frankl's work? He wrote about his experiences in the prison camp, for example in a profound book titled *Meaning of Life*. It was amazing what insignificant things he found, which gave meaning to a life of despair within those camps. We're trying to put a value on things that we probably can't fully value because it comes down to the individual. It's very much an epistemological thing that we're trying to attach a value to. I'm probably going to sit on the fence on this one.

DMa: We can get too carried away with hypothetical, philosophical conversations. What matters is the language of the conversation; we should reflect upon how language has evolved.

We've realised that there's something else to life, which is what the FAWC was getting at. Peter Sandøe is right about *the life worth living* and *life not worth living*, it is really about this extreme. The words in the FAWC report are *literally better off dead*. I don't think that definition moves the debate on much further. *A good life* means to have lived well. What are the measures? How can we show that animals live well? An animal that lives longer is better off, but it has to have positive aspects as well. It's about changing the language, moving just from the negatives to the positives.

RG: At the beginning of the debate, I abstained. After listening, I think the answer depends on the individual's belief. If you are looking from a selfish point of view, I would rather not live than lose, probably better never to have lived at all. If you think of it from an altruistic point of view and the actual benefit that you give to others or to society, then perhaps the answer is that it is better to have lived than lost. Actually, there are two answers rather than one and it depends on the individual.

For a selfish individual, the answer is the second part of the question; for an altruistic individual, it would be the first part. And we had various examples for that. If Benji is owned by an elderly person and is his only focus, then there might be a lot of value for that dog to continue living. You could argue both ways but I think my answer is probably still that I abstain because there are two answers.

MA: Socrates said '*Better an unhappy philosopher than a happy pig*'. In relation to the eminent scientist's argument, people have asked severely handicapped humans whether they think they should not have been born. Universally, they say no, no matter what condition they have lived in, they value their life.

C: It's not universal. There are quite a few people who say they wish they'd never been born.

MA: That must, of course, depend on the severity of the disability.

C: Yes.

MA: We have kept coming back to the question of whether we can take an animal's view. A primate expert said that he was quite sure that he could train a chimpanzee to understand death but that he would not remotely consider doing so.

DM: Someone mentioned that lambs don't have a [good] quality of life, it's all too neutral. I disagree. It's pretty obvious once a lamb is up and conscious that it can experience a quality of life, which can be good or bad.

AS: The question revolves around our consideration of what is the effect on us? The phrase 'animal welfare' comes to mind. What would happen if there was a world without animals? What would the world be like if there were no humans, would animal welfare be any different? We wouldn't know. To us it's important that animals should have lived and lost. It may resonate in some that a human's needs include happiness. Using the example of Happy Feet, a lot of people gained a lot of benefit from investing in the short-term happiness of one animal because it filled a need in the human population. If the human population wasn't there, whether that animal had a good welfare or not would not have been known. It's really a question of how humans perceive these attitudes.

CB: Moving the debate to a more pragmatic ethical question and focusing on Benji the dog. We have advanced our technology and abilities to cure disease. As an example, the European College of Veterinary Surgeons considers that veterinarians are akin to mechanics, not paediatricians. We're facing challenging questions, similar to the medical ethics question about neonates and how far to give life support to neonates. We have to make decisions not just about feral cats but about whether or not to treat, and how to treat and keep alive, a blind 15-year-old Labrador, or for example to replace a hip or elbow.

NW: I'm an optimist, who is always thinking that something better is round the corner. Animals, because of their simplicity are much more optimistic generally than are humans. The animal isn't necessarily always thinking about life always being like that. There's every little opportunity for something to be. Their ability to maintain optimism – you see it in animals in captivity mostly – is an incredible gift and is the thing that makes their *life worth living*, even though we don't necessarily think that the life that they have is of high quality as we would like it to be.

DW: I'm not sure that I can accept that in a broiler facility, where a bird is meeting a new bird every few minutes and is lame with the beginning of ascites, it has had a positive life.

SWO: Of course experimental animals are the classic example of ones that have lived and lost but the question is 'is it better to be an experimental animal and live and lose or never live at all?' This is fundamental to the ethical review process and the harm–benefit balance of using that animal. By definition, and in this case, it is better to have lived and lost.

But the other thing to think about with experimental animals is this question of the potential for living better. I've seen long-term experimental animals which are definitely losing but, because they're there long term, they have the potential for things to get better. I've also seen long-term animals in a 'not very good environment' in an experiment that's not particularly in their favour. Because they have the potential to do better, which is a principle of the 3Rs, there is the potential for their lives to improve so they do have *a life worth living* or even *a good life*. Those animals that do lose out, can contribute to the development of refinements to benefit other animals in future experiments.

NP: Like every veterinarian, I have had to euthanase a few animals for medical reasons. I coped with the act by thinking that the animal is going to be killed shortly and is in pain or is living in not very good conditions. Maybe I'm doing him a favour.

One day, I had a little calf suffering from arthritis. After many treatments, it couldn't move or get up. It was on an intensive farm and had lived in a box all its life. It was ending its life in such pain that I thought, well, I'm really doing him a favour so I injected him once, nothing happened, twice, nothing happened. I changed my bottle because I thought something is wrong with my product; I had to inject him six times before he died. I don't understand what happened but as I was doing it I thought, well, there is little value to the life of an animal in that condition; I'm doing him a favour by killing him. I looked at the others and they were all in their little boxes. They were quite old, so not far from being slaughtered and couldn't move in their boxes. I looked them in the eyes and thought that these animals want to live whatever happens, not waiting here for slaughter. They don't understand that they're going to be slaughtered shortly. They are living a life. We have put them in these conditions; the value of their life can't be so different to that of other animals. At that moment, I decided that instead of working as a practicing veterinarian, I'd be better off working in animal welfare, stopping practicing, to try to give animals a better life.

JH: If we take humans out of the equation, the answer is a no brainer it's yes. It's what the whole force of life is about. The confusion is when we add the human dimension then change the words slightly.

PJ: If an animal's life is short, nasty, brutish, waiting for that moment when it's going to be taken, for example a meerkat or rabbit thinking that any moment something is going to have it, it is questionable whether it's a very good life because it is expecting death almost constantly. What intrigues me is that come the spring, you can watch rabbits, which are running around and having a mad moment, which anthropomorphically looks like pleasure, knowing that death is instantaneous or very soon to arrive. The converse for the prey is rather different. It is dominant and doesn't go around fearing that moment in quite the same way. If I'm going to come back in the next life, I would like to come back not as the prey but the hunter.

C: I'm not sure you're right that the prey really do know what they can expect from their predators.

CG: Something is missing from this question. For animals to have lived and lost, the argument is predicated on the idea that something else has lived and won. So we may be being rather hard on ourselves by thinking only about animals that have lived and lost. There are always opportunities for improvement and betterment and we've heard some examples, which have made me feel a bit chirpier. For animals to have the opportunity to either lose or win, they need to live in the first place; this concludes the argument for me.

Vote:

In favour	35	Against	15
Abstentions	21	Changed their vote after the debate	4

Index

Veterinary & Animal Ethics: Proceedings of the First International Conference on Veterinary and Animal Ethics, September 2011, First Edition. Edited by Christopher M. Wathes, Sandra A. Corr, Stephen A. May, Steven P. McCulloch and Martin C. Whiting.
© 2013 Universities Federation for Animal Welfare. Published 2013 by Blackwell Publishing Ltd.